*CANDIDA

SILVER (mercury) FILLINGS

AND THE

IMMUNE SYSTEM

Edited by
Betsy Russell-Manning

***CAUSES:** Pesticides, Chemicals, Fluoride, Food Additives, Silver (mercury) Fillings, Antibiotics, Nickel Crowns, Radiation, Yeast, Sugar, Imbalance of the Electromagnetic Field, Acid/Alkaline Imbalance, Birth Control Pills, etc.

BY THE SAME EDITOR:

How Safe Are Silver (mercury) Fillings? —
Hidden Health Facts (1984)

How Silver•Mercury Fillings Affect Your Energy System (1984)

Wheatgrass Juice — Gift of Nature (1979)

CANDIDA, Silver (mercury) Fillings and the Immune System

Revised Edition - 1986

Library of Congress Catalog Card No. 85-80413

International Standard Book Number

0-930165-10-1

Greensward Press
1600 Larkin #104
San Francisco, California 94109

Spilman Printing Company
Sacramento, California

This book is dedicated to the memory of John Nicholas Morphy

and

The Twilight of Mankind

Destroy a man's mind, his reasoning ability, his imagination, and neither gold, silver, mansions, freedom, love, nor anything else will matter to him. This is EASILY ACCOMPLISHED, is BEING ACCOMPLISHED by simple means: the creation of disease in his body by toxic substances in his food; shattering his nervous system, hardening his muscles, and deteriorating his mind; making of man, the godly human, a sub-human creature, a lesser animal, a vegetation, Soulless - THE CRIME AGAINST HUMANITY.

From-

Cancer, The Destroyer
Cancer, Man's Most Fearful Enemy

This book is also dedicated to all light bearers of truth.

ACKNOWLEDGEMENTS

Those Who Contributed to this Edition

This book was researched by the reading of hundreds of Journals and many books and a close analysis of many more Journals and books not mentioned because of lack of space. Nevertheless, these Journals and papers are equally important to the subject Candida and its relation to silver (mercury) fillings and the immune system.

Dozens of people contributed their articles and advice to this book. Dr. James Ouye, D.D.S. always received my phone calls, giving me his time, knowledge and wonderful wisdom. Marie MacMartin, R.N. contributed her time, thoughtful advice and fine contributions. A few of the other names who contributed are: Dr. Luc De Schepper, M.D., Dr. Carlton Fredericks, Ph.D., Dr. John Lubecki, D.C., Alan Cantwell, M.D., Jeffrey Bland, Ph.D., Shirley Lorenzani, Ph.D., Orian Truss, M.D., Wm. Crook, M.D., Gail Nielsen, President Candida Research, Devaki Berkson, D.C., John Jaeckle, Roy Kupsinel, M.D., William Koch, M.D., Peter Ark, Ph.D., Professor Emeritas, U.C. Berkeley, D. Eggleston, D.D.S., Burton Silver, Ph.D., Jerry Mittelman, D.D.S. Walter Grotz, Fr. Richard Willhelm, Paul Keyes, D.D.S., John Ott, Ori Bachechi, S. Bursuk, N.D., Sol Silverman, D.D.S., John Gofman, M.D., Ph.D., Royal Lee, D.D.S., John Yiamouyiannis, Ph.D., Virginia Livingston, M.D., Otto Warburg, M.D., R. Voll, M.D., Roger J. Williams, Ph.D., Al Battista, N.D., Lorraine Rosenthal, Hanna Kroeger, Paul Lee, Ph.D., Zane Kime, M.D., William Tiller, Ph.D., Pat Flannagan, Ph.D., Roy Smudde, DDS, Ida Honorof, Winifred Wirth, Robert Cathcart, M.D., Hal Huggins, DDS, Dwight McKee, M.D., Abram Hoffer, M.D., Ph.D., Donald Barber, D.D.S., Marcia Smith, Dana Ullmann, M.P.H., and Mani, National Health Researcher.

I would like to thank Donald Barber, DDS of Williamsville, New York for his grammatical editing of the book. I would also like to thank my good friend Zak Mohammed for his help; without which this book would not have been possible. Last but not least, I would like to thank all my family for taking such loving care of my son, Kevin allowing me the time to reasearch this publication; thanks to Lynn and Bob, Tom and Stella, Grandma Russell, Missy, Bud, Mark, Tommy, Mary Ann, Kim and Ga Ga.

Cover by Kevin of
Apple Slide Productions
San Francisco, California

INTRODUCTION

This is a book that had to be written. Leaving much of the theory to other researchers, Betsy Russell-Manning has brought together a remarkable amount of logical, practical and clearly written information on Candida albicans, its previously underestimated effect on human biologic systems and its possible link to the person already immunologically compromised with mercury toxicity. Because of her own personal involvement with these adverse metabolic conditions, she has worked with zeal and perspicuity. Her book is real, totally understandable by the multitudes who suffer with chronic yeast infections and very alarming. It should appeal to health practitioners and patients alike and raise immediate concerns in anyone who suffers from diffuse mental and/or physical symptoms for which medicine has no definitive, identifying disease state.

Her cause is legitimate: public awareness of the magnitude of chronic Candida infection and its tie to diet and antibiotic usage has never been higher. In addition to its appeal to the bewildered and suffering patient, it is hoped that Russell-Manning's book will help also to answer the request recently sounded by the National Research Council when it asked publicly the medical schools of the nation to bring their nutrition programs at least up to the level of the lay public's knowledge. No nutrition program can ignore the food supply available to a microbial agent or the effect on the immune system of a heavy metal toxicity.

I applaud Betsy Russell-Manning for researching and compiling this extensive collection of biologic information on this vital subject. I believe you will thank her, too, when you have finished reading this book.

Helyn Luechauer, D.D.S.
President of the American Holistic Dental Assn.
Past President of California State Board of Dental Examiners;
Past President of the American Assn. of Women Dentists
Former Assistant Clinical Professor, Operative Dentistry
University of California, Los Angeles School of Dentistry;
and in private practice in Hollywood, California

PREFACE

This book is packed with references and sources of information and supplies. Since there is no objective information available on many of the problems discussed, an intelligent individual can sift through this information and be better educated about the options available when individuals have difficult problems of the immune system. Obviously, it is important whenever possible to be certain that one does not have a serious illness or one which is easily curable with a simple medical approach. Most of the illnesses discussed in this book certainly do not have such a treatment. When there is no standard medical treatment, then patients need to search carefully for the alternatives. CANDIDA, SILVER (MERCURY) FILLINGS AND THE IMMUNE SYSTEM offers such individuals an opportunity to examine the various alternatives.

C. Norman Shealy, M.D., Ph.D.
Founder and first President of the American Holistic Medical Association
Director of the Shealy Pain and Health Rehabilitation Institute-Springfield, Missouri

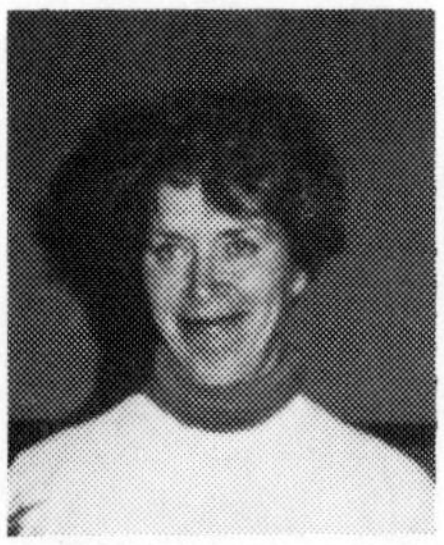

A MESSAGE TO THE READER FROM THE EDITOR

The handwriting is on the wall. Both the medical and scientific communities are using such terms as epidemic, catastrophic and impending doom as they are being alerted that there is a hidden epidemic in our midst--a fungal infection called Candidiasis. Leading immunologists estimate that 80 million Americans -- that's one out of every three persons -- are suffering with symptoms of this debilitating infection.

The health of this nation is in serious trouble. Our food is laced with pesticides and chemicals. The soil is depleted of minerals. Our cows are fed steroids. Three-fourths of the drinking water in this country is contaminated or radioactive. The air is polluted and many working places are unfit for humans to spend any extended time. Frequently we read of chemicals and pesticides which have been used for a number of years causing cancer or other types of degenerative disease/birth defects, and retardation. We also read of the psychological as well as the physical harm of radiation from T.V.,video terminals, microwaves, radar, etc.

Recently it has again surfaced in the scientific literature that amalgam fillings gas out mercury into the body, causing the Thymus (part of the immune system) to lower its production of T Cells (our body's defense). Journals warn world-wide of the harm of this poison. The literature also addresses nickel used in crowns as being cancer causing.

For the most part M.D.'s have been trained in allopathic medicine. For example, antibiotics are commonly prescribed. This takes care of the immediate symptoms but if the underlying problem is Candida, this only deepens the problem of the patient.

With the onset of Candidiasis raging in this country, causing serious illness, we need to know the alternatives if we are to survive. I have listed for you the reader references, sources of information (parasites, colon, acid/alkaline balance, etc.) and supplies so that you and your holistic physician may help the body to heal itself. If you decide to prescribe and treat yourself it is your constitutional right.

It is time to take responsibility for your own body, read, research and study the alternatives so that you will be a survivor.

It is my sincere desire that you the reader will have gained in understanding, knowledge and help in this most pervasive disease; after reading this compilation it is my wish that "each one teach one."

May you all be Light Bearers of Truth!

About the Editor

Betsy Russell-Manning has actively sought means to a healthier life for many years. After attending secretarial school, Ursuline College and the University of Louisville in Kentucky, Ms. Manning taught school in Chicago and co-oped at a grassroots nursery school in San Francisco. In the past Betsy has worked for Hippocrates Health Institute (California and Michigan Chapters) and is currently on the Executive Committee of Hippocrates Health Institute International Alumni Association in Boston. Ms. Manning has volunteered at the Gerson Clinic "Half-Way-House" in Chula Vista,California. Currently Betsy is a volunteer for Cancer Control Society (alternative health-care education) and an active member of the National Health Federation and a certified colonic hygienist. Ms. Manning is a free-lance writer and has contributed several articles to alternative health magazines and has been interviewed on several radio talk shows in San Francisco and Hawaii. Betsy has researched other books: How Safe Are Silver (mercury) Fillings? How Silver-Mercury Fillings Affect Your Energy System, Wheat Grass Juice - Gift of Nature and Mercury, A Poison In Your Mouth. Ms. Manning was nominated as one of the Outstanding Young Women of America for 1984 through the organization of "Outstanding Americans". Betsy resides in San Francisco and has one son Kevin Patrick, 17 years old.

CONTENTS

EDITOR'S NOTE: In making suggestions relating to nutrition, including vitamins, minerals and food supplements in general, the Editor has not diagnosed or prescribed, and none of the information offered or accepted is to be interpreted as pertaining either directly or indirectly to the treatment of any disease or condition. The information is offered to further public education and information and to assist individuals who request such information, to better cooperate with the doctors of their choice in building better health, and for balancing nutrition through nutrient intake. In the event the information is used without the supervision or approval of a doctor, you may be prescribing for yourself, which is your constitutional right, but the Editor assumes no responsibility. Since every person has different characteristics, nutritional results, if any, necessarily vary from individual to individual.

As the Editor of the Candida, Silver (mercury) Fillings and the Immune System book, I would like to ask your patience in any errors you may encounter as I am not a physician or dentist, but an Investigative Health Research Reporter.

In this book are suggestions by health professionals to eat meat. The San Francisco Vegetarian Society maintains there are health hazards related to eating any flesh foods including chicken and fish and that it is not necessary to include them in the diet for adequate protein.

For further information on the Vegetarian Society write: San Francisco Vegetarian Society, 1450 Broadway, San Francisco, California 94109 Telephone, (415) 775-6874.

Listings in this resource/reference book in no way constitutes an endorsement or recommendation.
Not all organizations or individuals in each field have been listed. Inevitably, the addresses of some of those listed may have changed since the publication of this book.

I

ANYONE CAN HAVE ACQUIRED IMMUNE DEFICIENCY SYNDROME (A.I.D.S.)

When we first began to hear of the term 'A.I.D.S.' we were told that it was strictly a homosexual disease that sometimes struck drug addicts and Haitians. Then we learned hemopheliacs were also coming down with it; those who required many blood transfusions. The nutritional state of the Haitians is usually very poor due to the almost starvation conditions in Haiti, so that when they are then subjected to the immune system destroyer, fluoride,in Miami and other fluoridated areas many of them succumb to the so-called AIDS even though this is very rare in unfluoridated Haiti. Since gays are more intimately in contact with disease organisms, and their lifestyle may not include proper nutrition, and since drug users have damaged body chemistry and exposure to germs from needles, these two sub-cultures are most often affected by AIDS.

Now we learn just recently through the San Francisco Chronicle, dated Monday, March 19, 1984 - AIDS FROM A BLOOD TRANSFUSION- Los Angeles
"The 38-year old woman went into the hospital for a hysterectomy. She came out with AIDS....It took a year before doctors could be certain that she was suffering from acquired immune deficiency syndrome, the often-fatal disorder that is considered rare among women. Still, neither she, her physician, the hospital nor Los Angeles County health officials were surprised-all had been watching and waiting since the man who donated the blood she received during surgery fell ill with AIDS.

Dr. Shirley Fannin, head of the county communicable disease program.... said there is no question about the source of this AIDS case; she said the patient is "an unmarried career woman with no contact with patients, no drug use, straight as an arrow, not homosexual, and with infrequent sexual contacts."

"Dr. Dennis Goldfinger, director of the Cedars-Sinai blood bank, said this case is extremely important to AIDS researchers."

According to Dr. Luc DeSchepper, M.D. the fungus Candida and AIDS travel the same highway. (While Candida continues down the same road, AIDS 'forks' off.)

Candida is caused by many different things. This fungus can be proliferated through the use of silver (mercury) fillings which cause electrical current &/or irritation along the gum line. Candida is drawn to live in this type of environment. (Dr. Carlton Fredericks, Ph.D., Director of Nutritional Services at the Atkins Center for Alternative Therapies, makes the hypothesis that amalgam filled teeth could be responsible for candidiasis in some patients).*

OTHER CANDIDA CAUSING FACTORS:Jaw Joint Syndrome,Fluoride,Pesticides,Chemicals, Birth Control Pills, Antibiotics, Nickel Crowns, Radiation and other environmental factors along with a diet high in sugar intake, pH Imbalance and Parasites.

According to Robert Picker, M.D., "There is evidence that up to 90 percent of this yeast is widespread, and is probably present in everybody."

Picker lists some of the most commonly reported symptoms of chronic candidiasis:

*See Dr. Fredericks' article in Chapter XII

Central Nervous System: depression, anxiety, irritability, lethargy and fatigue, agitation, inability to concentrate, memory loss, headaches.
Gastro-Intestinal Tract: heartburn, gastritis, colitis, bloating and gas, constipation and/or diarrhea, indigestion.
Genitourinary Tract: vaginal infections, menstrual irregularities, severe menstrual cramps and/or premenstrual tension, cystitis and/or urethritis (repeated urinary tract infections).
Allergic Manifestations: food and chemical sensitivities, sometimes severe, asthma, hives, sinusitis, hay fever, ear-aches, acne and possibly psoriasis.

In a medical journal there appeared a paper by Dr. R. Hurley of Queen Charlotte's Maternity Hospital in London: "Untreated systemic Candidiasis has a mortality rate approaching 100 percent. Delay in treatment is dangerous and will almost certainly end in death of the patient."

Dr. Sol Silverman, M.A., D.D.S., Professor and Chairman, Division of Oral Medicine, University of California, School of Dentistry, San Francisco, stated in his lecture on September 21, 1984 (18th annual John F. Gurley Lecture) that there are at least 100,000 people in the United States who will contract A.I.D.S. sometime in the near future.

This fungi which many of us give a home to can be transmitted sexually. Candida, or candidiasis lives at opposite ends of the gastrointestinal tract. It can live in the mouth, throat, esophagus and large bowel.

This fungi can proliferate in the throat area due to an acid/alkaline imbalance of the body due to improper function of the intestines, (infrequent bowel movements). The small intestine area is joined to the large intestine area by the 'ileocecal' valve. This valve sometimes becomes stuck in an open position. When this happens much of the waste matter which is on its way out through the large intestine of the body, re-enters the small intestinal area through this 'stuck' valve, thus polluting the blood stream and setting up an ideal spot for parasites to breed and for fungi to grow. (See Dr. John Lubecki's Book concerning the above, Better Health through Body Balancing, Chapter No. 11.
Also see Chapter No.3, "Changes in the Oral Flora in Sjogren's Syndrome"

When the fungus, Candida gains a foot-hold in the body (thus destroying the good bacteria & enzymes) through the use of chemicals, pesticides, birth control pills, antibiotics, yeast, sugar, silver (mercury) fillings, nickel crowns, radiation, fluoride, food additives; etc., the body can then succumb to any opportunistic organism, i.e., cancer, Kaposi's Sarcoma etc., as the immune system has been more or less paralyzed by the 79 different toxins given off by Candida; thus causing the Thymus's T cells to no longer mature. These T cells are the body's major defense against disease, bacteria, etc.

II

THE ENDOCRINE SYSTEM (THYMUS) AND THE CANDIDA CONNECTION

ENDOCRINE SYSTEM (THYMUS) AND THE CANDIDA CONNECTION

Hormones are essential to our understanding of the body's metabolism or normal functioning. Endocrine glands secrete hormones directly into the bloodstream, not just to a special organ; thus these secretions reach every part of the body. Hormones influence the flow of substances through cell membranes and often work together, which means that a hormonal imbalance may interfere with normal body functions.

The Endocrine System consists of the Thymus, Thyroid, Parathyroid, Pituitary, Pineal, Adrenal, Pancreas, Ovaries, and Testes.

In this Chapter concerning the Endocrine System and the hormones, I would like to again focus your attention on the fact that Candida in the tissues somehow inhibit the tissues to respond normally to hormones.

Dr. Truss, M.D. states, "When tests are done on estrogen levels, thyroid levels, or other hormone levels and people are suffering from these symptoms, the hormones are there in the blood stream, but they are not activating any response." Dr. Truss surmises that because of the presence of Candida in the tissues, these toxins somehow inhibit the tissues to respond normally to hormones. Cold hands and feet are a common symptom of candidiasis, and yet on a blood test a person will have a perfectly normal thyroid level.

This latter paragraph helps clarify the fact that the Thymus which produces the T Cells to fight disease in the body becomes inactivated by Candida albicans, subsequently shutting down the manufacturing of the T Cells, thus shutting down the immune system.

---

[1]MORBIDITY AND MORTALITY WEEKLY REPORT (Full report covered in Chapter VIII)

UPDATE ON ACQUIRED IMMUNE DEFICIENCY SYNDROME, the EDITORS NOTE: CDC "Center for Disease Control" defines a case of AIDS as a disease, at least moderately predictive of a defect in cell-mediated immunity, occurring in a person with no known cause for diminished resistance to that disease. Such diseases included KS, PCP, and serious *OOI. The foot note reads:

*"These infections include pneumonia, meninigitis, or encephalitis DUE to one or more of the following: ESOPHAGITIS DUE TO CANDIDIASIS..."

From the above report we can see that one of the ways in which the Thymus will shut down or lessen its production of T Cells is through inflammation of the esophagus due to the fungi, Candida, which inhibits the tissues through toxins, to respond normally to hormones,

---

[1]The MORBIDITY AND MORTALITY WEEKLY REPORT is published by the United States Department of Health and Human Services.

The following paragraphs explain the intimate connection between the Thymus (part of the Endocrine system) and the different systems of the body.

THE CONNECTION BETWEEN THE THYMUS, VERTEBRAE C1, C2 AND CANDIDA

C1 and C2 are the first two vertebrae in the neck area. The atlas and axis. The atlas is called the "King Pin" (most important vertebrae). If these vertebrae are out of alignment, the entire structure will be out of alignment. Both of these vertebrae supply the THYMUS. Through mis-alignmnet, nerve flow from C1 and C2 to the THYMUS will effect the function of the immune system.

THE CONNECTION BETWEEN THE VAGUS NERVE, THYMUS AND CANDIDA

The vagus nerve not only serves the larynx, trachea, bronchi, lungs, esophagus, stomach, large and small intestines but also the THYMUS. If the vagus nerve is in some way pressed upon or injured, the nerve flow from this 10th cranial nerve will be lessened, which in turn will cut down on the nerve stimulation it sends to the THYMUS, causing less production of the T Cells to fight disease within the body.

THE CONNECTION BETWEEN THE JAW JOINT, THYMUS AND CANDIDA

The jaw joint (temporamandibular joint) is in very close proximity to the vagus nerve. If the jaw joint is out of alignment either through heredity, accident or dentistry (noxious impulses from metal fillings, bridges, teeth being drilled too far down-malocclusion) this in turn can lessen the nerve stimulation to the THYMUS.

THE CONNECTION BETWEEN THE THYMUS, THE MERIDIAN SYSTEM AND CANDIDA

The THYMUS gland controls, monitors and regulates the energy flow throughout the meridian system.

The largest meridian which runs through the middle of the body, according to oriental medicine is weakened along with the other meridians when metal crosses this line, (e.g., dental bridges, fillings, metal glasses, etc.), especially in the concentrated areas of the head and neck region.

THE CONNECTION BETWEEN SILVER (mercury) FILLINGS, THE THYMUS AND CANDIDA

"The T-4 Cell is the helper cell. It identifies the cancer cells, foreign bodies, it identifies the bacteria, *fungus, virus. *(Candida? -Editor)

....Her T Cell level was 47. ....We took out the amalgams and prepared for gold inlays. ....We re-took the blood test. Her T Cell level went up to 73. ....The ideal T Cell level is somewhere in the 70's...." Dr. D. Eggleston's lecture to the Wholistic Dental Convention-1983.

THE CONNECTION BETWEEN FLUORIDATION, THE THYMUS AND CANDIDA

"The immune system is the body's major defense mechanism against disease. It is composed of white blood cells.... These cells serve as the body's surveillance system to recognize and destroy foreign agents such as bacteria, viruses, and chemicals as well as the body's own obsolete, damaged, or cancerous cells." Fluoride the Aging Factor

THE CONNECTION BETWEEN THE ENVIRONMENTAL FACTORS THAT DISTURB THE BODY, THE THYMUS AND CANDIDA

"The patient as well as the physician must become aware of the many things in the environment that serve to lower the body's resistance and the immune system." Dr. James Ouye, D.D.S.

THE CONNECTION BETWEEN THE ELECTROMAGNETIC FIELD, THE THYMUS & CANDIDA

Four main acupuncture circuits run through the jaw joint. If these circuits are interferred with through bacteria and infection in the jaw, this can in turn weaken the jaw causing Candida to proliferate (travelling down to the thymus and paralyzing the T Cells) and actually causing the joint to dis-engate from its proper functioning. If this joint is interferred with there are severe mental, emotional, physical and spiritual complications that will follow.

THE CONNECTION BETWEEN ARTIFICIAL LIGHT, THE THYMUS AND CANDIDA

According to Dr. R.J. Wurtman, of M.I.T., "....Recognition that levels of hormonal secretion vary markedly from day to night has triggered intensive investigation into the influence of environmental light upon endocrine function."

III

LECTURE AND INTERVIEW ON CANDIDA

ORAL CANDIDIASIS IN THE HEALTHY AND COMPROMISED PATIENT
Given by:
University of California-San Francisco: School of Dentistry - Postgraduate Education
(John Gurley Memorial Lecture)
Friday, September 21, 1984
Holiday Inn-Golden Gateway
San Francisco

Lecturer:
Dr. Sol Silverman, M.A., D.D.S.
Professor and Chairman, Division of Oral Medicine
University of California, School of Dentistry
San Francisco.

Candida in the mouth can look like cancer. Appliances in mouth increase risk of having Candida. According to Budtz Jorgensen (1970), "83%" of denture wearers have Candida.

Persons radiated for cancer in the neck and head area will have less saliva and be more inclined to harbor candida. (According to McFarlane 1974 and Berdicenesky 1980).

Where there is low hemoglobin + anemia you have glossitis and cheilitis, which will then harbor candida 100% of the time. Glossitis is a problem of iron deficiency.

Diabetic's have high blood sugar. First signs of diabetes is dry and burning mouth. Diabetic has dryness (less saliva) and this makes a good candidate for Candida.

There are at least 100,000 people within the United States at this time who will contact A.I.D.S.

Once you have Kaposi's Sarcoma you have A.I.D.S. *

Those that have more markers for A.I.D.S. are persons with allergies, hypoglycemia, G.I. problems, warts, Candida. These persons have the greatest risk. They have suppressed immune systems and are leaning towards A.I.D.S.

Candida is an opportunistic infection. If you are immune suppressed, you are at risk for developing A.I.D.S.

*See "Kaposi's Sarcoma" Abstract following this lecture.

Candida can increase Leukoplakia which can go into cancer.

Candidiasis can occur anywhere in the body. Candida is transmissible by food, faeces, cuts, sex, etc.

Candida can get in your blood stream and affect other organ systems.

50% of the population is carrying Candida.

Candida can grow in cells and between cells and on the surface of the body.

Candida a fungal organism, can invade in and between tissues.

Candida can invade surface epithelial.

Candida organisms can circulate in the blood.

Fungal organisms can get in to different organ systems when the immune system is suppressed.

Candida does circulate in the peripheral blood.

CANDIDA MANAGEMENT

Peroxide and Saline solution in water will interfere with Candida and be a good control for Candida.

The least expensive drug is Nystatin and it is effective for Candida. Mycolog cream and powder for corners of mouth.

Increase absorption of iron across mucosa for anemic patient with Candida,

CLINICAL CHARACTERISTICS - WAYS TO RECOGNIZE CANDIDA

No. 1 By smear
No. 2 By culture

SMEAR

A 30 or 60 second stain will tell if patient has Candida.

CULTURE

Within 72 hours white growth of fungal colonies will appear. You will be able to recognize species of fungus.

The white colony is then put on slide and it will show how candida sits on the oral mucosa growing and invading the epithelial cells.

It is a good idea to wear gloves and sterilize your hands as 50% of the population carry Candida.

DENTURE WEARERS-ORAL CANDIDA AND THE JOURNALS: Fletcher (1975), Berdicensky (1981) Epstein (1981)

WHAT TYPE OF SOLUTION TO BE USED BY DENTIST WHEN HE REMOVES FULL OR PARTIAL DENTURES & OTHER APPLIANCES

Use diluted clorox solution for hygiene purposes.

DIETARY CONTROL OF CANDIDA

Use wheat free crackers & less sugar.

QUESTION & ANSWER TIME

QUESTION: Does diet have any part to play in healing the body of Candida?
ANSWER: No, diet has no significant role in curing the body of Candida.

I would like to refer to the above answer whereby Dr. Silverman states, "Food plays no significant role in curing the body of Candida". Perhaps Dr. Silverman meant food plays no significant part in Candida when there is no overgrowth in the body. Certainly after there is Candida overgrowth in the body, different foods feed Candida; subsequently these particular foods must be avoided in order to cure oneself of this fungus. (See Chapter VII on "Questionnaires & Remedies for Candida") - Editor.

(Notes taken at this lecture by Editor)

KAPOSI'S SARCOMA & VARIABLY ACID-FAST BACTERIA IN VIVO IN TWO HOMOSEXUAL MEN

by Alan R. Cantwell, Jr., M.D. (Excerpts-Reprinted with Permission)

"Current epidemiologic data suggest that a possible infectious and contagious microbial agent is responsible for the recent outbreak of kaposi's sarcoma and the acquired immunodeficiency syndrome affecting young homosexual men. In this histopathologic study, rare foci of acid-fast, and Giemsa-stained coccoid forms, and more rare foci of Gram-variable coccoid forms, were observed within the microscopic skin biopsy specimens from two young homosexual men with Kaposi's sarcoma. These findings, in addition to other previously reported histopathologic findings of similar bacteria in vivo in "typical" cases of Kaposi's sarcoma occurring in elderly Jewish men, suggest that bacteria may be implicated in the pathogenesis of Kaposi's Sarcoma."

(From the Department of Dermatology, Southern California Permanente Medical Center, 4900 Sunset Boulevard, Los Angeles, California)

For Reprint Requests- Write to: Department of Dermatology
Southern California Permanente Medical
Center, 4900 Sunset Boulevard
Los Angeles, California 90027

Please Note: The following (4) articles were mentioned in Dr. Silverman's Lecture.

ORAL CANDIDIASIS IN HIGH-RISK PATIENTS AS THE INITIAL MANIFESTATION OF THE ACQUIRED IMMUNODEFICIENCY SYNDROME

ROBERT S. KLEIN, M.D., CAROL A. HARRIS, M.D., CATHERINE BUTKUS SMALL, M.D., BERNICE MOLL, PH.D., MARTIN LESSER, PH.D., AND GERALD H. FRIEDLAND, M.D.

Abstract We studied the frequency with which unexplained oral candidiasis led to unequivocal acquired immunodeficiency syndrome (AIDS) in patients at risk. Twenty-two previously healthy adults with unexplained oral candidiasis, of whom the 19 tested had a reversed T4/T8 ratio and 20 had generalized lymphadenopathy, were compared with 20 similar patients with a reversed T4/T8 ratio and generalized lymphadenopathy who did not have oral candidiasis. All were intravenous-drug abusers, homosexual or bisexual men, or both. Thirteen of the 22 patients with oral candidiasis (59 per cent) acquired a major opportunistic infection or Kaposi's sarcoma at a median of three months (range, 1 to 23) as compared with none of 20 patients with generalized lymphadenopathy and immunodeficiency but without candidiasis who were followed for a median of 12 months (range, 5 to 21) ($P<0.001$). AIDS developed in 12 of 15 patients with candidiasis and T4/T8 ratios less than or equal to 0.51, as compared with none of four with ratios equal to or greater than 0.60 ($P<0.01$). We conclude that in patients at high risk for AIDS, the presence of unexplained oral candidiasis predicts the development of serious opportunistic infections more than 50 per cent of the time. Whether the remainder will have AIDS is not yet known. (N Engl J Med 1984; 311: 354-8.)

Table 2. Outcome in Patients with Unexplained Oral Candidiasis.

Patient No.	Age/ Sex	Initial T4/T8 Ratio	Outcome
1	33/M	0.05	*Pneumocystis carinii* pneumonia at 3 mo
2	21/M	0.06	Central-nervous-system toxoplasmosis at 5 mo
3	31/M	0.06	*P. carinii* pneumonia at 1 mo
4	33/M	0.06	No opportunistic infection at 7 mo
5	27/M	0.08	*P. carinii* pneumonia at 1 mo
6	35/M	0.08	Probable *P. carinii* pneumonia at 2 mo *
7	30/M	0.18	*P. carinii* pneumonia at 12 mo
8	30/M	0.20	*P. carinii* pneumonia at 3 mo
9	37/M	0.27	Probable *P. carinii* pneumonia at 6 mo *
10	29/F	0.40	*P. carinii* pneumonia at 1 mo
11	26/F	0.45	Probable central-nervous-system toxoplasmosis at 4 mo *
12	24/M	0.47	No opportunistic infection at 12 mo
13	34/M	0.48	No opportunistic infection at 13 mo
14	26/M	0.50 †	Cryptococcal meningitis at 4 mo
15	38/M	0.51	Kaposi's sarcoma at 23 mo
16	36/M	0.60	No opportunistic infection at 4 mo
17	31/M	0.62	No opportunistic infection at 8 mo
18	19/M	0.70	No opportunistic infection at 19 mo
19	34/M	0.80	No opportunistic infection at 13 mo
20	23/F	Not tested	No opportunistic infection at 6 mo
21	31/F	Not tested	No opportunistic infection at 11 mo
22	31/M	Not tested	*P. carinii* pneumonia at 3 mo

*See text. †Performed at another institution.

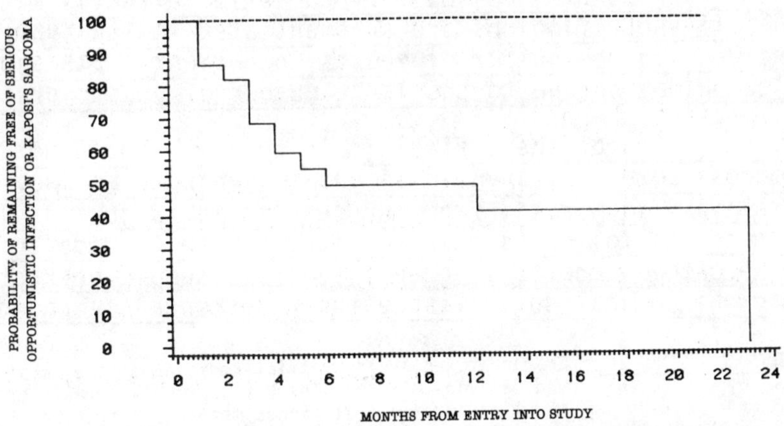

Figure 1. Estimated Probability of Remaining Free of Serious Opportunistic Infection or Kaposi's Sarcoma (AIDS) over Time among Patients with Unexplained Oral Candidiasis (Solid Line) or AIDS-Related Complex without Candidiasis (Broken Line). Probability is expressed as a percentage.

CANDIDA EXISTS IN THE ORAL CAVITY IN PATIENTS WITH LOW SALIVARY pH & IN PATIENTS WITH SJOGREN'S SYNDROME & XEROSTOMIA*.

CHANGES IN THE ORAL FLORA IN SJOGREN'S SYNDROME (Excerpt)
T.W. MacFarlane and D.K. Mason-Dept. of Oral Medicine and Pathology, Glasgow Dental Hospital and School, Glasgow
J. Clin. Path., 1974, 27, 416-419

Synopsis: The oral flora of 10 patients with Sjogren's syndrome was compared with that of 10 healthy control subjects. Significantly greater numbers of Candida albicans, Staphylococcus aureus, and coliform bacilli were present in the Sjogren's group. Possible reasons for these changes are discussed.

Many strains of Staphylococcus aureus are inhibited by saliva (Bibby et al, 1938) but the nature of the inhibitory factor is not known. In contrast to E. coli and Staphylococcus aureus, saliva from normal healthy adults appears to have no inhibitory effect on yeasts. Lehner (1965) has shown that patients with candidosis secrete antibodies against the yeast in their saliva. The loss of these inhibitory factors, together with the malfunction of the mechanical washing action of saliva, may partially explain our findings. Llory, Dammron, and Frank (1971) reported changes in the salivary and dental plaque microbial flora of patients whose salivary glands had been irradiated in the treatment of cervico-facial carcinoma. The numbers of cariogenic lactic bacteria (streptococci and lactobacilli) were increased but no quantitative increase in Staphylococcus aureus or coliform bacilli was noted. Yeasts were not mentioned at any stage of their investigations, which contrast with the present study where all the patients with xerostomia had yeasts present in the oral flora.

In relation to the number of yeasts present in the Sjogren's group, it is interesting to note that Young, Resca, and Sullivan (1951), investigating the number of yeasts in the mouths of healthy young adults, found that the numbers of yeasts isolated varied inversely with salivary pH. For example, the few subjects with a salivary pH of 5 to 5.5 had a 91% carrier rate for yeasts compared with a 52% carrier rate at salivary pH 6.5. It is known that patients with xerostomia due to irradiation for carcinoma have low salivary pH values (Frank, Herdly, and Philippe, 1965). Similar pH values for patients with severe Sjogren's syndrome are not available. However, preliminary studies carried out on four patients suggest that the salivary pH of patients with Sjogren's syndrome, all of whom had very low flow rates, was 4.5-5.5. These findings are not surprising since salivary pH varies directly with flow rate (Jenkins 1960). If these findings are substantiated low salivary pH may explain the increase in the number of yeasts in patients with Sjogren's syndrome, although the low pH may be due to the large number of yeasts present in the mouth.

The clinical implication of these findings is that we should not accept the inflamed dry mucosa sometimes seen in Sjogren's syndrome as inevitable due to decreased salivary flow rate; from our results it is just as likely that the inflammation is due to, or associated with, active Candida infection. Thus patients with xerostomia due to Sjogren's syndrome should be kept under regular clinical and microbiological surveillance for recurrence of candidosis.

* SJOGREN'S SYNDROME: Characterized by chronic inflammation of the lacrimal and salivary glands. There is commonly dryness of the lips and the oral mucosa with the secretion of thick, ropy saliva. The symptoms may be sufficiently severe to interfere with mastication and produce angular cheilitis and atrophy of the oral mucosa.

XEROSTOMIA: Excessive dryness of the mouth due to insufficient secretion of the salivary glands.

ORAL CANDIDA IN ASYMPTOMATIC DENTURE WEARERS (Excerpt)

Berdicevsky, I.:Dept. of Microbiology, Faculty of Medicine
Dept. of Oral and Maxillofacial Surger, Laboratory of Oral Biology,
Rambam Medical Center, Faculty of Medicine, Technion, Haifa, Israel:1980

ABSTRACT - The presence of Candida in the oral cavity of denture wearers was compared to a control group. A significantly higher percentage (88%) of Candida "carriers" was found among the denture wearers in comparison to the control group (52%). No difference between the sialochemistry of denture wearers and controls was found in oral Candida "carriers".

It is known that the alteration from commensalism to parasitism in Candida albicans is a result of changes in the host rather than in the fungi.

Table 1. Incidence of Candida in the oral cavity

	No. of patients	Candida (+)	%	Average titer
Controls	30	16	52	1×10^3/ml
Denture wearers	26	23	88	2.7×10^4/ml

(Excerpt)

ORAL CANDIDIASIS: EFFECTS OF ANTIFUNGAL THERAPY UPON CLINICAL SIGNS AND SYMPTOMS, SALIVARY ANTIBODY, AND MUCOSAL ADHERENCE OF CANDIDA ALBICANS

Epstein, Joel B., D.M.D.: University of Washington, Seattle, Washington: 1981

"A human study of the effects of topical nystatin (Mycostatin) therapy of oral candidiasis showed that effects of treatment were limited to the time in which the drug was used. Two weeks of therapy resulted in significant reduction in number of organisms and marked improvement in signs and symptoms of candidiasis. The condition recurred rapidly following cessation of treatment. No change in specific anticandida antibody in saliva or in adherence of Candida albicans to mucosal epithelium (in vitro) was seen with treatment."

...."Candidiasis often causes significant problems in patients with blood dyscrasias and in patients undergoing chemotherapy, radiotherapy, or bone marrow transplantation. Oral candidiasis in these patients may be very difficult to control, and the potential for systemic candidiasis is greater; thus, control of the infection is imperative. Antifungal agents are available as relatively specific therapy. However, even when the agent is effective, recurrences are common soon after cessation of medication."

Table II. Study population

Subject group	*No.*	*Mean age (yrs.)*
Control	16	58
Carrier	13	49
Chronic candidiasis	13	64
Acute candidiasis	10	55
Total	52	56.5

*SYMPTOMS OF SIDE EFFECTS THROUGH THE USE OF MATERIALS FOR PROTHESES (Stomatitis)

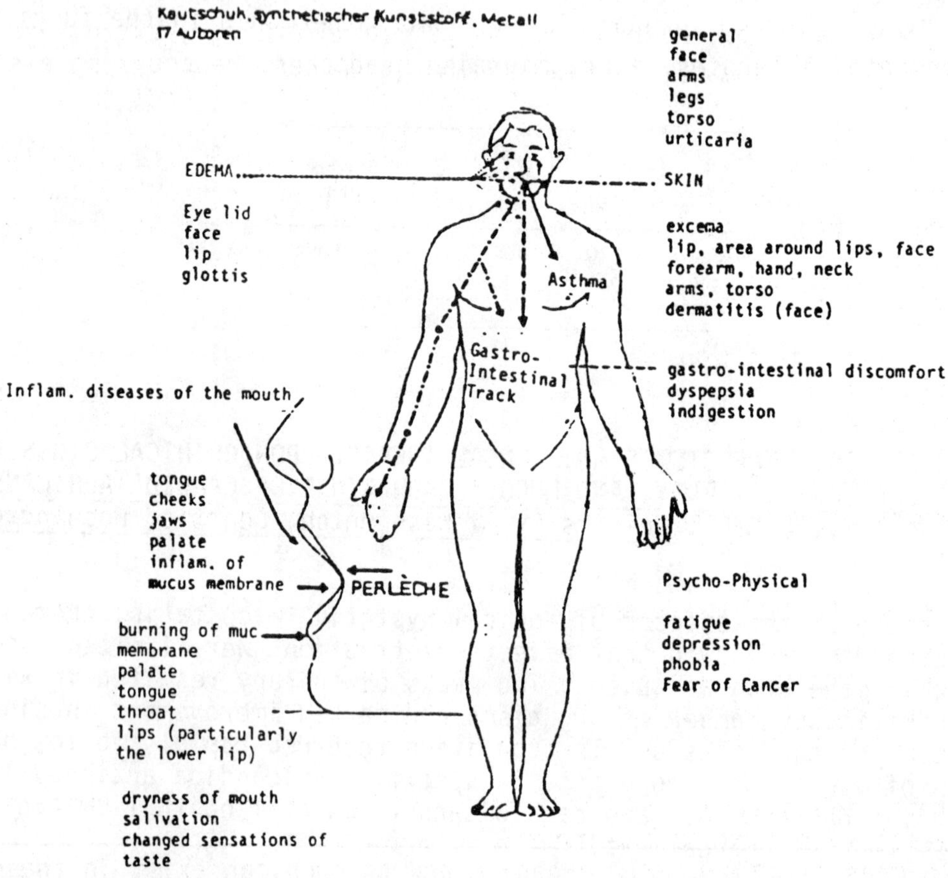

Diagram of symptoms of side effects through the use of materials for Protheses

*Translated from the German:

Gasser, Von F.: Concerning foreign bodies in the mouth in research and practice. Schweizerische Monatsschrift Fuer Zahnheilkunde (SSO) 77(4): 307-323. April 1967

*Robert Staat, Ph.D., University of Louisville School of Dentistry states the hard plastic (pink part) supporting the dentures, harbors yeast and in some people causes irritation known as 'stomatitis'.

Refer to Page No. 20, article titled, Oral Candida in Asymptomatic Dental Wearers.

(Excerpts)

CANDIDA ALBICANS: AN UNSUSPECTED PROBLEM

by: Jeffrey Bland, Ph.D. - Director, Linus Pauling Institute
Nutritional Biochemistry Laboratory for Nutritional Supplement Analysis
Univeristy of Puget Sound
Tacoma, Washington

Patients may have heard many times from doctors that they are suffering from "neurotic anxiety syndrome" when they complain of depression, anxiety, reoccurring irritability, heartburn, indigestion, lethargy, extreme food and environmental allergies, acne, migraine headaches, reoccurring cystitis, or vaginal infections, premenstrual tension, or menstrual problems, all of which have not been identified with any disease entity. Yet recently, thanks to the pioneering work of Dr. C. Orian Truss of Birmingham, Alabama in the United States, considerable progress has been made in understanding the origin of this symptom constellation in many individuals. The explanation is locked into understanding the life cycle of a symbiotic yeast become a *PARASITE called Candida albicans.

Candida albicans is present in all of us not long after birth. It lives in our intestinal tract and is a yeast-like organism which in the infective phase produces a condition called thrush, or candidiasis. Most medical practitioners feel that in the absence of the overt signs of candidiasis, which is the acute infection stage of Candida albicans, there is no concern about this organism and that chronic Candida overgrowth has not been well recognized.

Dr. Truss points out, however, that the Candida organism can increase its numbers during periods of stress or lowered immune potential of the individual. It is well known that the use of antibiotics for a long period of time can increase the Candida population in the intestinal tract, as well as the regular use of oral contraceptive medication.

As Candida proliferates in the intestines, it can change its anatomy and physiology from the yeast-like form to the mycelial fungal form. It is well recognized that Candida albicans is a*DIMORPHIC organism and as such can exist in these two states. The yeast-like state is noninvasive, sugar-fermenting organism, whereas the fungal state produces *RHIZOIDS, or very long root-like structures, which can penetrate the mucosa, and it is invasive.

Recent work from Dr. W.A. Hemmings in England and from the National Institutes of Health in the United States has indicated that some of these incomplete protein-breakdown products, if absorbed, may have endorphin-like activity and can change mood, mind, memory, and behavior.

One of the common side effects of chronic Candida infection is reoccurring vaginal infections or cystitis. We all harbor the organism in our bodies, but it is when the body loses its proper immune protection, or the intestinal pH is altered unfavorably, that the organism can then proliferate and change its state from the yeast form to the fungal form.

Dr. Truss has found that the classic test for *Candida albicans* overgrowth, a stool culture, does not always pinpoint the chronic infection problem. His experience is that a clinical trial of an anti-Candida program is best administered when there are symptoms suggesting Candida overgrowth. Relying upon stool culture information alone to assess the problem many times leads to a missed diagnosis.

....A program which would prevent the conversion of the yeast form to the fungal form of the organism would help to reduce the symptoms of chronic *Candida* infection. Dr. Truss has used the anti-yeast medication nystatin and finds that sometimes the program needs to be continued for six to nine months before successful alleviation of symptoms is achieved.

We have been very excited about an alternative therapy for the management of Candida infection, which avoids the use of the anti-yeast medication. It is well recognized that a disturbed flora of the gastrointestinal tract can establish a proper environment for the yeast proliferation. By reinocculating the bowel with proper symbiotic acid producing bacteria, there is a reduction in the compatibility of the intestinal environment for yeast proliferation. We have recently used an oral supplement of *Lactobacillus acidophilus*, cultured from mother's milk, to reinnoculate the bowel. This has been extremely successful in reducing *Candida albicans* in the intestinal tract. The *Lactobacilus acidophilus* mixture is given as a dry culture (1 teaspoon taken three times daily).

The second portion of the program, which is extremely important, is the recognition that the conversion of the yeast form to the fungal form of *Candida* is partially dependent upon biotin deficiency. Dr. Yamaguchi and colleagues have recently found that when biotin is added to the medium in high levels, it can prevent the conversion of the yeast form of *Candida* to its fungal form. They have also found that the fatty acid oleic acid seems to prevent this same conversion.

This concept has been used very successfully in conjunction with the *Lactobacillus acidophilus* culture to treat *Candida albicans*. Biotin is given orally (300m cg taken three times daily) along with two teaspoons of olive oil taken three times daily, as a source of oleic acid. This is done along with a higher than normal fiber diet, using oat bran fiber, to increase the absorptive surface area of the fecal material and to hasten the elimination of metabolic by-products. This may have to be continued for a period of one to six months depending upon the severity of the infection and the length of time htat there has been a Candida problem.

Once the organism is arrested in its growth and has been coverted back to the yeast form, a program is then instituted to facilitate the healing of the gastrointestinal mucosa. This program includes higher levels of zinc (30 to 50mg a day), vitamin A (25,000 to 30,000 units a day), vitamin E (400 to 800 I.U. per day), and calcium pantothenate (200 to 1000 mg per day). The success of this program is determined by the improvement of symptoms, which could be everything from panallergic syndrome to headaches, to acne, or menstrual irregularities.

Although not entirely successful, this program has been helpful in well in excess of 50 percent of the patients who have employed it to alleviate symptoms of chronic conditions that were otherwise ill-defined and seemingly untreatable. Cases such as 10- to 15-year recurrent migraine headaches have been alleviated by the use of this program, as well as long standing adult acne and joint pain resembling arthritis, which may really be a result of the build-up of immunochemically reactive materials from the direct or indirect effects of Candida.

There still may exist food hypersensitivities even after the control of Candida albicans, so the patient may additionally need to be put on a food rotation or elimination diet, depending upon the degree of sensitivity to to certain foods.

The prevalence of the Candida infection problem may be a result of the widespread use of antibiotics, particularly in animal feed, which end up in our meats, and may expose us to long-term, low-levels of antibiotics. Secondly, it may come from the widespread use of various medications, such as oral contraceptives, which have the ability to stimulate Candida growth; and thirdly it may be the nutrient-poor, low-residue diets that we eat, which alter the gastrointestinal pH and the mucosal integrity and set up the environment for Candida albicans hyperproliferation. These factors may then explain why so many people seem now to have chronic Candida infections and to be in need of the Candida control program.

Published in Preventive Medicine
Vol. 9, No. 2 - February, 1984
Reprinted With Permission

Suggested Reading on Candida-Editor

A Physician's Handbook on Orthomolecular Medicine- Edited by R.J. Williams with introduction by Abram Hoffer, M.D., Keats Publishing 1977

> "However, chronic infections are by and large ignored and undiagnosed or even unsuspected. ....I cultured 29 infections including bacteria and fungi. I have found that fungi such as Candida albicans,....& so forth are important infecting agents. ....A 20 year old catatonic schizophrenic developed catatonia on sublingual exposure to Candida albicans. She had a history episodic Candida albicans vaginal infection."
>
> From pages 151-152

Medical Mycology (2nd Edition) Rippon, J.W Philadelpha, Pennsylvania, W.B. Saunders, 1982

> "....Candida albicans accounts for the vast majority of diseases caused by the yeast."

Candida and Candidosis, Odds, F.C.: Baltimore, Maryland, U. Park Press 1979

> According to Dr. Odds, 200 to 300 scientific articles on candida appear annually, and his book lists 2,265 references.

The Missing Diagnosis, Truss, C.O. P.O. Box 26508, Birmingham, Al 35226

> "Virtually any organ can function improperly in this condition which we call chronic candidiasis".

Candida, A Twentieth Century Disease, Shirley S. Lorenzani, Ph.D., Keats Pub. 1986

INTERVIEW WITH DR. LUC DE SCHEPPER, M.D.

ON CANDIDA

Dr. Luc De Schepper, M.D. D.AC., C.A.
Certified Acupuncturist, Holland
Doctorate in Acupuncture, France
Certified Acupuncturist, State of Calif.
2901 Wilshire Blvd. Suite 435
Santa Monica, California 90403

Dr. Luc De Schepper, M.D. received his degree from Ghent University in Belgium. He studied in France receiving a degree in Acupuncture and and practiced there for 10 years. Dr. De Schepper will complete his residency at Veterans Hospital in Los Angeles, California.

Dr. De Schepper treats Candida through Acupuncture and tests for allergies through the use of the Voll machine.

"Mugwort", a dry ash from China, is used by De Schepper and is lighted and held over the acupuncture point while treating patients with Candida. This ash warms up the meridian being treated and the patient then begins to feel a sense of well-being and warmth throughout his/her body.

According to De Schepper all skin is dominated by the lung. The inner skin or mucosa is dominated by the spleen. The spleen point is in the foot. The eyelids, lips and "sleep" mechanism are all under the control of the spleen. The spleen is the master of the Immune System and the producer of the blood, while the liver stocks the blood and the heart and vessels pump this blood throughout the body.

Dr. De Schepper feels Candida is a spleen deficiency along with an entire 'web' of other symptoms. Some of these symptoms are: Low hereditory energy of the spleen; Gas problems (cellulitis); Tendency to get ulcers

General Diet for Candida Patients: No cold or raw foods; Small amount of sweets; Vegetables steamed; Brown Rice; Meats, fish and chicken.

Environment: Stay out of damp, cold or moldy climates.

Psychological symptoms: Emotional; Analytical (Intelligent); Serious; Worry (thinks a lot); Stubborn;

Dr. De Schepper states Candida and AIDS are on the same highway, however AIDS takes a different "fork" in the road. He feels what causes Candida (antibiotics) can also cause worms which in turn drain energy. According to De Schepper, "Dr. Adler of Switzerland states teeth No. 4 and 5 are connected with the spleen and stomach meridians." In Oriential medicine the spleen is (Yin-storing) and the stomach is (Yang-carrying).

Dr. De Schepper states that Candida patients have no energy against pesticides and if they are inadvertently exposed, they can become very ill and some almost to the point of death.

IV

CANDIDA, ANTIBIOTICS & A.I.D.S.

Dr. Orian Truss, M.D.:*THE MISSING DIAGNOSIS, 1982

Dr. Truss is a graduate of Birmingham-Southern College and of Cornell University Medical College. His post-graduate training was on the Cornell Division of Bellevue Hospital in New York City, where he completed successive years as Intern, Assistant Resident, and Chief Resident in Internal Medicine. He later held the positions of Chief of Cardiology and Assistant Chief of Medicine at the U.S. Air Force Hospital at Maxwell Field, Alabama. There followed a year devoted to study of the female endocrine system as a Fellow in Pharmacology at the University of Alabama Medical College in Birmingham.

Dr. Truss served as Instructor in Medicine at Cornell Medical College and as Instructor in Clinical Medicine at the University of Alabama Medical College prior to devoting full time to private practice. Dr. Truss is a certified specialist (Diplomate) of the American Board of Internal Medicine and a member of numerous medical organizations.

For many years his private practice has focused on the relationship of allergy and infection to many of the problems dealt with by internists. In particular this interest has centered on the role of the yeast Candida albicans in human illness...."

Dr. Truss has just published his book, THE MISSING DIAGNOSIS concerning Candida Albicans and its relationship to other diseases. Following are excerpts from the book:

"Already a number of patients have benefited greatly from treatment based on suppressing this yeast and endeavoring to restore competence to the immune system. ...."patients with autoimmune disease deserve to have their yeast problem treated. If it is not the cause of their illness, treating it should do no harm, and if it IS the cause, then that is what we are looking for."

CASES PRESENTED WHEREBY THE AUTOIMMUNE SYSTEM RETURNED TO NORMAL WITH TREATMENT

1) The first case is that of a three year old boy who developed severe autoimmune hemolytic anemia at 11 months of age. His immune system attacked his own red blood cells, destroying them in massive amounts in crises that continued until institution of therapy with the anti-yeast drug nystatin. On one occasion heart failure had occurred when his immune system destroyed two thirds of his red blood cells and he had so little hemoglobin to carry oxygen to his tissues that his heart could no longer function properly. Only massive therapy with predisone had kept him alive. With nystatin his multiple

*To order Dr. Truss' book, The Missing Diagnosis on Candida see address in Bibliography.

loose bowel movements immediately dropped to normal and his extreme hyperactivity abruptly ceased; within eight weeks his red blood count was climbing toward normal. It reached adult levels in 14 weeks and he is well now two years after treatment was started, having been off nystatin for three months with as yet no recurrence.

2) The next case of myasthenia gravis in a 22 year-old woman with severe yeast vaginitis from age eight years and chronic diarrhea for many years. Myasthenia developed at age 21 and was very severe despite maximum doses of Mestenon, the drug used in its treatment. This disease is thought to be an autoimmune response represented by an abnormal antibody that forms to a normal protein located on the end of individual muscle fibers.

After 12 weeks on Nystatin a young woman who could hardly talk, and could not wrinkle her forehead, was jogging three miles, working regularly, had reduced her Mestenon from two tablets every hour to one-half table every three hours, and was having one or two bowel movements per day instead of five or six.

3-4) Two men in their mid-thirties have Multiple Sclerosis that started in their early twenties. In each several manifestations have improved after 12 and six weeks of treatment with nystatin.

5) One case of Crohn's disease of the lower colon has cleared. In addition I know of two additional different autoimmune diseases, systemic lupus erthematosus and thrombocytopenic purpura, that have responded, and of a published case report of sarcoidosis, (yet another autoimmune disease) that recovered completely with anti-Candida treatment.

Dr. Truss goes on to say, "I have saved until last a statement regarding the autoimmune diseases. It is impossible not to feel excited about the possibility that Candida albicans is able to release into the bloodstream products that can alter cells of the immune system in a way that prevents it from exerting its normal suppressing effect on immunologic attacks of normal tissues."

"The thought that a number of diseases of such prominence, differing so markedly in their clinical pictures, could share a common underlying basis, at first seems totally incomprehensible. But perhaps just as difficult to comprehend, if each of these many diseases has its own separate cause, is the failure of even one of these diseases to yield to the massive expenditure of money and energy in research funded by the government, and often by national societies, for the past 35 years."

"This thought, together with the knowledge that these diseases share the abnormality of loss of immunologic tolerance to normal tissues, lends some support to the concept of a common etiology based on distortions in the cells of the immune system. That this agent could be Candida albicans is plausible in view of its presence in the body from soon after birth until death."

THE HOUSTON POST/Fri., March 30, 1984
by Barbara Boughton

"DO YOU FEEL BAD ALL OVER? Physician believes 'harmless' yeast at root of ailments."

"We endure everything. The pollen in the air, the chemicals in our food and cleaning stuffs, the diesel fumes that we sniff as we travel the highways. Now, it seems that these things are not just mere annoyances. They're things that can make us sick-horribly sick.

*Dr. William Crook, a Tennessee physician, says that pollen, chemicals and diesel fumes are among the things that can cause the growth of yeast in our bodies. And an over-abundance of yeast, usually a harmless germ, can cause any number of devastating health problems-everything from premenstrual tension to depression to arthritis and schizophrenia, he says."

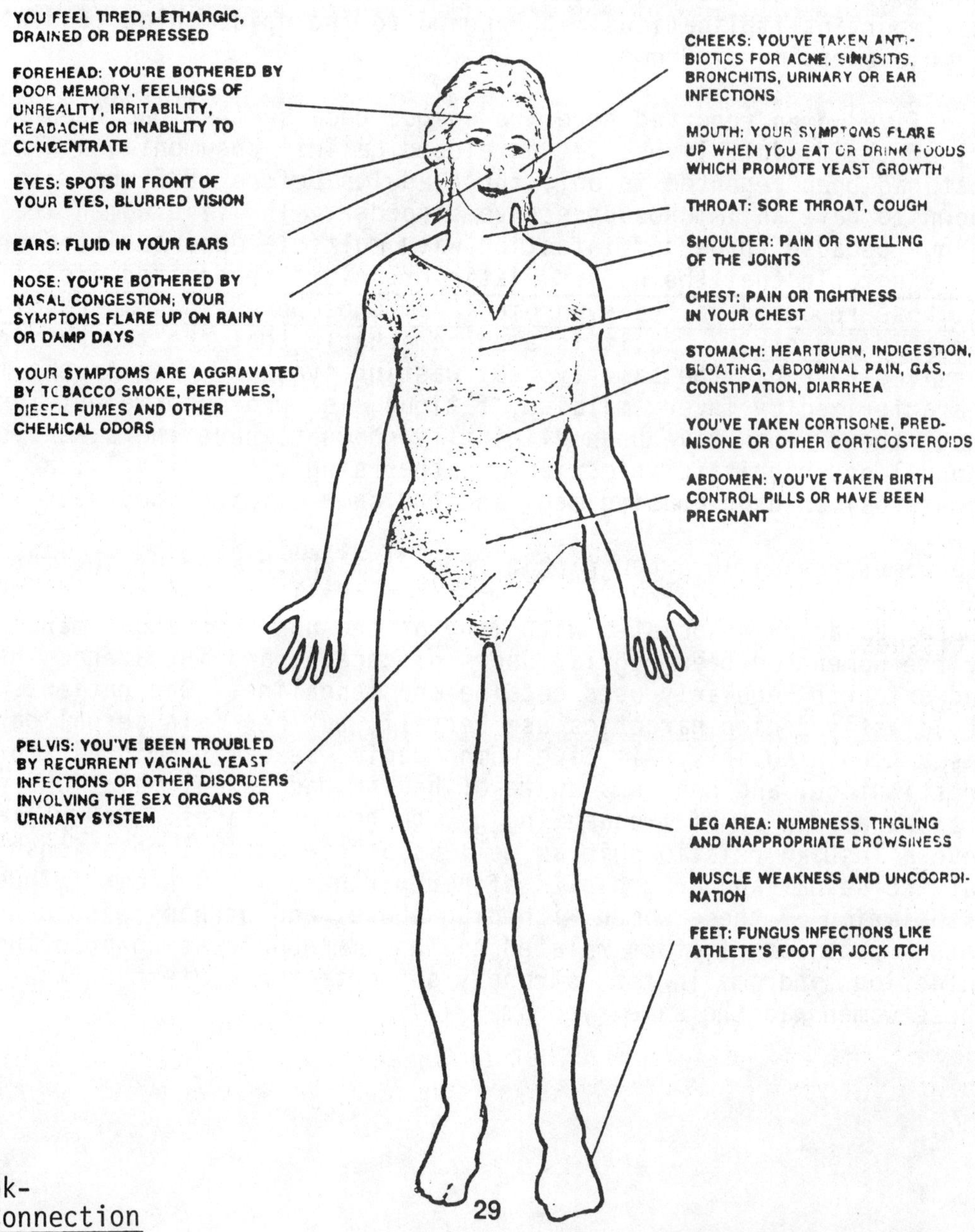

*New Book-
Yeast Connection

Post Illustration by Court Smith

AIDS REPORTED IN WOMEN

OPPORTUNISTIC INFECTION IN PREVIOUSLY HEALTHY WOMEN
Initial Manifestations of a Community-Acquired Cellular Immunodeficiency
Henry Masur, M.D.: Mary Ann Michelis, M.D.: Gary P. Wormser, M.D.: Sharon Lewin, M.D.: Etc. Annals of Internal Medicine Vol 97, No. 4, 10/82

Opportunistic infections and unusual tumors have been reported in an unprecedented outbreak of community-acquired cellular immune deficiency among homosexual and drug-abusing men. We report five women with the same syndrome. The women were residents of metropolitan New York City closely associated with drug abuse either by personal use (four patients) or close sexual contact with an abuser (one patient). One patient was bisexual. All five patients developed Pneumocystis carinii pneumonia as well as combinations of other opportunistic infections including oral candida,.... All patients had marked depression of cellular immune function. Three patients died The appearance of this syndrome in women has important implications with regard to the epidemiology and etiology of this emerging syndrome.

The five women reported here are unique because they had been healthy all of their adult lives, yet developed carinii pneumonia, a disease that had been reported in only three adults before 1978 who were not known to have an immunosuppressive disorder. The five women are also unique because three had infection with multiple opportunistic organisms. It is notable that the opportunistic organisms recognized are similar to those reported in the syndrome in immunosuppressed homosexual men or narcotic abusers. .....It is also remarkable that the two patients who survived have had the same type of wasting syndrome seen in the men, characterized by fever, malaise, fatigue, and profound weight loss. Thus, these women have been clinically shown to have the same types of unusual opportunistic infections, either singly or multiply, as the homosexual or drug-abusing men, and the same clinical course.

The women reside in a geographic area from which many of the men have been reported. Moreover, these women were all associated with drug abuse, a factor associated with many of the non-homosexual men. Three of the women had been regular users of cocaine and intravenous heroin and a fourth regularly used cocaine and mescaline. One patient, however, steadfastly denied narcotics use herself, but her male sexual partner was a heroin addict. All five women denied sexual promiscuity or prostitution, and none was aware of having had sexual relations with a bisexual man or of frequenting gay gathering places. One patient did have a lesbian relationship as well as a heterosexual relationship, but the sexual and drug habits of her partners are unknown. Thus, the association of these women with drug abuse, and perhaps with unusual sexual practice, factors related to the immunodepression-opportunistic infection syndrome in men, strongly supports the contention that these women had the same syndrome.

These women all had defects in cell-mediated immune response that were similar to the defects described in the syndrome in men.

The possibility that the syndrome can be acquired by intimate heterosexual contact is raised by the observation that the only apparent risk factor for Patient 2 was regular sexual contact with a heroin addict who, although clinically well, had depressed lymphoproliferative response. This factor raises the possibility that susceptibility to this syndrome may involve a transmissible infectious agent, although it would appear that multiple factors in addition to exposure determine development of the clinical disorder.

The development of this syndrome in women should clearly show the need for clinicians to consider the presence of community-acquired immunodeficiency in new patient populations. The occurrence of the syndrome in homosexual men or drug abusers as well as the potential for transmission into new groups should further the urgency to investigate this disorder so that transmission can be prevented and so a treatment can be discovered to reverse the current dismal prospects for survival that face patients who have acuqired this syndrome.

This paper is from the Clinical Center, National Institutes of Health, Bethesda, Maryland: The New York Hospital-Cornell Medical Center, Memorial-Sloan Kettering Cancer Center, Queens Hospital Center Affiliation Long Island Jewish-Hillside Medical Center, Lenox Hill Hospital, and the Mount Sinai Medical Center, New York, New York; Hackensack Medical Center, Hackensack, New Jersey; Westchester County Medical Center, Hackensack New Jersey; Westchester County Medical Center, Valhalla, New York; and the City Hospital Center, Elmhurst, New York.

CHRONIC MUCOCUTANEOUS CANDIDIASIS: Ann. Rev. Med. Vol. 32: 1981.

The fungus Candida albicans, lives within the intestinal flora of man and may remain harmless, when its growth is limited by our normal intestinal bacterial flora..... Chronic mucocutaneous candidiasis is a syndrome characterized by proliferation of the Candida in the skin, nails, as well as oral, esophageal, and genital mucosa. Many reports of this syndrome document the association of a wide spectrum of endocrine and nonendocrine organ dysfunction. Hypothyroidism is the most common endocrine defect followed by adrenal failure. Other associations include chronic lymphocytic thyroiditis, diabetes mellitus, ovarian failure, and ACTH deficiency. Susceptibility can be familial due to abnormalities in immuno-regulatory T cells. Iron deficiency is a constant finding associated with the syndrome. Treatment involves use of anti-fungal antibiotics, avoidance of yeast containing foods, and in some cases a diet low in carbohydrates.

ANTIBIOTICS, CANDIDA AND A.I.D.S.

PLAYING ANTIBIOTIC POOL: TIME TO TALLY THE SCORE
by Stuart B. Levy, M.D., Tufts University School of Medicine, New England Medical Center, Boston, Massachusetts
Source: The New England Journal of Medicine, Vol. 311, No. 10, Sept. 6, 1984, Editorials.

For more than 30 years in this country, subtherapeutic amounts of broad-spectrum antibiotics have been added to animal feeds to promote growth. The amount of feed additives in the United States has risen from thousands of pounds of antibiotics in the 1950s to millions of pounds today. But concern has been mounting about the relation of this use to the emergence of increasing numbers of antibiotic-resistant bacteria that threaten human health. ...There is general agreement that antibiotic use is responsible for the rise in resistant bacteria, but controversy continues over whether antibiotic use in people or animals has contributed most to the environmental pool. This issue is complicated by the facts that both groups receive the same kind of antibiotics and each receives about half of the more than 35 million pounds of antibiotics produced in the United States. ...Bacteria originating in the animal gut can find their way into the human intestinal tract. When pathogenic, they can cause human disease. Spread of multiply resistant salmonella from calves to human beings has been reported.

In England in the 1960s, serious human disease caused by the same multiply resistant Salmonella typhimurium type 29 originally found in cattle was important in establishing the Swann Committee. The committee's report, which attributed the rise in resistant organisms to low-level use of antibiotics in animals, resulted in the removal of therapeutic antibiotics from subtherapeutic use in England. Later other countries of the European Economic Community followed suit. Here in the United States, lawmakers have repeatedly asked for more data.

To date, all cases of animal-to-human spread of disease from resistant bacteria have originated in livestock in which antibiotic use has been either at therapeutic levels or ill-defined. A clear association between subtherapeutic use and human disease had not been shown. This important missing link is now provided by the elegant detective work of Holmberg and colleagues in this week's issue of the Journal. They show that a multiply resistant Salmonella newport strain in calves fed subtherapeutic doses of chlortetracycline caused illness in 18 people; some were hospitalized and one died. The article also shows how probable inappropriate use of antibiotics by the people involved increased the disease potential of the cattle-borne resistant salmonella once ingested. ...Antibiotic use disrupts the normal competition between the resident flora and a newly ingested organism.

Every animal or person taking an antibiotic (therapeutically or subtherapeutically) becomes a factory producing resistant strains through selection of existing and newly emerging resistant organisms. Since there are two to three times more livestock than people in the United States, the number of animals fed antibiotics at subtherapeutic levels (almost all poultry, pigs, and calves) is enormously greater than the number of people taking antibiotics in therapeutic amounts. Depending on the animal's size, its daily fecal excretion can be 5 to 400 times greater than the 100 to 200g excreted daily by adult human beings, and dispersal of animal feces is not well controlled. Therefore, one can understand why many consider the use of antibiotics in animals to be a more important contributor to the environmental pool of resistant strains than their use in human beings.

Surely, the time has come to stop gambling with antibiotics. Although their use as feed additives had a major role in advancing livestock production in the past, the consequences of this practice are now too evident to overlook. Alternatives for growth promotion are available and should be employed. However, looking solely at animal use as the cause of antibiotic resistance neglects the role and misuse and overuse in human beings.

ROLE OF ANTIBIOTIC IN THE PATHOGENESIS OF CANDIDA INFECTIONS.
Excerpted from: American Journal of Medicine, Vol. 40, pgs. 887-917, 1966
Mildred Seelig, M.D., M.P.H.

Candida albicans is a saprophytic organism under normal circumstances, and a limited pathogen when present in large numbers, but distinctly pathogenic in a host with depressed defense mechanisms. The increased incidence of Candidiasis in recent years has been shown to be clearly related to the increased use of antibiotics. ...In particular, the increased incidence of disseminated Candidiases and localized visceral candidal infections has been convincingly correlated with the administration of combined antibiotic therapy or broad-spectrum antibiotic administration, with or without corticosteroid treatment.

EFFECT OF ANTIBIOTICS ON THE IMMUNE RESPONSE
Excerpted from: The American Journal of Medicine, Vol. 72, No. 5, May 1982, Editorial by William E. Hauser, Jr., M.D. and Jack S. Remington, M.D.

The occurrence of serious bacterial, fungal and opportunistic infections in patients whose immune responses have been suppressed has led to the use of intensive and prolonged prophylactic and therapeutic antimicrobial regimens which often are administered in conjunction with corticosteroids and/or cytotoxic chemotherapy. Important to the clinical approach to such patients then, is an understanding of the potential beneficial and deleterious effects of antibiotic therapy on the host's immune response.

TABLE I Antibiotics That Have an Adverse Effect on the Immune Response

Chemotaxis	Lymphocyte Transformation	Delayed Hypersensitivity	Antibody Production	Miscellaneous
Gentamicin	Trimethoprim	Rifampin	Chloramphenicol	Phagocytosis
Tobramycin	Sulfamethoxazole	Amphotericin B*	Trimethoprim-sulfamethoxazole	Tetracycline
Amikacin	Trimethoprim-sulfamethoxazole	Metronidazole*	Rifampin	Doxycycline
Tetracycline	Amphotericin B	Doxycycline*	Doxycycline	Amphotericin B
Doxycycline	Tetracycline	Tetracycline*		Microbicidal activity of phagocytes
Lymecycline	Doxycycline			Sulfonamides
Rifampin	Minocycline			Amikacin
Amphotericin B	Lymecycline			Gentamicin
	Cephalothin			Tobramycin
	Chloramphenicol			Oxidative metabolism of PMN
	Clindamycin			Chloramphenicol
	Nitrofurantoin			Trimethoprim
				Sulfamethoxazole
				Trimethoprim-sulfamethoxazole
				Amphotericin B
				Allograft survival
				Rifampin*
				Trimethoprim*

Studies performed in human subjects or with cells from human subjects unless otherwise indicated; PMN = polymorphonuclear neutrophil.
* Effect seen in animal studies only.

CANDIDIASIS: AN INFECTIOUS DISEASE OF INCREASING IMPORTANCE
By Maxwell G. Shepherd
New Zealand Dental Journal 78:89, July 1982

Since the introduction of antibiotics and with the use of corticosteroids and immunosuppressive agents, there has been an increase in the prevalence of both superficial and systematic Candidiasis. An indication of the prevalence of fungal infections in the community can be gleaned from the amount spent on anti-fungal agents. In 1978, the wholesale value of anti-fungal drugs in the USA was $104 million; this compares with the $220 million spent on penicillins.

QUINTESSENCE INTERNATIONAL DENTAL DIGEST Vol 15, February 1984
Drug Administration

It is now known that the placenta does not act as a barrier against transfer of toxic substances from the maternal to the fetal circulation. Because some drugs are definitely dangerous when taken during pregnancy, and many others are suspect the prescription of any medication, especially during the first trimester, should be discussed with the patient's medical advisor. This is particularly important when administering steroids, which are known to cause congenital malformations such as cleft lip and cleft palate, or antibiotics such as tetrcycline, which cause discoloration of the enamel of the teeth, Candidal vaginitis, and kidney disturbances in pregnant women.

EDITOR'S NOTE: If you are on antibiotics have your doctor give you Vitamin C

METHOD OF DETERMINING PROPER DOSES OF VITAMIN C FOR THE TREATMENT OF DISEASE BY TITRATING TO BOWEL TOLERANCE-
Robert Cathcart, M.D.
Journal of Orthomolecular Psychiatry: Vol. 10, No. 2, 1982

Dr. Cathcart's experience in utilizing vitamin C in large doses has extended over a 9 year period and has involved over 9000 patients. The purpose of this paper is to describe a method which maximizes the effectiveness of ascorbic acid taken orally for various diseases and stress processes.

Candida albicans, Candida infections occur less frequently in patients being treated with antibiotics if bowel tolerance doses of ascorbic acid are simutaneously used. Ascorbic acid seems to have little effect on established Candida infections. It may be found that appropriate antifungal agents will penetrate tissues saturated in ascorbate better.

SOME THOUGHTS ON THE ACQUIRED IMMUNODEFICIENCY SYNDROME (AIDS).
Excerpted from: Nutrition Research, Vol 5, pgs. 3-7, 1985 Pergamon Press Ltd., by Gurdip S. Sidhu, M.D., Wafas El-Sadr, M.D., Depts. of Pathology and Medicine, New York University School of Medicine, New York, and New York V.A. Medical Center, New York 10010.

It has been recently proposed by Jain and Chandra that AIDS may be the result of an opportunistic infection by a retrovirus occurring in the context of nutritional deficits that compromise immunological competence. They cite evidence to show that protein-energy malnutrition is associated with alterations of the T,B and natural killer lymphocyte populations that very closely mimic the changes seen in A.ID.S. Victims of A.I.D.S. are generally wasted and malnourished at the time they present themselves to a hospital. Another association they point out is the effect of zinc deficiency on T Cell and natural killer cell populations, both of which are adversely affected. They cite preliminary evidence for the presence of zinc deficiency in A.I.D.S.

NUTRITION RESEARCH, Vol 5, pp. 9-19, 1985 - HYPOTHESIS

INTESTINAL INFECTION AND MALNUTRITION INITIATE ACQUIRED IMMUNE DEFICIENCY SYNDROME (AIDS)
Nutrition Research, Volume 5, pp. 9-19, 1985. Hypothesis
by Douglas L. Archer, Ph.D., and Walter H. Glinsmann, M.D., Division of Microbiology and Division of Nutrition, Food and Drug Administration, Department of Health and Human Services, Washington, D.C.

In our review of factors that might contribute casually to A.I.D.S., including the establishment of HTLV-III infections, and might provide preventive and therapeutic approaches, we were impressed that the following observations could be linked to a potentially causal, or at least predisposing, mechanism. 1. The occurrence of immunologic defects characteristic of A.I.D.S. in asymptomatic homosexuals in proportion to the number of sexual partners; 2. The presence of polymicrobial enteric infections in asymptomatic homosexuals, and 3, known relationships between enteric infections, malabsorption, intestinal permeability, and immune dysfunctions.

...in another study, enteric pathogens were found in 80 percent of homosexual men without such symptoms; the colitis/enteritis-associated pathogens included: Campylobacter jejuni, Campylobacter fetus, Shigella flexneri, Chlamidia trachomatis, Entamoeba histolytica, Clostridium difficile and Giardia lambia. Intestinal infection with enteric pathogens, such as the aforementioned, has long been known to cause nutrient malabsorption. ...Malabsorption with resultant malnutrition due to enteric infections and loss of endogenous nutrients due to diarrhea or otherwise altered gastrointestinal permeability has been shown to lead to immune dysfunction, including reversed T4/T8 ratios. Malnutrition has likewise been shown to predispose an individual to opportunistic infections such as Pneumocystis carinii, and to lead to a nutrition-immunity-infection nexus which further debilitates and predisposes the host to additional infections.

Intestinal infections and associated diarrhea are known to cause malabsorption. The types of enteric pathogens that are positively associated with malabsorption include bacteria, viruses, protozoa, fungi, and parasitic worms. ....Mucosal Candidiasis frequently is present in A.I.D.S. victims. As pointed out by Gracey, yeasts are often overlooked as harmless passers-by in the gut, but there is evidence that they may be toxigenic.

It is suggested that detailed gastroenterologic and nutritional studies may provide important clues to the pathogenesis of A.I.D.S. and that early identification and intervention should be considered for the purpose of maintaining the integrity of the intestine and the stability of the normal bowel flora. Education of the homosexual population pertaining to the risks of pathogen transfer associated with lifestyle and sexual practice also would be necessary in any prevention strategy.

SEMINARS IN MEDICINE OF THE BETH ISRAEL HOSPITAL, BOSTON

PATHOGENESIS OF VIRAL-INFECTIONS-BASIC CONCEPTS DERIVED FROM REOVIRUS MODEL.
The New England Journal of Medicine, February 21, 1985
by Arlene H. Sharpe, M.D., Ph.D. and Bernard N. Fields, M.D.

Infectious agents such as bacteria, viruses, fungi and protozoa are the most frequent causes of acute illnesses. However, only a small proportion of the microorganisms associated with human beings give rise to pathologic changes. To produce disease, many microorganisms must enter the host, multiply locally in host tissues, spread from the site of entry, and overcome host immune defenses.

The reoviruses are widely disseminated in nature and are found in vertebrates, invertebrates, and plants. The mammalian reoviruses are divided into serotypes 1, 2, and 3 on the basis of hemagglutination-inhibition and
By the age of 16 years, 50 to 80 percent of the general population has reovirus antibodies.

Some members of the reoviridae family are known pathogens in human beings. ...However, the importance of mammalian reoviruses in disease is difficult to acertain

Reoviruses are thought to enter the host primarily through the gastrointestinal tract.

The upper alimentary tract is the natural portal for reoviruses and other "enteric" viruses. To initiate infection in the gastrointestinal tract, reovirus must survive the harsh acidic environment of the stomach; withstand direct contact with proteolytic enzymes, bile, and other constituents of the intestinal lumen; and penetrate the intestinal mucosa.

After successfully traversing the enteric environment, viruses such as the rotavirus can enter intestinal epithelial cells and cause local inflammation and diarrhea.

...In addition to causing acute infections, viruses can produce infections that persist for months or years. Fenner et. al, have divided persistent infections that persist for months or years. Fenner et. al. have divided persistent infections into three categories: latent infections characterized by intermittent episodes of acute disease between which virus is not actually seen, chronic infections in which virus is always demonstrable but disease is either absent or associated with an immunologic disorder, and slow infections characterized by a long incubation period.

STUDIES ON THE CELLULAR NATURE OF CANDIDA ALBICANS-INDUCED SUPPRESSION
Excerpted from: The Journal of Immunology, Vol. 130, No. 1, Jan. 1983, by Victor Rivas and Thomas J. Rogers, from the Department of Microbiology and Immunology, Temple University School of Medicine, Philadelphia, Pennsylvania 19140 and the Department of Microbiology, Oregon State University, Uorvallis, Oregon 97331.

Animals treated with formalinized Candida albicans manifest depressed cellular immune activity. ...Human chronic mucocutaneous Candidiasis has been associated with a depressed cellular immune system. ...It has previously been shown that rodents infected with Candida albicans manifest a transient decline in the ability to respond to various T Cell-dependent mitogens. We report data here that show that mice treated with nonviable Candida also manifest depressed T Cell-dependent activity.

PNEUMOCYSTIC CARINII PNEUMONIA AND MUCOSAL CANDIDIASIS IN PREVIOUSLY HEALTHY HOMOSEXUAL MEN-Evidence of a New ACQUIRED CELLULAR IMMUNODEFICIENCY.
Excerpted from: The New England Journal of Medicine, Vol. 350, No. 24, Dec. 10, 1981, by Michael S. Gottlieb, M.D., etc.

Abstract: Four previously healthy homosexual men contacted Pneumocystis carinii pneumonia, extensive mucosal Candidiasis, and multiple viral infections. In three of the patients these infections followed prolonged fevers of unknown origin. In all four cytomegalovirus was recovered from secretions. Kaposi's sarcoma developed in one patient eight months after he presented with esophageal Candidiasis.

ECOLOGY OF CANDIDA ALBICANS GUT COLONIZATION: INHIBITION OF CANDIDA ADHESION, COLONIZATION, AND DISSEMINATION FROM THE GASTROINTESTINAL TRACT BY BACTERIAL ANTAGONISM.
Excerpted from: Infection and Immunity, Sept. 1985, pgs. 654-663, by Michael J. Kennedy and Paul A. Volz.

Systemic Candida infections are important causes of morbidity and mortality among patients who are compromised immunologically or who are undergroing prolonged antibiotic therapy. The passage of viable Candida albicans through the gastrointestinal (GI) mucosa into the host bloodstream is believed to be an important mechanism leading to systemic Candidosis particularly in patients with acute leukemia. Patient and animal studies support this hypothesis and indicate that a number of opportunistic fungal pathogens can spread systemically from the intestinal lumen to invade visceral organs.

DOES NUTRITIONAL DEFICIENCY PREDISPOSE TO ACQUIRED IMMUNE DEFICIENCY SYNDROME?
Excerpted from: Nutrition Research, Vol 4, pgs. 537-543, 1984, by V.K. Jain, M.B., B.S., etc., Department of Pediatrics, Medicine and Biochemistry, Memorial University of Newfoundland, Sh. John's, Newfoundland, CAnada

Abstract: The immunologic abnormalities seen with acquired immune deficiency syndrome (A.I.D.S.) are reminiscent of the immune changes seen in various nutritional deficiency states. It is proposed that A.I.D.S. is an opportunistic infection with a retrovirus, such as the human T Cell leukemia virus, that predominantly affects people at high risk due to a variety of underlying factors, including nutritional deficits.

Zinc deficiency also causes depression of cell-mediated immune responses. Hypothesis: We suggest that nutritional deficiencies play an important role in the pathogenesis of A.I.D.S. Once the patient develops the major manifestations of A.I.D.S., there may be mutually detrimental interactions between nutrition, immunity and infection. Malnutrition will cause suboptimal immunity which will permit infection by the A.I.D.S. agent, which in turn will cause severe impairment of immunity.

Equal attention has not been paid to the third side of the triangle, the nutritional status of the patient. We suggest that appropriate supplementation of calories, protein and trace elements would go some way in improving the immune status of the patients and, if given prophylactically to the high risk groups, might even prevent the development of the syndrome.

NUTRITION AND THE ACQUIRED IMMUNODEFICIENCY SYNDROME.
Excerpted from: Annals of Internal Medicine, Vol. 99, No. 4, Oct. 1983, by Richard S. Beach, Ph.D., Peter F. Laura, University of California, Davis, California 95616.

Nutritional status markedly influences immunocompetence. ...Deficiencies of specific nutrients such as zinc profoundly influence immunocompetence. We have shown that zinc deficiency during gestation results in an immunodeficiency syndrome that is passed on through three generations.

Exposure to toxic chemicals and heavy metals, stress, and superimposed infection may also predispose to immunodeficiency and facilitate the development of the syndrome.

ESSENTIAL TRACE ELEMENTS IN HUMAN HEALTH AND DISEASE
Excerpted from: Journal of the American College of Nutrition 4:1-2, 1985, by Ananda S. Prasad, M.D., Ph.D., Department of Medicine, Wayne State University School of Medicine, Detroit, Michigan

The most exciting development in recent years has been the recognition that zinc is essential for the functions of the thymic-dependent lymphocytes (T Cells). The essentiality of chromium for glucose metabolism in animal and human nutrition is now well recognized.

Selenium is an integral part of the essential enzyme glutathione peroxidase, as such, there is no doubt that this trace element is important for human health. Although magnesium is usually not considered to be a trace element, its bio-chemical role in enzymatic functions is similar to that of other trace elements. For this reason it has been included in this symposium.

Final Remarks: On the other hand, very large amounts of zinc may suppress immune responses.

ENTERIC INFECTIONS AND OTHER COFACTORS IN A.I.D.S.
Excerpted from Immunology Today, Vol. VI, No. 10, 1985
Douglas L. Archer and Walter H. Glinsmann

Editor's Note: In this article Douglas Archer and Walter Glinsmann discuss the history of A.I.D.S. and propose a link between HTLV-III infection and gastrointestinal disease processes with attendant malabsorption. They further propose that maximizing the nutritional status and minimizing the incidence of gastrointestinal infection of individuals infected with HTLV-III may prevent development of the full-blown A.I.D.S.

Abstract: "Similarities between symptoms of A.I.D.S. and nutritional deficiencies, particularly protein-calorie malnutrition, have been discussed by several groups. Others have suggested the possible role of parasitic and gastrointestinal infections in predisposing to A.I.D.S. or acting in concert with HTLV-III to cause the catastrophic loss of immune function. From the historical perspective of the A.I.D.S. epidemic in the U.S., little has been said about parasitic/gastrointestinal infections except as sequellae to A.I.D.S. although historically, the gastrointestinal infections of epidemic proportion involving Shigella Giardia and Entameoba preceded introduction of HTLV-III."

The clinical evidence suggests a role for intestinal pathogens and bowel dysfunction in predisposition to A.I.D.S., as a possible trigger mechanism or cofactor for HTLV-III infections and in the pathogenic process of A.I.D.S. itself. Considerable hope can be derived from the variety of intervention points in which the progression to full-blown A.I.D.S. may be altered by prevention/cure of bowel infections, nutritional support, and immunologic modulation.

Lecture given on May 14, 1986 - On Homeopathy - This section on A.I.D.S.
by Dana Ullmann, M.P.H.
Author of Everybody's Guide to Homeopathic Medicines*

Editor's Note: Mr. Ullman spoke on homeopathy. He touched on A.I.D.S. and the following is a short synopsis of this section. The ideas presented here are Mr. Ullmann's, however, in taking notes I was unable to capture word for word his exact statements.

Some of the areas Mr. Ullmann spoke about were the gay communities, drug addicts, A.I.D.S. in Africa, and Haiti.

Gays use recreational drugs. Gays get veneral disease more often then other populations and therefore receive more antibiotics for this problem. Also, because of anal intercourse it is easier for them to proliferate the fungus. Doctors prescribe high doses of antibiotics for this problem.

One of the things not talked about is the iatrogenic side of A.I.D.S. The doctors recommend immunosuppressors, ignoring the fact that many of these conventional drugs do in fact inhibit the immune system.

Penicillium is not an immunosuppressor. It does reduce white blood cell count. It does inhibit our ability to defend ourselves.

In central Africia where A.I.D.S. is prevalent, Mr. Ullmann indicated this is so because they are not using sterile needles when injecting penicillium. Patients are not only getting infected by needles but also subjected to the drug of penicillium, which stresses the defense system so patients can't heal;with increasing infection then they get the disease.

Haiti-Antibiotics

Antibiotics are distributed over-the-counter in massive doses in Haiti.

In New York gays are getting AIDS, also intravenous drug users from shared needles. Suppressed immune systems get infections, thus this population goes to the doctor and gets antibiotics, thus becoming more and more ill.

A book Mr. Ullman recommended: Mirage of Health by DeBose

Mr. Ullman's final comment at this time concerning A.I.D.S. was, "Look for ways to stimulate host defense through homeopathy of similars."

A book mentioned by Mr. Ullmann, Logic of Figures; concerns tables on morbidity or mortality rate in comparison of homeopathy to allopathic death rates.

For every homeopathic death there were two, four, six or eight allopathic deaths.

*This book is published by Jeremy P. Tarcher, Inc., Los Angeles, California.

Editor's Note: Homeopathic Educational Services, (books,tapes, homeopathic kits, etc.) 2124 Kittredge St., Berkeley, Calif. 94704

SUGGESTED READING

Conquering A.I.D.S. NOW! by Scott J. Gregory, M.S. Bianca Leonardo, Ph.D. Tree of Life Publications 513 Wilshire Blvd., #244 Santa Monica, Ca. 90401	$15.95 + $2.00 postage
Maximum Immunity by Michael Weiner Aurora Book Companions P.O. Box 5852 Denver, Colorado 80217	$16.95
AIDS Prevention and Healing With Nutrition Aurora Book Companions P.O. Box 5852 Denver, Colorado 80217	$ 7.95
When Someone you Love has AIDS by Betty Clare Moffatt IBS Press 2339 28th Street Santa Monica, Ca. 90405	$ 9.95
A.I.D.S., Cancer & The Medical Establishment by Raymond Keith Brown, M.D. Robert Speller Publishers New York, New York 10010	$16.95

V

CANDIDA RESEARCH & INFORMATION FOUNDATION

—

CHEMICALS & PESTICIDES

The Candida Research and Information Foundation has been formed by patients for the purpose of educating people on the subject of Candida and its effects on human health, providing research and information which may help patients to get the help necessary to regain health and to aid in ultimately irradicating Candida as a problem in human health.

GAIL NIELSEN, PRESIDENT
ADDRESS: CANDIDA RESEARCH AND INFORMATION FOUNDATION
31111 Palomares Road
Castro Valley, California 94552

TEL: (415) 582 2179

NEWSLETTER- July 1984 (CANDIDA RESEARCH & INFORMATION FOUNDATION)

"Research Update: Candida Albicans was found to be a highly toxin producing strain. Three days after infected, the T cells were obviously decreased and B cells gradually decreased in laboratory animals."

"Dr. Kazuo Iwata of Japan reported the results of extensive Candida research done in that country. In laboratory studies, the animals receiving isolated Candida Albicans toxins developed severe symptoms: paralysis of the extremities, lesions in various organs, edema and changes in the cerebrum, and in some cases, even death. Certain immune factors were found effective in neutralizing the effects of the toxins."

"Rabbits infected with Candida were found to have increased hypersensitivity. Changes in the brain were reported as well as lesions in the central nervous system. Although the mechanism was not known, it was reported possible that impairment by the toxins produced by the fungi allowed the infection to invade the central nervous system."

"Drunken symptoms caused by fermentation of the yeasts in the stomach of patients ranging in age from 1 1/2 years to 75 years - listed the following in order of severity are: flushed face, dizziness, euphoria, headache, palpitation, staggering, high fever, nausea, vomiting, excitation, delirium."

TAPE: DIET AND THE CANDIDA PATIENT by Dr. Devaki Berkson (2 tapes-$12.00)
CANDIDA-AN EPIDEMIC? by Gail Nielsen (1 tape- $ 6.00)

Address: Same as above.

To become a member of CRIF send a check for $20.00 and you will receive the Newsletter along with other information on Candida.

ENVIRONMENTAL HEALTH ASSOCIATION

The environmental Health Association (EHA) is a statewide non-profit tax deductible corporation whose purpose is to:

Network chemically-sensitive individuals and environmental organizations throughout California.
- provide information, education and research on toxic chemicals as they relate to human health
- provide assistance to chemically-sensitive individuals on matters relating to social services (social security), legal, housing, medical and other needs.

They are currently working to organize testimony for a hearing on "Indoor Pollution and Hypersensitivity to Toxics." The hearing is currently scheduled for Tuesday, November 15th, in Los Angeles before assemblywoman Sally Tanner's Consumer Protection and Toxic Materials Committee.

HOW TO JOIN EHA- Send $15.00 for a yearly membership or $5.00 for disabled or low income. Make checks payable to: Environmental Health Assn., 3609 Folsom Boulevard, Sacramento, California 95816. Phone No. 457-2098.

NOTE: THE CANDIDA FOUNDATION has affiliated with this umbrella organization.

Mr. John Jaeckle who has been involved with the Environmental Health Issue and the Chemically sensitive person for some time now has mounds of information on these subjects and is willing to help guide the patient to the latest medical help concerning these issues and the fungus, Candida. Mr. Jaeckle's address is:

Mr. John Jaeckle
Rt 1-78
Campo, California 92006

Mr. Jaeckle heads a Candida Study Group in San Diego which meets monthly at the Price Pottinger Foundation. Mr. Jaeckle states that "You can form a similar group finding like minded patients through your local doctors. The mutual learning and living support gained through such an effort can be of great assistance especially to those who suffer emotional impairments." Address for this group:

San Diego Area Candida Study Group
c/o Price Pottinger Foundation
5871 El Cajon Blvd.
San Diego, California 92115

REFERRING ORGANIZATIONS

Huxley Institute for Biosocial Research
219 E. 31 St.
New York, New York 10016

Society for Clinical Ecology
2005 Franklin Street #490
Denver, Co. 80205

HEAL
505 N. Lakeshore Dr. #6506
Chicago, Ill. 60611

TAPES ON CANDIDA

The NEW ENGLAND JOURNAL OF MEDICINE notes the Candida Albicans Conference, 1982 in Dallas on July 10, 1982, in Vol. 308, #2, page 101, Jan. 13, 1983 edition. The Conference is on tapes (8) available from:

Creative Audio 8751 Osborne Highland, Indiana 46322	$58.00 + $ 3.00 shipping & handling. $61.00 Total

IMPORTANT NOTE: Since 1978, when Dr. Truss' paper appeared in the Journal of Orthomolecular Psychiatry, the word about the link between chronic yeast illness has been spreading. Because no simple syndrome represents the expression of this link, the information about it tended to spread informally among a network of invironmentally and nutritionally minded physicians. The Dallas Conference formed an exchange of information among doctors who have been struck by the frequency of the "Yeast" problem. This meeting helped to form a consensus about what we do and don't know, based on clinical experience and basic immunology. Those attending the conference enthusiastically expressed that its purpose was fulfilled beyond expectation.

One of the speakers, Dr. A. Levin, M.D. of San Francisco, lectured on "The Interaction of Candida with the Immune System" and Experiences in Earlier Studies on Mucocutaneous Candidiasis."

Doctors who participated in the Dallas Candida Conference

Sidney Baker, M.D.
310 Prospect St.
New Haven, Ct. 06511

C. Orian Truss, M.D.
2614 Highland Ave.
Birmingham, Al. 35205

J. O'Shea, M.D.
50 Prospect St.
Lawrence, Ma. 01841

Kendall Gerdes, M.D.
1889 York St.
Denver, Co. 80206

Joseph Miller
273 Azalea Rd.
Mobile, Ala. 36609

Phyllis Saifer, M.D.
3031 Telegraph Ave. #144
Berkeley, Ca. 94705

Aubrey Worrell, Jr., M.D.
1600 Hickory St.
Pine Bluff, Ar. 71603

R. Mabray, M.D.
4204 N. Laurent St.
Victoria, Tx. 77901

Robert Marshall, M.D.
Theron Randolph, M.D.
505 N. Lakeshore Dr. #6506
Chicago, Ill. 60611

Alan Levin, M.D.
326 6th St.
San Francisco, Ca. 94103

F. Waickman, M.D.
1625 W. Portage Trail
Cayahoga Falls, Oh 44223

M. Teich, M.D.
930 Park Ave.
N.Y., N.Y. 10028

Robert Stroud, M.D.
722 North Brown St.
Chadbourn, N.C. 28413

Howard Hagglund, M.D.
2227 W. Lindsey #401
Norman, Ok. 73069

*A NATION-WIDE LIST OF PHYSICIANS IN YOUR AREA WHO TREAT CANDIDA

Write to Nutri-Cology, Inc., 2336-C Stanwell Circle, Concord, California 94520 and ask for a COMPUTERIZED LIST of physicians in your area who treat Candida. (The list of doctors will be according to your ZIP CODE AREA. Remember to include your zip code.

A LIST OF PROFESSIONALS IN CALIFORNIA WHO TREAT CANDIDA

Dr. Robert Cathcart, M.D.
San Mateo, California

Dr. Peter Madill, M.D.
Sebastopol, California

Dr. M. Rosenbaum, M.D.
Mill Valley, California

Dr. Richard Kunin, M.D.
San Francisco, California

Dr. Geary Ross, M.D.
San Francisco, California

Saram Singh Kahalsa, M.D.
Los Angeles, California

Dr. P. Saifer, M.D.
Berkeley, California

Dr. Miriam Yost, M.D.
Half Moon Bay, California

Dr. Robert Krakovitz, M.D.
Marina del Rey, California

Dr. Devaki Berkson, D.C.
Los Altos, California

Dr. Alan Levin, M.D.
San Francisco, California

---

*A partial list of physicians who treat Candida across the United States

Alan Gaby, M.D.
Washington, D.C.

R.G. Oberg, M.D.
Crystal Lake, Illinois

Donald Mannerberg, M.D.
Richardson, Texas

Jonathan Wright, M.D.
Kent, Washington, 98042

David Busher, M.D.
Kirkland, Washington

John Argabrite, M.D.
Watertown, South Dakota

* See previous page for list of physicians at the Dallas "Candida" conference who also treat this fungus.

A PUBLICATION FOR PEOPLE WITH IMMUNE SYSTEM DYSREGULATION & CHEMICAL SENSITIVITY

NON TOXIC & NATURAL NEWSLETTER

$10.00 per year (bi-monthly)
6 issues

- Feature story
- Update on product listings
- Recipes-dessert column
- Alternative sweetners
- Question & answer column
- *Update on book

Write to:
Non Toxic Lifestyles
P.O. Box 210019
San Francisco, Ca. 94121

FREE SAMPLE NEWSLETTER
WITH SASE.

---

*NEW BOOK - NON TOXIC AND NATURAL by Debra Lynn Dadd

An encyclopedia for the chemically sensitive. This is an excellent book. No home should be without it!

A complete guide on such necessities as: air, water, food, personal hygiene, household maintenance, natural fibers & stuffing, reading & writing, workplace, home, immunotoxic chemicals, food additives, cosmetic ingredients, manufactures and distributors, mail order businesses. It is jammed full of lots of information. It is available through

Cancer Control Society
2043 North Berendo St.
Los Angeles, California 90027

Price: $9.95 + $1.50 shipping - .98 Tax for California Residents.

PLEASE NOTE:

A Kodak copy of the book may be ordered through the writer. (Reproduced without printer's ink)

Price: $15.00 + $1.50 shipping .98 Tax for California Residents.

Address for Kodak copy:

Debra Lynn Dadd
P.O. Box 210019
San Francisco, California 94121

NEW BOOK AVAILABLE

Nurse who cured herself of Candida

Lady of Gray
Elizabeth Rose
Butterfly Publishing Company
2210 Wilshire Blvd., Suite 845
Santa Monica, Ca. 90403

$16.50 + $1.50 Shipping + Calif. Tax.

PESTICIDES AND CHEMICALS

"The new environmental health problems are multiple-created by radiation in all its forms, born of the never-ending stream of chemicals of which pesticides are a part...."

a quote from- SILENT SPRING
by Raychel Carson

When you suffer from an immune-system disorder and your health problems are yeast related, you will then have pesticide and chemical sensitivities.

Dr. William Rea and others state that chemical/pesticide exposure adversely affects many parts of the immune system.

When Candida is treated these adverse symptoms of chemical/pesticide sensitivities will disappear.

Some of the ways in which we ingest chemicals and pesticides is through our water supply, as insecticides and weed killers get into the water supply through use in fields, farms and homes.

Another way in which we can ingest a pesticide is through the skin and through breathing it in.

I would like to give an example of a chemical that was sprayed in California and what it does to the human anatomy.

MALATHION

"Malathion often kills insects in the same way that it and other nerve gases affect humans-by acting on their nervous system. This is what made the chemical attractive to the Nazis when they developed it as a chemical warfare agent during World War II. Dr. Frank H. Duffy, of Harvard Medical School, reports that his studies show that small amounts of malathion cause long-term alteration in brain waves, resulting in insomnia, irritability and other abnormalities.

One highly publicized use of malathion began in the summer of 1981, when an infestation of Mediterranean fruit flies was discovered in California and Florida. Despite the opposition of environmentalists and initially of California Governor Jerry Brown, huge amounts of the chemical were repeatedly sprayed over large areas of these states, including residential counties adjacent to San Francisco, comprising over 100 square miles and populated by almost 800,000 people... ....By August, over 1,300 square miles were being sprayed every week...

Additional evidence of malathion's toxicity has been ignored or suppressed. in 1981, pathologist Dr. Melvin Reuber was forced to resign from a federally funded research laboratory after he insisted that three National Cancer Institute studies supposedly showing the safety of the pesticide, actually demonstrated that it caused cancer. And after California state pathologist Marc Lappe released an internal study showing that malathion was more dangerous than the state's health services department claimed, he was removed as chief of its hazard evaluation office.

....the deadly nerve gas sarin is quite closely related to malathion, one of the most widely-used ingredients in household insecticides and mosquito spraying programs... Some 20 years ago, Rachel Carson, in Silent Spring, described the dangers of malathion, pointing out that it causes severe muscular weakness, among other ailments. Moreover, its effects are multiplied when it is combined with other chemicals.

....Dr. Adrian Gross, chief scientist for EPA's hazards evaluation division, charged that in approving this use of the chemical, EPA "could mislead the public about the dangers involved," and called EDB probably the most potent and toxic carcinogenic substance used as a pesticide today. Low level exposure to EDB causes cancer in 80 to 90 percent of the animals tested, and in a very short time period. During nation-side testing, EPA found the chemical in almost all samples of grain analyzed, so it can be assumed to be present in bread and other food products.

....Despite the overwhelming evidence that many pesticides cause cancer and are extremely damaging to humans and the environment, almost none of these chemicals has ever been "banned" by the government in the true sense of the word.

....even a single exposure to some common organophosphate pesticides (such as malathion, ...) can alter brain electrical activity for years....Some preliminary studies suggest altered learning patterns and behavior.

A study of the long term effect of such common organophosphates as malathion, ...upon human electro-encephalograms shows that just one exposure can alter the electrical activity of an infant's brain for years and possibly cause abnormal behavior and learning patterns. Other studies at Harvard Medical School on the tendency of organophosphates to cause insomnia, irritability memory loss, difficulty in concentrating and decreased libido, have concluded that "there is a dangerous possibility that organophosphate pesticides have the potential for causing long-term brain damage."

by Lewis Regenstein
America the Poisoned
Acropolis

-On Pesticide Poisoning-

Notes taken from Lecture by
Dr. Fuller Royal at the 1982
National Health Federation Convention
San Jose, California

"DDT and other pesticides-we are finding a lot of people have pesticide poisoning. We tell patients before they come to the clinic, to do something that sounds very strange. We tell them that they must soak in a tub of water with two tablespoons of clorox for 20 minutes at least 2 or 3 times before they come in. The reason for this is, that pesticides deposit in the fat of the body. There is a lot of fat in the skin, and so what happens is you will detoxify the pesticide that's in the skin. This reduces the toxic load, sometimes the patient doesn't feel well. They say, "I am allergic to the clorox, I am allergic to clorine." Usually what happens is there is a mobilization or a shifting of the pesticides and the moving of it around the body, the patient doesn't feel well. We are finding allot of pesticides in people today.

Some of them are saying, "I don't know where I could have gotten it, because I have never been out working on a farm", or this or that. We are finding so much of it. Patients do respond when you treat them homeopathically to eliminate it."

(For further information on Clorox bath write to: Hazel R. Parcells, D.C., N.D., Ph.D 111 Cardenas Dr., NE., Albuquerque, N.M.)

PESTICIDES

PESTICIDES MAY ALTER BRAIN FUNCTION
Science News, Vol. 129, February 8th, 1986

A recently released study funded by the Environmental Protection Agency indicated that there is a link between exposure to poisonous doses of agricultural pesticides known as organophosphates and a number of neuropsychological problems including depression, irritability and difficulties in thinking, memory and communication.

Organophosphates such as parathion and malathion have been used in agriculture and other industries for several decades says study director Eldon P. Savage of Colorado State University in Ft. Collins.

More Than You Ever Thought You Would Know About Food Additives

By Phyllis Lehmann, Reprinted From the *FDA Consumer*

Food additives are so much a part of the American way of eating today that most of us would find it difficult to put together a meal that did not include them.

Take a typical lunch, for example: sandwich, instant soup, gelatin dessert and a cola drink. The bread has been fortified with vitamins and also contains an additive to keep it fresh. The margarine has been colored pale yellow—or, if you use salad dresing, it has been made with emulsifiers to keep it from "separating." The luncheon meat contains nitrite; the soup, an additive to keep it from becoming rancid; the gelatin, red coloring to make it pretty. Finally, the cola to wash it all down; without coloring, flavoring, sweeteners or artificial carbonation, the pause that refreshes is nothing more than plain water!

Changing lifestyles in this century have resulted in more additives than former generations could have imagined. As Americans moved from farms to cities, there was a need for foods that could be mass produced, distributed over considerable distances and stored for long periods. The exodus of women from the home into the outside work place created a demand for more pre-prepared convenience foods. Greater sophistication increased demand for year-round supplies of seasonal products. Greater buying power gave industry a bigger market to please. So today we have a wider variety of foods available—and more additives in all foods.

By broadest definition, a food additive is any substance that becomes part of a food product when added either directly or indirectly. Today, some 2,800 substances are intentionally added to foods to produce a desired effect. As many as 10,000 other compounds or combinations of compounds find their way into various foods during processing, packaging or storage.

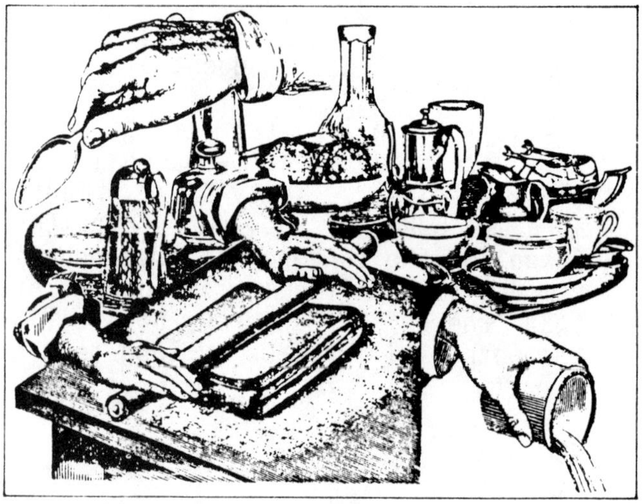

Editor's Note: In order to maintain freshness and to preserve the food shippers are spraying fruits and vegetables with Bipnenyl, a chemical used to embalm the body after death. This chemical is most harmful to the human body.

On the crate that comes into the grocery store the label might read:
Protected with Biphenyl, 2,4-Dichlorophenoxyacetate and sodium o-phenylphenate

Diet Coke and Pepsi contain "Aspertain" (Nutri Sweet). According to Amer. J. of Clinical Nutrition, March 1986, it causes depression, mood alterations, insommia and fatigue.

I ask you the reader, could this be the culpret in the many teen suicides happening around the country today?

SAUNAS, ETC. TO RID ONESELF OF TOXIC CHEMICALS, ETC.

TOXIC BIO-ACCUMULATION - The Waste Dump Within
by Bob Warner
The Beacon, Official Publication of the Sacramento Area Fire Fighters Local 522
Volume 6, No. 1

"Research literature tells us that toxic chemicals can weaken the human immune system which protects us against everything from colds to, perhaps, even cancer. The brain and nervous system, which have a high fat content, can suffer a serious impairment in functioning. Persons who have suffered toxic exposures often complain for months or years later of headaches, impaired memory, irritability and clouded thought processes. Chronic diseases, such as cancer, are of concern to everyone...

With this in mind, researchers with the Foundation for Advancements in Science and Education for the past 3 years have been testing a technique designed to reduce bodily accumulations of toxic chemicals. The technique, known as the Hubbard method after its developer, researcher L. Ron Hubbard, consists of a precise integration of seven components:

a) aerobic exercise
b) two-to-five hours daily of low-heat sauna with periodic breaks to avoid over-heating
c) gradually increasing doses of Niacin (vitamin B3), which promotes the release of toxins from the body fat;
d) polyunsaturated oil supplements, which help the body to exchange toxic for clean fat;
e) vitamin and mineral supplements; and
f) water and salts taken to avert dehydration of salt depletion due to sweating, and to increase perspiration. The program length varies from person to person, but averages two to three weeks.

A report in Ambio, the International Journal published by the Royal Swedish Academy of Sciences, states that followup tests of persons treated showed an average reduction of 21% for all chemicals studied which included PCS, PBB (a related substance) and three pesticides.

Four month post-treatment examinations revealed that a further reduction (to 42%) had taken place, a fact, which has led some physicians to speculate that the program may rehabilitate or enhance natural bodily mechanisms for throwing off toxic elements.

The Health-Med Clinic, a medical facility with offices in Los Angeles and Sacramento, has now treated over 1,000 persons using the Hubbard method. Many of those treated were sent by various Worker Compensation Insurance carriers who have found the treatment effective in the handling of their low-level chemical exposure cases."

Dr. Zane Gard, M.D., San Diego has a clinic for detoxifying chemicals and metals in San Diego, California. Dr. Vincent Mark, M.D., Soquel, California helps detoxify the patient of heavy metals and chemicals. Dr. George Mitchel, M.D. Washington, D.C. and Dr. Wm. Rhea, M.D. of Texas also help the chemically sensitive patient to detox. Dr. Craig Foster, D.D.S. and Nutritionist has also just opened up a detox center for chemically sensitive in Redding, California.

FURTHER READING ON CANDIDA, PESTICIDES & CHEMICALS

The Yeast Connection
Wm. Crook, M.D.
Professional Books

Food Pollution
Gene Marine
Holt

Silent Spring
Rachel Carson
Houghton

The Missing Diagnosis
C. Orian Truss, M.D.
Birmingham, Alabama

America the Poisoned
Lewis Regenstein
Acropolis

A Report to the Consumer
Newsletter-published monthly
Ida Honorof
P.O. Box 5449
Sherman Oaks, Ca. 91403

Keeping Healthy in A Polluted World
Harold J. Taub
Harper & Row

Consumer Beware!
Beatrice Trum Hunter
Touchstone

How to Survive Modern Technology
Charles T. McGee, M.D.
Ecology Press

How to Get Rid of the Poison in Your Body
Gary Null
Arco Press

Coping with your Allergies
N. Golos
Simon & Schuster

Lady of Gray
Elizabeth Rose
Butterfly Publishing Company
2210 Wilshire Blvd., Suite 845
Santa Monica, Ca. 90403

Non Toxic and Natural
Debra Lynn Dadd
P.O. Box 210019
San Francisco, Ca. 94121

Ms. Magazine
"Medical Expose"
A New American Nightmare?
-- For seven years, their work was breaking down their immune system --- They have a high-tech disease with no name, and we know that one million American women... are now working with chemicals whose combined effects are still unknown.
March 1986, page 35, by Amanda Spake

VI

CANDIDA, CANCER, CHEMOTHERAPY, & REFERENCES

CANDIDA CAN MAKE YOU DRUNK

CANDIDA IN THE CANCER PATIENT &* REFERENCES

....This early infection may or may not lead to later problems, but research reveals a growing population that suffers from diseases involving the immune system or that require therapies which adversely affect immune competence, that are treated intensively with anti-bacterial agents (antibiotics, penicillin, sulfa drugs) or have been innoculated intravenously with Candida, thus bypassing normal defenses. 1,2,5,7,11,13,14.

....Several studies revealed chemotherapy and antibiotic use as more commonly preceding the development of invasive disseminated Candidiasis. 1,2,11,14.

....It was reported that the sequence of events leading to disseminated Candida infection in surgery patients differs from that of patients with blood malignancies (leukemia). 11,14.

....Tests for detecting Candida cell constituents such as mannan [12], or a metabolite, arabinatol[8], may be promising for early diagnosis. Gas-liquid chromotography is reported to appear promising although unproven in the early detection of systemic Candida infection. [8,12].

....In the past there was concern about the potential renal toxicity associated with the use of amphotericin B therapy, but findings reported are that the clinically relevant determinant of organ failure was uncontrolled infection not amphotericin therapy.[2,6,14]. ....Nystatin as a treatment to prevent dissemination of Candida infection in cancer patients having had both chemotherapy and antibiotic treatment was not found to be effective.[2]
....It was reported that prolonged use (Ketoconazole) may cause: nausea and gastrointestinal distress, skin rashes, loss of libido, enlarged mammary glands in males, and hepatitis. [6,7,10]. Although this does not occur as the rule, prolonged use may pose a problem.

De Gregorio and others report the connection between antibiotic use, disturbance of the balance of microbial flora in various parts of the body and the removal of normal inhibitors of Candida overgrowth. They also report a connection between chemotherapy induced disturbance of mucosal integrity which may allow superficial invasion by opportunistic pathogens such as Candida.[2]

In view of the research, it appears important to begin anti-fungal therapy rather than wait until positive blood cultures are obtained. Autopsies have revealed disseminated Candidiasis in patients with neoplastic (cancer) diseases even though negative blood cultures had previously been obtained. 2.11.14. There is evidence to support that early or preventative therapy appeared to prevent dissemination of fungal infection.

Courtesy of the Candida Research & Information Foundation Newsletter- October 1984.

* References-See next page

REFERENCES

1. Carter, S.K., Glatstein, E.,Livingston, R.B., Principles of Cancer Treatment. McGraw Hill Book Co., N.Y. 1982, 193-194.
2. De Gregorio, M.W., Lee, Wm., Ries, C.A., Candida Infection in Patients with Acute Leukemia: Ineffectiveness of Nystation Prophyloxis and Relationship Between Oropharyneal and Systemic Candidiasis. Cancer. Dec. 15, 1982; 50: 2780-2784.
3. Felice, G., Yu B, Armstrong D., Immodiffusion and Agglutination Tests for Candida in Patients With Neoplastic Diseases. J Infect Dis. 1977; 135: 349-357
4. Glew, R.H., Buckley, H.R., Rosen, H.M., et al, Serologic Tests in the Diagnosis of Systemic Candidiasis. Am J Med. 1978: 64: 586-591.
5. Goldstein, E., Hoeprich, P.D., Problems in the Diagnosis and Treatment of Systemic Candidiasis. J. Infect. Dis. 1972: 125: 190-192.
6. Hermans, P.E., Keys, T.F., Antifungal Agents Used for Deep-Seated Mycotic Infections. Mayo Clin Proc. April 1983: 58: 223-231.
7. Hoeprich, P.D., Ranaldi, M.G., Infectious Diseases. Harper and Row, Philadelphia, 1983. 436-450.
8. Kiehn T., Bernard, E.M., Gold J.W., Armstrong, D., Candidiasis: Detection by Gas-Liquid Chromotrography of D - Anobinitol, A Fungal Metabolite in Human Serum. Science. 1979; 206: 577-580.
9. Kozinn, P.J., Galen, R.S., Tachdjian C.L., et al, The Precipitin Test in Systemic Candidiasis. JAMA. 1976; 124: 628-629.
10. Meunier-Carpentier, F., Treatment of Mycoses in Cancer Patients. Am J of Med. Jan. 24, 1983, 74-79.
11. Meunier-Carpentier, F., Kiehn, T.E., Armstrong, D., Fungemia in the Immuno-compromised Host. Am J of Med. Sept. 1981; 71: 363-370.
12. Miller, G.G., Wativer, M.W., Braude, A.L., Davis, C.E., Rapid Identification of Candida Albicans Septicemia in Man by Gas Liquid Chromotography. J. Clin Invest 1974; 54: 1235-1944.
13. Parker, J.C., Jr., McCloskey, J.J., Kanuer, K.A., Pathobiologic Features of Human Candidiasis. Am J. Clin Pathol. 1976; 65: 991-1000.
14. Solomkin, J.S., Flohr, A., Simmons, R. L., Candida Infections in Surgical Patients. Annuals of Surgery, Feb. 1982, 177-185.
15. Taschdjian, C.L., Kozinn, P.F., Cuesta, M.B., et al, Serodiagnosis of Candida Infections. Am J Clin Pathol. 1972: 57: 195-205

CANDIDA CAN MAKE YOU DRUNK!

An article in the Seattle Times, dated Saturday, January 8, 1983 -
DRUNK WITHOUT DRINKS: MAN'S BODY MADE HIM INTOXICATED

"It was in the spring of 1954, though," he recalls, "that I realized I could get drunk without so much as a short beer. I was in Lankenau Hospital for a month recovering from a severe attack of virus hepatitis and I got drunk there. And then, when my personal physician, the late Dr. Edwin A. Bortz, warned me that, because of severe liver damage, I must not touch anything alcoholic for at least two years, I followed his advice to the letter. And I still got drunk."

....Subsequent research on the subject, Swaart recalls, established that about 60 percent of the population has some yeast embedded in its alimentary canal (any of about 20 to 30 strains) and that this yeast is capable of producing some alcohol in the stomach,...

Swaart was exhilarated that mycostatin, a drug used in the United States to treat yeast infestation, mitigated his situation.

But in 1970, the mycostatin began losing its punch and the symptoms returned, with a vengeance this time. There also was cause for further alarm on Swaart's part. In a medical journal he had run across a paper written by Dr. R. Hurley of Queen Charlotte's Maternity Hospital in London: "Untreated systemic candidosis has a mortality rate approaching 100 percent. Delay in treatment is dangerous and will almost certainly end in death of the patient."

Crestfallen, the couple returned to Phoenix to find a letter from Dr. Kazuo Iwata, the professor of microbiology at the University of Tokyo School of Medicine that enclosed a sheaf of medical journal reprints detailing 30 Candida cases identical to Swaart's - all of them Japanese and ranging in age from 3 to 74.

Intrigued by the first non-Japanese to be stricken with the Japanese drunkenness disease, Iwata visited the Swaarts' home in Phoenix en route to a medical convention, consulted with Charlie's own Dr. Sierakowski and recommended drugs found effective on his Japanese patients. Armed with translations from the Japanese medical journals, doctors at Phoenix's St. Joseph's Medical Center tested Swaart for Candida, sending the cultures to Dr. Iwata in Tokyo. It was found to be a raging case; the attacks were now coming like clockwork.

The insurmountable block: The drugs recommended by Iwata and found effective in Tokyo had not been approved by the Federal Drug Administration and were not available in the United States.

The Swaarts flew to Tokyo. Hiding the medicine in her furs, Betty Swaart smuggled a year's supply into the States. Shortly after their return, the drug, known as Roche Ancobon 500mg, became legally available. "From that day to this," Swaart smiles broadly," ..I haven't had one symptom of intoxication."

IF CANDIDA CAN MAKE YOU DRUNK, IS IT POSSIBLE THE BIZARRE PHENOMENON OF SPONTANEOUS HUMAN COMBUSTION (Human Fireballs) IS ALSO CAUSED BY CANDIDA WHICH CREATES SO MUCH ALCOHOL IN THE BODY THUS CAUSING IT TO IGNITE AND BURN THE BODY TO ASHES?

I found the following article interesting in relation to the past article on DRUNK WITHOUT DRINKS-MAN'S BODY MADE HIM INTOXICATED

HUMAN FIREBALLS - Science Digest October 1981
by Larry Arnold

Subatomic Pyrotrons

Generations of scientists have speculated about the causes of spontaneous human combustion-and questioned whether the phenomenon existed.

....Some theorists traced the problem to excess flammable body fat that was thought to burn like the tallow of a candle with the clothes acting as a wick. Other explanations have included some kind of natural "electric fluid" in the body that ignited combustible elements and "internal decomposition" leading to the formation of highly flammable substances. The buildup of phosphorus ("not duly discharged" by habitual drunkards) or "carbonic oxide" (carbon monoxide) gas was thought to produce the "luminous flame" seen in some bodies undergoing SHC (spontaneous human combustion).

More recent explanations have drawn upon new discoveries in physics. For example, this writer has hypothesized the existence of a subatomic particle-the pyrotron-that perhaps vaporized a human being not by oxidizing combustion, as has always been assumed, but by the fire of an internal subatomic chain reaction.

While scientists tend to find all of these explanations unacceptable even preposterous, science has not been able to account for the facts with traditional theories.

VII
PARASITES AND COLON HEALTH

IS THERE A PARASITE THAT NOT ONLY CAUSES CANCER BUT KAPOSI'S SARCOMA AND A.I.D.S. AS WELL?

For almost 40 years, the leading proponent of the bacterial cause of cancer has been Virginia Livingston, a physician from San Diego, California. Livingston, not only showed the cancer microbe both within (in vivo) and outside the human body (in vitro), but also described the appearance of the microbe within the blood of cancer patients, by use of the "dark-field" microscope. By means of electron microscopy, she and her co-workers, were the first to photograph the submicroscopic, "filtrable" virus-like forms of the microbe.

Livingston showed the cancer microbe could be identified both in vivo and in vit.ro, by its "acid-fast" staining quality. The "red-stained (acid-fast) appearance of the cancer microbe indicates that this microbe might be related to other acid-fast bacteria, such as the mycobacteria that cause tuberculosis and leprosy.

Livingston was the first to demonstrate that cancer microbes could secrete a "growth" hormone, similar to human choriogonadotropic hormone HCG.

Bacteriologist have had great difficulty accepting the idea of "pleomorphic" microbes, and question the existence of the many different growth-forms claimed for the so-called cancer microbe. Most microbiologists believe a coçcus always remains a coccus.

The idea of a bacterium changing from a coccus to a rod, or to a fungus, or to virus-size forms, is completely unacceptable.

According to Livingston, the cancer microbe is a specific, and highly adaptable microbe, which she has name *Progenitor cryptocides. Depending on its environment, the microbe may attain large size, even larger than a red blood cell. Other forms are submicroscopic and virus-sized.

Microbiologists, such as Lida Mattman, and Gerald Domingue, have emphasized the possible role of these long-neglected cell wall bacteria, as pathognic agents in human diseases.

Despite the century-long history of the cancer microbe, the idea of a cancer bacterium remains unacceptable to modern medical scientists. However, medical history is studded with examples of medical truths which have taken decades, and even centuries, to be understood and accepted as truths. In general, great advances in medical thought have occurred very slowly, especially in the area of infectious disease.

Perhaps with the A.I.D.S. crisis, scientists will again be stimulated to search for bacteria. We now suggest that the cancer "parasite" is the long-sought-after microbe which causes, not only cancer & (1) Kaposi's Sarcoma, but A.I.D.S. as well!

*The organism is "pleomorphic", which means it may appear in many different forms. These forms range in size from submicroscopic forms resembling viruses, up to the size of much larger forms resembling yeast, fungi, and parasites.

(1) See Chapter III (paper on Kaposi's Sarcoma)

The above paper on the Cancer Research of Virginia Livingston, M.D. presents her findings of microorganisms as being one of the causes of cancer and other degenerative diseases. This summary may help the reader see more clearly how hydrogen peroxide once taken internally will flood the body, releasing oxygen and thus destroying these microorganisms, yeasts and fungi which live without oxygen.

Parasites

Worms are Still a Health Hazard: What You Can Do About Them Naturally
By Martin Zucker; Excerpted from Let's Live Magazine, May 1984

At a recent California Medical Association meeting, one expert speaker told his professional audience that worms are the unsuspected and unrecognized causes of a remarkable number of illnesses. What's more, he said, most physicians are unaware of this fact and the public, well, they know even less.

Ann Louise Gittleman, M.S., is a health professional very much concerned with these possibilities. In fact she looks for them, and often finds them.

In more than ten years as a practicing nutritionist, she has found worm infestations in a large percentage of patients. "It surprised me at first but no longer," she says.

Miss Gittleman, who practices in Santa Monica, California*, was formerly director of the nutrition department at the Pritikin Longevity Center, and also staff nutritionist of the pediatric clinic at New York's Bellevue Hospital and the Yale Hill Health Center in New Haven, Connecticut.

"It has not been a situation where people come to me for their worm infestations" says Gittleman. "Most have no ideal they are carrying worms at all. Most come for nutritional therapy for a wide variety of problems -- anything from diabetes to diverticulosis -- and frequently what we find are parasites aggravating conditions or even causing them.

The toxicity produced by these worms can be significant enough to create symptoms anywhere in the body. By no means are symptoms limited to the intestines. These toxins put a heavy burdon on the liver which is already working overtime to neutralize the contaminants brought into the body via food and air.

Tapeworms can grow up to 50 feet long. That means you are not only feeding a monster within you but also absorbing the toxicity of its waste products.

The eggs of tapeworms can also imbed themselves in body tissue and cause physiologic disturbances."

Gittleman says that digestive disorders are frequently involved with owrms. "Often there is constipation or diarrhea, bloating, inability to lose weight, gas, burping after meals and sensitivity to foods. I have traced a lot of food allergy problems to worms. There can be sleep problems, nervousness, and often difficulties with skin such as acne, oily skin, pustules, eczema, seborrhea, and cystic conditions.

Note: Ann Louise Gittleman is now living in San Francisco, California where she is currently writing and counseling. She is a nutritional consultant

Often there is a craving for sugar and a ravenous appetite that no amount of eating seems to satisfy. Remember you have another living organism -- or many living organisms -- in your system and this infestation needs sustenance. The food it preempts is food that your body would normally be utilizing. So your body demands more.

Once the intestines are cleansed and the worms and eggs eliminated, many of the symptoms disappear."

If worms are determined, Gittleman's therapy approach included a colonic irrigation to rid the body of toxic residue, and then an individual herbal cleansing program.

For many mild infestations she will use a combination of wormwood, black walnut and cloves. For more serious situations she employs pumpkin seeds, cranberry, garlic, capsicum and thyme, plus a combination of goldenrod and goldenseal for liver detoxification.

This herbal attack is followed by two months on comfrey-pepsin supplements to eliminate eggs or any other parasitical residue. Patients are also recommended to take a garlic supplement throughout the treatment. A fast is used in some cases as well.

Editor's Note: We recommend you consult your nutritionally-oriented physician if you suspect you suffer from this health problem.

WORMS: THE UNSUSPECTED CAUSE OF DISEASE, by Ann Louise Gittleman, M.S. and John Maxwell Desgrey, N.D.

Worms may very well be the missing diagnosis underlying many contemporary maladies. Symptoms as diverse as Candidiasis, allergies, diabetes, hypoglycemia, anemia, constipation, diarrhea, ulcers and tumors often disappear when parasites are cleared from the system.

In a survey taken in 1976 by the Center for Disease Control in Atlanta, it was revealed that one in every six people has one or more parasites living somewhere in the body.

According to other estimates worldwide, one out of every four people is infected. And these parasites -- ranging in size from microscopic single cells to foot long tape worms -- annually kill many more people than cancer does.

Roundworm, hookworm, malaria, trichuriasis, amebiasis, filariasis, and giardiasis are diseases afflicting over millions of people worldwide. The United States is not immune from these conditions as every known parasitic disease has been diagnosed in America over the past few years. These parasites may be the key to many diseases that baffle doctors every day, and are now being connected with the current auto immune problems such as A.I.D.S

Roundworm, hookworm, malaria, trichuriasis, amebiasis, filariasis, and giardiasis are diseases afflicting over millions of people worldwide. The United States is not immune from these conditions as every known parasitic disease has been diagnosed in America over the past few years. These parasites may be the key to many diseases that baffle doctors every day, and are now being connected with the current auto immune problems such as A.I.D.S.

Often an underlying factor in many of our contemporary health problems, when these infections are in people of "middle" or "upper class", often doctors don't consider the possibility of worms as a problem in these people; thus do not include a stool purge examination.

Where They are Coming From

Parasites can be picked up from public or private toilets, door-knobs, and handrails, as well as in contaminated dirt, water, food and dust. Hookworm can be acquired by walking barefoot on infected soil or sand. Although prevalent in the southeastern part of the U.S., who would suspect that a vacationer to a warm, tropical climate could get hookworm infection from simply walking on sand while sunbathing? Yet, according to Dr. Jerrold Turner, Chief Parasitologist at the Harbor UCLA Medical Center in Torrance, California, Americans are bringing back parasites from vacation hot spots all over the world.

Tapeworms come from improperly cooked or raw beef, pork and fish. In Finland where raw smoked fish is common, tapeworm anemia is a major problem in that country. In the United States, due to the popularity of sushi bars where eating raw fish has become common, tapeworm has increased over 200% in the past 15 years.

Household pets can also cause health problems as they carry more than 150 virus, bacterial, and parasitic infections that can infect man. Dogs transmit approximately 65 known diseases, cats 39, and horses 35. Ringworm, cat scratch, and toxoplasmosis are the most common but usually unrecognized because animal-transmitted diseases are so often unsuspected. Dog heartworm which has lodged in the lung of man has even been mistaken for cancer and there is a strong medical hypothesis that multiple sclerosis can be caused by canine distemper virus.

A popular health magazine reported in April of 1984 that in families bothered by repeated strep throat infection, 40% of the family pets turned out to be harboring strep organisms.

The current most popular protozoan parasite is known as Giardia lamblia, the number one water borne disease in the country today. It has caused epidemic outbreaks in upstate New York, Colorado and Washington. Once considered nonpathogenic, it is now recognized as being pathogenic and is very prevalent in gay men as well in those who have drunk contaminated water both here and abroad. Travelers to Russia have evidenced a high rate of infection, as well as children visiting South America. While some people remain asymptomatic, others show gastrointestinal symptoms such as abdominal pain, diarrhea, weight loss, nausea, and overall weakness.

According to experts in the field of parasitology, many protozoan can be transmitted through oral sex and so caution should be observed in that area.

Probably because of their association with poor sanitation and poverty, worms are regarded as unmentionable, uncomfortable, secret diseases. Most people don't like to think about the possibility of uninvited visitors living inside the body. And so they ignore them. But more and more today parasites are becoming an increasing problem taking a large toll on human health

Fortunately, in Europe people have a much more open attitude towards parasites. In Germany, dietary spring cleaning twice a year is accepted as desirable. In Europe it is commonly accepted that if one has dogs or horses, then there is a strong possibility that the owner has parasites and systematic purges are encouraged.

Since so many of us can unknowingly ingest contaminated food or water, we must change our attitudes and accept the probability that parasites do exist. Practical measures can be taken such as:

1. Drink only bottled spring water from a reliable source. Small water systems throughout the country may not adequately purify tap water and thus spread contamination. When in doubt, boil the water for at least 20 minutes. Make sure you also peel and cook fruits and vegetables.
2. Clorox questionable fruits, vegetables, meat, fish, and poultry in a special purifying bath. Soak your produce or protein in about 1/2 tsp. Clorox bleach to a gallon of regular water for about 15 minutes. Then wash thoroughly and soak in a fresh bath of plain water. Store or cook.
3. Keep your pets wormed and cat litter changed daily -- not randomly dumped.
4. Do not allow your children to play in sand or dirt where your dog or cat also frequents.
5. Keep your dog vaccinated yearly against distemper.
6. A stool purge test for ova, parasites and culture. This test must be taken after drinking a buffered saline laxative which thoroughly cleans out the colon and mucosal lining where most parasites live. A watery specimen is then analyzed using a specifically designed microscope.
7. Keep up your resistance. Parasites don't like a sugar-free diet or a strong immune system. Clean intestines -- free of mucous -- are also a good preventative.

In conclusion, parasites are alive and well and thriving in the American system. It therefore behooves every health conscious person to know the variety of symptoms worms can cause and be in touch with qualified diagnosticians for routine check-ups. Anyone who has traveled out of the country and has experienced problems in the GI tract should be checked immediately. Most parasites don't go away, they just remain in the body like a low grade infection and come to life again when the resistance is low.

Periodic cleansing should be a part of everyone's health maintenance program. In this way we can purify our internal environment so that nothing foreign can take up residence. Parasites cause more toxicity than most any other ailments many can suffer. In this case, most definitely... ignorance is not bliss.

AMOEBA, A PRIMARY SOURCE-CAUSE OF A LIST OF SO-CALLED INCURABLE DISEASES

RHEUMATOID DISEASES CURED AT LAST, by Anthony D. Fabio, Rheumatoid Disease Foundation, Old Harding Road, Box 137, Franklin, Tennessee 37064, (615) 646-1030. Non-Profit and tax exempt foundation. Price $10.95

Summary and Addenda: CAUSATION OF RHEUMATOID DISEASE AND MANY HUMAN CANCERS, by Professor Roger Wyburn-Mason, Rheumatoid Disease Foundation, Old Harding Road, Box 137, Franklin, Tennessee 37064, (615) 646-1030. Price $8.50

Free Protocol on Rheumatoid Diseases upon request, and other free literature. Physician Referral list upon request.

FROM THE RHEUMATOID DISEASE FOUNDATION

That bacteria are a primary source of disease is not really considered a theory any longer, but rather a fact; and so it is also a fact that viruses and yeasts and fungi can cause disease. One aspect of our bio-sphere that has not been fully explored is that protozoa -- microscopic forms of animal life - also cause disease. Until relatively recently it was thought by many in the medical profession that, excepting for a small number of exceptional diseases, the amoeba did not particularly bother man.

Now we have another of those earth-shaking findings by Professor Roger Wyburn-Mason (Oct. 2, 1911 - June 16, 1983), an Englishman, who has shown that the amoeba not only invades man's body, but is the primary source-cause of a list of so-called incurable diseases so long that their naming would seem to make up a catalog by themselves.

Must it be said that such findings ar mind-boggling, and that the implications will not be fully realized for generations?

LETTER TO THE EDITOR

Dear Betsy:

The Crook-Truss dietary plan for Candida only covers one-half of the ideal plan which would more effectively deal with Cindida.

Then entire basis of the Crook-Truss theory hinges on the fact that Candida feeds on certain foods and therefore if that fuel is removed, the Candida will then die off. Let's examine that theory briefly, and list its inadequacies -- in particular with reference to the cleansing program of Robert Gray.

Actually, some of the Candida may die as a result of the Crook diet but not all, because without an intestinal cleansing program, encrustations of mucoid and other waste material will provide a haven for the Candida and other molds which may tend to grow in a putrefactive environment of toxins.

According to Gray's theory, most diseases are a result of colon toxemia. To deal with Candida, 3 measures are required:

1. Change diet to reduce fuel needed by molds
2. Introduce Lactobacillus by taking cabbage,rejuvelac (see page 76 of Gray's book THE COLON-HEALTH HANDBOOK).
3. Eliminate the toxins. The Crook-Truss plan does not include a program for eliminating toxins. Candida and other mods produce hundreds of toxins. The Robert Gray plan must be followed. This is composed of four measures.
    a. Skin brushing to facilitate lymph system cleansing

a. skin brushing to facilitate lymph system cleansing
b. herbs-lymph and blood purifiers
c. psyllium husks
d. introduction of lactobacillus, via cabbage, rejuvelac.

Therefore, in fiew of the above, we see that theJ Crook-Truss diet is only one-half complete. A colon cleansing program patterned after Robert Gray's recommendations is of the utmost importance to rid the body of toxins. Remember, toxins are a product of Candida, and also feed the Candida. The source of the initial toxins are constipation, lack of fiber, and eating the wrong food.

Crook & Truss address only the question of eating the right food. In fact, the food they recommend is the wrong food, because (if you read Gray's book), you will see that meat is a mucoid forming food. Although mucoid encrustations in the colon do not directly feed the Candida, they produce toxins which cause putrefaction in the colon. And (this is the point) a TOXIC colon provides a haven for Candida!

Don't forget lymph cleansing! This is facilitated by skin-brushing.

The Crook-Truss diet errors in the relative proportions of meats, grains, and vegetables for an ideal anti-Candida plan - too much meat causes putrefaction in the colon - Dr. Richard Dahout's plan of 80% fruit and vegetables, 10 to 15% grains and only 5 to 10% animal protein.

Gray's plan eliminates all meat and dairy products, and is thus even more effective for Candida control.

Contrary to what Crook and Truss say, fruits are not a major problem because fruits are non-mucoid forming (see Gray's book). The only problem with some fruits is that molds tend to grow on them. Therefore, more emphasis should be placed on vegetables.

Next, I recommend Sonne's bentonite to detoxify the colon. You may find the product in your local health food store listed under the name Sonne's #7.

Another factor to consider is the endocrine support. Candida would not develop in the first place unless the endocrine system were weak. Strengthening the endocrine system and proper nutrition will kill the Candida. Live Cell injections aregood for this and may be obtained through Dr. W. Kuhnau, M.D. of American Biologics Hospital, Tijuana, Mexico. The address: P.O. Box 2014, San Ysidro, California 92073, Tel: 1-706-686-1909 & 686-1945.

Sincerely,

Mani
National Health Researcher

Source for The Colon Health Handbook by Robert Gray. Emerald Publishing Company, P.O. Box 11830, Reno, Nevada 89510 Cost $3.95 plus $1. shipping.

Robert Gray's Intestinal Cleansing Products may be purchased through Holistic Horizons, Box 2868, Oaklnad, California 94618-0068, (415) 652-4975.

Send for your free copy of Mr. Gray's Newsletter, "The Friends of Robert Gray Bulletin", c/o Holistic Horizons address.

LIFE IN THE 21st CENTURY by Viktoras Kulvinskas, Omangod Press, P.O. Box 64, Woodstock Valley, Connecticut 06282. Excerpts reprinted with permission

Evidence for Intestinal Toxemia. In 1933, Dr. Anthony Bassler, a professor of Gastroenterology in Fordham University Medical College and New York Polyclinic Medical College, and consulting gastroenterologist of Christs Polyclinic and Peoples Hospitals in New York states, after 25-year study of over 5000 cases, that: "Every physician should realize that the intestinal toxemias are the most important primary and contributing causes of many disorders and diseases of the human body." Dr. H.Y. Boeker, in 1928, went so far as to say, "It is now universally conceded that autointoxication is the underlying cause of an exceptionally large group of symptom complexes."

A thorough review of the literature was undertaken in the preparation of this paper. "Index Medicus," from the years 1879 to 1978, was checked under multiple listings: many medical texts were perused to find leads to articles; the "Citation Index" was also checked. The result of this search was tofind that almost no clinically-orientated articles have been written in the English language about intestinal toxemia since late 1950s. In fact, few papers have been published since 1940 which directly address this subject. It is for this reason that most of the clinically-oriented papers reviewed in this paper are dated from before 1940.

The reader may wonder why the theory of intestinal toxemia has not been discussed in recent times, and is not well known today. The fact is that a change in opinion over the years, not based on any new scientific research, has led to the abandoning of this idea by the medical profession. It is important to emphasize that this has not resulted from new scientific research proving the error of the theory of intestinal toxemia. It is well known that certain ideas fall into and out of favor as the years pass, regardless of thier validity, which has been the present case. An analogy may be drawn from the theory of chiropractic which, despite its great clinical usefulness, has been repeatedly "discovered" then abandoned or forgotten since ancient times; D.D. Palmer was the most recent individual to revive this old healing practice and bring ti to our attention.

Allergy: Dr. Sm. Lintz, M.D., successfully treated 472 patients suffering from "gastrointestinal allergy, a condition of hypersensitivity of the digestive tract, by eliminating the following allergens from the gastrointestinal tract: "bacteria and their toxins, foods and their split products. The most frequent symptoms were endocrine gland disturbances of many types such as hypothyroidism, pituitary malfunction, etc., heart disease, hypertension, and many others.

Asthma: Dr. Allan Eustis, M.D., instructor at Tulane University of Medicine in 1912, reports that 121 cases of bronchial asthma were relieved by eliminating the intestinal toxemia universally present. Dr. D. Rochester, M.D., of the University of Buffalo School of Medicine in 1906, stated that it was his conclusion, after 23 years of observation, that toxemia of gastrointestinal tract origin is the underlying cause of asthma. He stated, "I believe the results of treatment justify my position."

Arthritis: Dr. Anthony Bassler treated 44 arthritis patients by relieving intestinal toxemia, and observed marked improvement in 21, moderate in 19, none in 4.

Cardiac Arrhythmias: Guyton states that "Toxic conditions of the heart can cause arrhythmias. Dr. Bassler rdports 100 percent success in eliminating such heart irregularities in 43 patients treated by reducing intestinal toxémia.

Ear, nose, and throat problems: The experience of three doctors is neatly summed up by Dr. J.A. Stucky, M.D., "In several hundreds of cases of diseases of the nasal accessory sinuses, middle and internal ear, ...I have found unmistakable and marked evidence of toxemia of intestinal origin as evidenced by excessive indican in the urine, and when the condition causing this was remaoved there was marked amelioration or entire relief of the disease.

Eye Problems: Dr. C.W. Hawley, M.D. treated many cases of eye strain and disease with success once again by relieving intestinal toxemia

Thyroid gland disease: Dr. W.W. Reveno, M.D., theoretically links exophthalmic goiter to "A toxic process in the intestinal tract."

Nervous System: Many disorders of the nervous system are involved. Dr. Carl Von Noorden, M.D., professor of the first Medical Clinic, Vienna, Austria, in 1913, described a condition of diffuse sensory polyneuritis with pronounced vagal irritation treated with positive results by relieving inestinal toxemia. He and his assistant extracted a "poisonous substance from the feces, which in animal experiments produced quite similar symptoms.

Senility: The following should be mentioned: "Auto-intoxication from intestinal stasis or from constipation dye to lessened peristaltic activity, undoubtedly plays a contributing part in the process of senescence."

Low Back Pain and Sciatica:Dr. R.B. Osgood, M.D., cites six cases of patients suffering from these conditions. A few had also received chiropractive manipulative care with no improvement. In these cases, the cause was a toxemic state of the intestine; the pain completely left upon elimination of the toxemia, and returned upon return of toxemia because of dietary errors.

Dermatoses: Dr. Hans J. Schwartz, M.D., in a statistical analysis of 900 patients suffering from acne, eczema, and many other skin conditions, concluded that intestinal toxemia is an important etiologic factor in the production of many dermatoses, especially those of the inflammatory type."

Breast pathology: Changes in the breast resulting from intestinal toxemia have been described by many doctors. The views of three can be summarized a such: "The breasts undergo degenerative changes, manifested in the first instance

Cancer: There is no claim that intestinal toxemia is the cause of cancer. However, some physicians believe that "Even the beginning of malignant disease of various organs comes within the wide range of intestinal stasis."

BACTERIAL INHABITANTS IN OUR INTESTINES

(Excerpts)

What goes on in Our Compost Heap?- A Physician's Handbook on Orthomolecular Medicine, Edited by Roger J. Williams-1977, Keats Publishing, Inc.

In addition to their function in the cholesterol-biliary system, our intestinal bacteria make significant quantities of vitamins: niacin, riboflavin, K, B_{12}, folic acid, biotin and paraaminobenzoic acid. It has been shown that antibiotics like penicillin may kill off so many of these useful bacteria that a vitamin deficiency develops and persists until the flora re-establishes itself or supplementary vitamins are given.

by Miles H. Robinson, M.D.

INTESTINAL PARASITES

Vitamin C in the Treatment of Acquired Immune Deficiency Syndrome (AIDS)
Robert F. Cathcart, III, Medical Hypotheses 14: 423-433, 1984

If the AIDS patient has intestinal parasites, he must be treated for them. There is a very high percentage of male homosexuals infected with intestinal parasites. These intestinal parasites are themselves very immunosuppressive. The prognosis for for an AIDS patient is greatly enhanced by proper treatment of these parasites. Entamoeba histolytica, especially, and Giardia lamblia must be treated. Intestinal parasites, ordinarily considered non-pathogens, should be treated. If negative, repeated stool examinations for ova and parasites should be taken if there is the slightest clinical sign of intestinal parasite infection. Samples should be fresh, not over 1/2 hour old. Laxatives may increase chances of discovering the parasites. Additional samples may have to be taken through a sigmoidoscope if other specimens are negative for ova and parasites. With treatment, Herxheimer's reactions should be expected frequently. Symptoms, incuding Kaposi's lesions, may be exacerbated, despite the ascorbate, during treatment for intestinal parasites.

BACILLUS SOURCES

U.A.S. Lab - D.D.S.I. Strain
U.A.S. Lab. 7864 -12th Ave. So.
Minneapolis, Minn. 95420 (612) 854-2233

Univ. of Nebraska -L. Acidophilus-
Devine Tree-Box 5062 (Rice Base)
So. San Francisco,Ca.94083 (415) 661-4222

NATURAL LACTOBACILLUS RESTORES NORMAL COLON FLORA

LACTO-B The bacteria in LACTO-B has been preserved by the freeze drying method and stabilized with Vitamin C and the amino acid, Glutamic Acid, to ensure proper pH. LACTO-B is formulated in non-fat milk solids and calcium lactate, and contains 3 million beneficial bacteria per capsule that normally reside in the colon. These bacteria are referred to as intestinal flora. They are often destroyed from taking antibiotics and for other reasons. Symptoms of having too low of a level of flora are: bad breath, cold sores, constipation, diarrhea, toxemia, vaginitis, yeast infections, and chronic infections such as acne. LACTO-B helps replenish the normal flora which will naturally control these conditions. See Multiway Products 3 pages over to order.

Why Lactobacillus Acidophilus is Vitally Important Not Only to the Colon, but the Entire Body

Acidophilus is a species of bacteria belonging to the genus Lactobacillus, i.e. Lactobacillus acidophilus. All of the lactobacilli are so named because they ferment carbohydrates, especially sugars, with the production of large quantities of lactic acid. This lowers the pH and creates an acidic environment which inhibits the growth of many other microorganisms, including some pathogenic to man.

The species of Lactobacillus useful to man include L. bulgaricus (used in the preparation of yogurt and other fermented foods, L. Bifidus found in human breast milk (which colonized the GI tract of the infant), and L. acidophilus, part of our normal bacterial flora. In humans, acidophilus is found in the distal small intestine, colon, rectum, oral cavity, and vagina.

The first published report of the healthful effects of lactobacilli was that of Metchnikov in 1908. Since that time numerous reports have been published concerning the beneficial effects of acidophilus and of foods which have been fermeted by acidophilus. The ingestion of lactobacillus acidophilus colonized in the gastrointestinal tract has been reported to effect the following results.

1. replacement and balancing of the beneficial flora of the digestive tract whichis frequently destroyed or greatly decreased by anti biotic therapies or other medications
2. production of the enzyme, lactose, which is essential for digestion of lactose (milk sugar)
3. production of Vitamin K which is necessary for the formation of prothrombin, a chemical required to aid in blood clotting
4. improves intestinal function to correct faulty elimination
5. production of essential B Vitamins, Folic Acid and B-12, needed for proper body functions
6. aids in the assimilation of calcium
7. reduction of blood cholesterol levels
8. production of anti-bacterial agents that inhibit the growth of pathogenic organisms
9. production of anti-bacterial agents that inhibit the growth of pathogenic organisms
10. production of digestive enzymes, aiding in the digestion of food
11. reduction of bad breath and flatulence (intestinal gas)
12. counteraction of toxic and hazardous substances.

LACTOBACILLUS ACIDOPHILUS PRODUCES NATURAL ANTIBIOTICS

Antibiotics have been reported to be effective against many life threatening organisms. In the past few years, however, health professionals have discovered that over-prescribing and over-medicating with antibiotics may be the cause of other health problems. Thus the question: "Are there alternative ways to help the body fight disease?"

Dr. Khem M. Shahani, Professor, Department of Food Science and Technology, University of Nebraska, Lincoln, Nebraska, states in his paper, "Nutritional Impact of Lactobacilli Fermented Foods": Recently, a number of studies have established that the lactobacilli used in the fermentation process may improve the nutritional quality as well as the nutritional quantity of the cultured products by increasing the B-Vitamin and enzyme contents. In addition, during fermentation the lactobacilli can also produce natural antibiotics, natural anticarcinogenic compounds which retard or inactivate toxins and poisons.

In another paper, "Properties of and Prospects for Cultured Dairy Foods," Dr. Shahani reports that the natural antibiotics, like acidophilin, produced by the lactobacillus acidophilus, can be effective against a large number of important pathogenic organisms.

PRODUCT: VITAL-DOPHILUS

The only acidophilus free of all common allergens: milk and yeast is Vital-Dophilus. Vital-Dophilus is free of the common dietary allergens that may be present in many other acidophilus products: milk, milk components such as lactose, whole grains and soy, yeast and apple pectin. Each gram (approximately 1/4 teaspoon) of Vital-Dophilus contains a minimum of ten billion plus live lactobacillus bacteria which are free of common allergens

Vital-Dophilus has an increased stability and shelf life and a count of ten billion plus of live bacteria, per gram, constituting a highly potent acidophilus product. The most modern, scientific techniques have been utilized in order that these lactobacillus organisms could be grown, stabilized and preserved for full retention of vitality, activity and reproducibility. Vital-Dophilus does not need special handling or refrigeration during shipping, therefore making it more convenient and economical. After opening, however, refrigeration is suggested.

NON-MILK: Formulation: Because of the name Lactobacillus it is commonly assumed that the organism can grow best in a milk base. Many individuals because of milk-intolerance, have been unable to benefit from the antibiotic and nutritional properties of Lactobacillus acidophilus, due to the milk base. However, with proper modification of the growth medium and appropriate strain selection, adaptation to modified media, genetic manipulation and bioengineering, suitable strains of Lactobacillus acidophilus can be developed, which could grow on a non-milk media. Vital-Dophilus is that strain.

Vital-Dophilus' medical and scientific consultants for Klaire Laboratories: Wm. H. Philpott, M.D., Jon B. Pangborn, Ph.D., Khem Shahani, Ph.D.

Address: Vital-Dophilus, P.O. Box 618, Carlsbad, California 92008-0110 (619) 744-9680.

Note: Vital-Dophilus may be ordered only through your physician. However, the health food stores carry the same product under the name Prime-Dophilus.

ECOLOGY NO. 3 by MULTIWAY

Ecology No. 3 is a concentrated form of Bio-Cultures from Lactobacillus Acidophilus, Lactobacillus Bulgaricus, and Lactobacillus Bifidus. In addition to these important cultures, Ecology No. 3 contains Streptococcus Faecalis, a special form of bacteria. Strepococcus Faecalis will multiply three to four times faster than other strains of bacteria and is more resistant to antibiotic therapy.

This formula may be individually purchases or purchased as part of the Ecology Pak Nutritional support program for Candida

To order: Marcia Smith, Multiway Distributor
8 Muriel Place
Fairfax, California 94930, (415) 459-5013

COLON PRODUCTS

Fiber and Colon Cleanser This product contains natural fiber, herbs, and lactobacillus that promotes the healthy colon. Because of the modern low-fiber diet, it is a fantastic supplement to provide proper elimination.

To Order: Charlotte Blacburn
P.O. Box 4130
San Rafael, California 94903, (415) 897-2028

Price: $14.00
Size: 11oz

Hydrated Bentonite: Nature's Age Old Aid to Intestinal Detoxification

The primitives used clay. The use of volcanic ashes internally is almost older than civilization itself. Primitive tribes of various continents have used various types of clay for conditions of toxicity. Dr. Weston Price's book NUTRITION AND PHYSICAL DEGENERATION, referred to the following; "In Chapter 15 I presented data regarding the treatment used by several primitive races for preventing and correcting serious disturbances in the digestive tract. This consisted in the use of clay or aluminum silicate which modern science has learned has the important quality of being able to absorb and thus collect toxic substances and other products.

TO ORDER: Vit-Ra-Tox #16 or Sonne's #7 or Veico #77 can be purchased through your health food store.

SUGGESTED READING

New journal by Cancer Control Society: STOP COLON-RECTAL CANCER BEFORE IT STOPS YOU! $6.00 plus $1.50 mailing. Address: 2043 N. Berendo St. Los Angeles, California 90027

PARASITE REMOVER

K-MIN: K-Min is made from a natural diatamacious earht and natural, untreated soft rock phosphate. K-Min and worms are enemies. The diatamacious earth acts like ground glass and cuts the seqments and eggs that are released as well as samaging the worm itself causing it to let go. Worms finding themselves surrounded by K-Min move out. Worms cause anyone to be more susceptible to disease. Parasites have been said to cause over/weight and underweight problems. Statistics show that in certain areas more than 80% of the people have worms.

Scientists believe that diatamacious is a de-ionizer or de-energyizer for the worms and parasites.

Directions: Take with meals. Repeat course of treatment after six months.

1/2 capsule a day for children under 4 years, for 4 days. One capsule a day for children under 10 years, for 60 days. All over 10 years should take 2 capsules 3X a day for 12 days, then take one per meal until the bottle of 100 tablets is taken.

Price $8.00 per 100 capsules + $2.00 shipping

Address: Daily Manufacturing, Inc.
Rt. 2, Box 223 - Pless Road
Rockwell, North Carolina 28138
(704) 782-0700

Editor's Note: Farmers are aware of the plain diatamacious earth for animals in divesting them of worms. This combination is an excellent product for parasite problems.

Caution: Do not give to pregnant women or pregnant animals.

PARASITE FORMULAS

Systemic Formulas of Calif.
P.O. Box 782
San Mateo, Ca. 94401
(415) 349-5144

Three different formulas effective against parasites

VRM 1 Formula 30 Capsules per bottle $19.00
VRM 2 Formula (for children & animals) 30 capsules $19.00 per bottle
"WO" 1/2 oz. bottle $12.00 retail.

SELF HELP IN CLEANSING THE COLON

The Ultimate Colonic Board: Fact and Benefits

Facts:
1. The table is made of one-piece fiberglass.
2. The catch basin is a rounded sloping area gradually turning down into a toilet.
3. The edges of the table are raised.
4. The water into the body is gravity flow
5. A single clamp valve controls the flow of the water
6. Attaches easily to any toilet
7. It is 42" long by 22" wide and weighs only 12 1/2 lbs.
8. Protel is flexible with a blunt end.

Benefits:
1. No cracks or crevices for bacteria to migrate from
2. Will last indefinitely
3. Should it become damaged it is easily repaired.
4. Weatherproof
5 Does not delaminate or deteriorate
6. The slope causes the fecal matter to glance downward into the toilet away from the user. (Some flat bulkheads on other colonic boards cause the fecal matter to splash back onto the user)
7. Unwanted waste water is guided into the toilet, spill-proof
8. Easy to sterilize and rinse
9. No siphoning to start water flow.
10. No gadgets or fixtures necessary.
11. It is small enough to fit in almost any bathroom, but large enough to comfortably rest your arms on the table or roll from side to side, if necessary (some tables are so narrow there is no place to rest your arms.
12. It's more comfortable

A five-gallon bucket is necessary but not included.

If your are contemplating purchasing a personal colonic board, utmost in your mind should be cleanliness, comfort and durability. Compare and you will see this is truly the ultimate colonic board.

Price $175. plus freight and handling
5 gallon bucket (plumbed), $17.00, freight free.
Address: Charlotte Blachbourn, P.O. Box 4130, San Rafael, Ca. 94903
(415) 897-2028

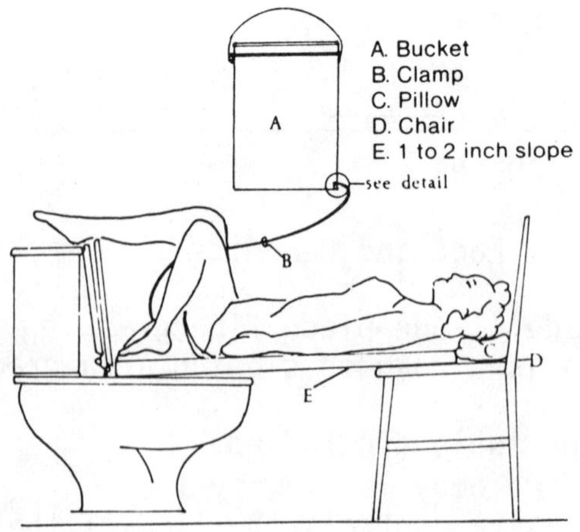

SUGGESTED READING: "Stop Colon-Rectal Cancer, Before it stops You!"
Cancer Control Society Journal- 1985 203 p.
2043 N. Berendo St. Los Angeles, Ca. 90027 $6.00 + $2.00 shipping

ROY KUPSINEL, M.D.
SHANGRI-LA LANE
P. O. BOX 550
OVIEDO, FL 32765
PHONE: (305) 365-6681

Lost Horizon Health Awareness Center

VIII

QUESTIONNAIRES AND REMEDIES FOR CANDIDA

SCORE: ______ NAME: ______________________________ DATE: ____________

In answering the following questions, indicate "yes" by a check mark. Be sure to enter your name and date above! The questions apply to your entire life -- past and present!

PAST	NOW	
____	____	1. Depression
____	____	2. Draggy
____	____	3. Lethargy
____	____	4. No energy
____	____	5. Body aches
____	____	6. Agitation
____	____	7. Hyper-irritability
____	____	8. Loss of memory
____	____	9. Loss of concentration
____	____	10. Headaches
____	____	11. Migraine headaches
____	____	12. Schizophrenia
____	____	13. Electric shock therapy
____	____	14. Dizziness
____	____	15. Insomnia
____	____	16. Hyperactivity
____	____	17. Disturbance in smell
____	____	18. Taste
____	____	19. Vision
____	____	20. Hearing
____	____	21. Psychoneurotic
____	____	22. Stuttering
____	____	23. "Learning disabled"
____	____	24. Sensitivity to chemicals
____	____	25. Odors
____	____	26. Fragrances
____	____	27. Foods
____	____	28. Gas heat
____	____	29. Gas stove
____	____	30. Weight loss
____	____	31. Asthma
____	____	32. Bronchitis
____	____	33. Hay Fever
____	____	34. Ear aches
____	____	35. Hives
____	____	36. Swelling
____	____	37. Endometriosis
____	____	38. Yeast vaginal infections
____	____	39. Menstrual irregularities
____	____	40. Menstrual cramping
____	____	41. Pre-menstrual depression
____	____	42. Pre-menstrual anxiety
____	____	43. Pre-menstrual cramping

PAST	NOW	
____	____	44. Repeated pregnancies
____	____	45. Loss of libido
____	____	46. Impotence
____	____	47. Birth Control Pill
____	____	48. Urethritis
____	____	49. Cystitis
____	____	50. Urinary infection
____	____	51. Gastritis
____	____	52. Colitis
____	____	53. Stomach distention
____	____	54. Bloating
____	____	55. Chronic heartburn
____	____	56. Diarrhea
____	____	47. Constipation
____	____	48. Crohn's disease
____	____	49. Anorexia nervosa
____	____	50. Hodgkin's Disease
____	____	51. Systemic Lupus Erythematosis
____	____	52. Multiple Sclerosis
____	____	53. Sarcoidosis
____	____	54. Rheumatoid arthritis
____	____	55. Myasthenia gravis
____	____	56. Scleroderma
____	____	57. Thrombocytopenic purpura
____	____	58. Alcoholic
____	____	59. Taken Valium
____	____	60. Taken other psychiatric drugs
____	____	61. Drug Addiction
____	____	62. Chronic infection
____	____	63. Chronic eye inflammation
____	____	64. Oral thrush
____	____	65. Diaper rash
____	____	66. High sugar/carbohydrate diet
____	____	67. High yeast foods, (breads, pastries, cookies cheeses, vinegar, whiskey, malted pro-ducts, vitamins from yeast
____	____	68. Treated with antibiotics or sulfa drugs, e.g., acne, sinus bronchitis, flu, urinary problem

Lost Horizon Health Awareness Center
ROY KUPSINEL, M.D.
SHANGRI-LA LANE
P. O. BOX 550
OVIEDO, FL 32765
PHONE: (305) 365-6681

PAST NOW

____ ___69. Taken immunosuppressant drugs, e.g. e.g., cortisone, other steroids, chemotherapy.

____ ___70. Prolonged exposure to molds in old moldy house, living near water, or at work.

____ ___71. Fungus infections between fingers, under breasts, in groin, in fatty tissue folds, on penis or scrotum

____ ___72. Onset of symptoms related to antibiotic therapy, birth control pill, pregnancy, cortisone or chemotherapy

If you answer yes to 40% of the above questions, there is a possibility you have Candida. If you answer yes to 50%, check with doctor for treatment of Candida.

DIETARY SUPPRESSION OF CANDIDA ALBICANS

A. The yeast grows on sugar and starch and is fed by gluten-containing grains. Gluten grains include wheat, oats, rye, and barley.

1. Do not eat sugar or sweets. This includes products made with honey. or molasses as well as sugar.
2. Do not eat wheat, oats, rye, or barley, Corn, rice potatoes, buckwheat, and millet may be eaten in very small quantities by most individuals. Some people, however, must temporarily exclude all of these starchy foods from the diet.
3. Pasteurized milk encourages Candida growth. Avoid milk and milk products except sweet butter.

B. Yeast, molds, and fungi cross-react. When taken in food or even breathed in high concentrations, they trigger symptoms and diminish the body's resistance to Candida. Bathrooms and air vents should be kept clean and dry. Yeast, mold and fungus should be minimized in foods.

1. Yeast is used in food preparation and flavoring.
   a) commercial breads, rolls, coffee cakes, pastries, etc.
   b) beer, wine, and all alcoholic beverages.
   c) most commercial soups, barbecue potato chips, and dry roasted nuts.
   d) vinegar and vinegar containing foods such as pickled vegetables, sauerkraut, relishes, green olives, and salad dressing. Lemon juice with oil may be used as a salad dressing.
   e) soy sauce, cider and natural root beer.

2. Yeast is the basis for many vitamin and mineral preparations, Tryptophan is often derived from yeast.

Lost Horizon Health Awareness Center

ROY KUPSINEL, M.D.
SHANGRI-LA LANE
P. O. BOX 550
OVIEDO, FL 32765
PHONE: (305) 365-6681

3. Molds build up on foods while drying, smoking, curing and fermenting.
   a) Avoid pickled, smoked, or dried meats, fish, and poultry, including sausages, salami, hot dogs, pickled tongue, corned beef, pastrami, smoked sardines and other fish that have been dried or smoked.
   b) Bacon should be avoided. Country style cured pork of all kinds is loaded with mold.
   c) Dried fruits such as prunes, raisins, dates, figs, citrus peels, candied cherries, currants, peaches, apples, and apricots should be avoided.
   d) All cheeses (including cottage cheese), sour cream, buttermilk and milk should be avoided.
   e) Chocolate, honey, maple syrup and nuts accumulate mold and should not be eaten.

4. Melons (especially cantaloupe) and the skins of fleshy vetetables or fruits accumulate mold during growth.

5. Avoid canned or frozen citrus, grape, and tomato juice. Avoid all canned or frozen foods which contain citric acid.

6. Mushrooms are fungi. Do not eat them.

C. Eating fruit will boost blood sugar levels and encourage yeast growth. Fruits and fruit juices must be temporarily omitted from the diet.

D. Teas, including herb teas, and spices are dried foods and accumulate molds. Avoid teas and dried spices.

WHAT IS LEFT TO EAT?

Proteins -- fish, chicken, beef, pork, turkey, duck, seafood of all kinds, eggs, goat, venison, rabbit, frog legs, pheasant, quail, lamb, veal. In other words, animals of all kinds if the meat is fresh instead of dried, smoked, pickled, or cured.

Vegetables -- All vegetables are potentially acceptable. Only starchy ones such as potatoes and sweet potatoes must be avoided by some people.

IS IT POSSIBLE TO EAT OUT?

YES! Just order carefully. Skip the cocktail. Have oil and lemon juice on your salad. Order meat, chicken, or other animal protein that is prepared without sauces which might contain sugar, mushrooms, wheat as a thickener, and other harmful ingredients. Broiled or plain items are obviously the safest choice. Steamed vegetables are perfect. Skip bread, crackers and dessert.

EDITOR'S NOTE: The Grains Quinoa and Amaranth from South America are as high in protein as meat. (Meat has antibiotics in it) The taste is a cross between rice & millet. These grains may be ordered through Arrowhead Mills, Box 2059, Hereford, Texas 79045 or through your health food store.

Lost Horizon Health Awareness Center

*ROY KUPSINEL, M.D.
SHANGRI-LA LANE
P. O. BOX 550
OVIEDO, FL 32765
PHONE: (305) 365-6681

FOODS CONTAINING YEAST

Breads
Crackers
Pastries
Pretzels
Hamburger and hot dog buns
Cookies
Flour enriched with vitamins from yeast
Rolls, homemade and canned
Canned Ice Box Cookies
Milk fortified with vitamins and yeast
Meat fried in cracker crumbs

Other yeast containing foods because of their nature of manufacture or preparation:

Mushrooms
Truffles
Cheese of all kinds
Buttermilk
Cottage cheese
Vinegar
- Apple
- Bin
- Pear
- Grape
- Distilled

Catsup
Mayonnaise
Olives
Pickles
Sauerkraut
Condiments
Horse radish
French dressing
Salad dressing
Barbeque sauce
Tomato sauce
Chili peppers
Mince pie
Gerbers oatmeal
Barley cereal
Whiskey
- Wine
- Brandy
- Rum
- Vodka

Root beer
Malted products:
- Cereals
- Candy
- Malted milk drinks

Frozen canned citrus fruit juices
Many of the vitamin products are, in fact derived from yeast or have their source from yeast

PLEASE NOTE: After reading this partial list of foods containing yeast products you now have a much better idea of the rather formidable task ahead of you. It is absolutely imperative while on the rotary diversification and avoidance diet that you carefully look at all labels on the canned and packaged foods and consult the list above constantly, or you will continue to suffer needlessly the consequences of allergic reactions.

CREDIT: The above skeletal outline of C.O. Truss, M.D., Birmingham, Alabama was incorporated with other suggestion to Dr. Roy Kupsinel, M.D. of Florida who uses this chart in his practice for patients with Candida. I wish to thank Dr. Truss and Dr. Kupsinel.

*Dr. Kupsinel has telephone Nutritional Consultation Services: General Evaluation, Candidiasis, or Mercury/Amalgam Toxicity. Call the above number.

Lost Horizon Health Awareness Center

*

ROY KUPSINEL, M.D.
SHANGRI-LA LANE
P. O. BOX 550
OVIEDO, FL 32765
PHONE: (305) 365-6681

CANDIDA ALBICAN TREATMENT PROTOCOL

I. DIET

A. VITAL LIFE DIET combined with avoidance of foods containing yeast (see list of yeast containing foods)

B. YEAST FREE DIET. This is the ideal diet but difficult for the average patient to follow.

II. AVOID USE OF BIRTH CONTROL PILLS

III. AVOID USE OF ANTIBIOTICS, CORTISONE, CORTISONE-LIKE DRUGS, AND IMMUNOSUPPRESSANT DRUGS.

IV. NYSTATIN

THE CANDIDA ALBICANS PROTOCOL - ACCORDING TO THE PAGE CLINIC

The Page Clinic and the Price-Pottinger Foundation are the two major references for this protocol.

1. The prescription drug NYSTATIN should be mixed in Bio Water and used to wash all body cavities and also used as a drink.
2. Many medical doctors practicing clinical ecology recommend two cups of the anti-fungal tea known as Pau D'Arco or Ipe Roxo be consumed daily.
3. Do not exceed 60 to 80 grams of carbohydrates in your diet per day. Buy a carbohydrate guide so you can keep track of your carbohydrate intake per day.
4. Avoid antibiotics and steroids unless absolutely necessary.
5. Ladies, do not use the birth control pill. The pill upsets your hormones, thus interfering with your body's ability to fight Candida.
6. Take at least three tablets or capsules of live lacto bacillus acidophilus, bulgaris and bifidis each meal. Since dairy products are contraindicated in Candidiasis, we have found LACTOZYME, a milk-free lacto bacillus & bifidus to be most effective.
7. Use garlic. If you cannot eat the whole garlic, take six to eight capsules daily of KYOLIC.
8. At least 300,000 IU of Vitamin A should be used for the first two weeks of this program. Thereafter, you can cut the dosage down to 25,000 IU per day. (Use the Emulsified form of A for the high dosage segment. It will not accumulate in your liver).
9. Essential Fatty Acids hasten the restoration of the auto-immune system. Take four to eight drops with each meal of a preparation containing essential fatty acids from various sources, but 20% of which is from Evening Primrose Oil.

10. A substance sometimes called B-15 also seems to be effective. We have found Organic 15 to work very well.
11. Approximately two weeks into the program add two tablets per meal of THYMUS tissue. After 10 days, the patient can cut the dosage down to 2 or 3 per day.
12. A supervised three or four day fast repeated every one to three months should be part of the program, until the Candida is cleared up.
13. Biotin, while a food for Candida is also necessary to fight it. Take 5-100 mcg. tablets several hours before eating with KYOLIC or NYSTATIN, so the Biotin will not feed the fungus.
14. Zinc tablets at a strength of 15 mg. each was found useful by taking 3 to 6 per day.
15. Proteolytic Enzymes: Take four tablets of Intenzyme after each meal and again at bedtime. You may get by with B10 6 PLUS.
16. Use CATALYST ACTIVATED WATER (B10 WATER) to mix your NYSTATIN and PAU D'ARCO tea. You can make 5 gallons from 4 ounces.
17. Exercise at least 20 minutes each day.
18. Train yourself to eat light meals.
19. Moderate sunlight is beneficial to kill Candida overgrowth.

POINTS TO BE AWARE OF:

Several years of therapy might be necessary to restore the auto-immune system.

Some people feel real grand when they start the program, (probably not very advanced with the overgrowth); others feel very ill, and often blame the supplements. However, the ill-feeling is due to Candida die-off and the program must be continued if you wish to regain your health.

The above article appeared in HEALTH EXPRESS under the title "YOU CAN STOP FUNGUS INFECTIONS", by Al Battista, N.D., (1983) *

Dr. Battista has lectured before large audiences of "A.I.D.S." patients on Candida. Battista is not only well known for his varied lectures in the health field, but he also writes for many of the popular health magazines. Dr. Battista is a member of the "Board of Governers" in the National Health Federation.

In the early spring of 1985 Dr. Battista will be available for telephone consultation and at this time he will be able to supply the various items necessary for the Candida protocol. Write to Dr. Battista at the following address; include your area code and phone number and he will call you.

Al Battista, N.D.,
211 So. State College Blvd., Suite 301
Anaheim, California 92806

*This protocol has been updated since the 1983 article.

PAC D'ARCO USED TO FIGHT CANCER AND CANDIDA

Dr. Duke, Ph.D. a former researcher of the United Stated Drug Administration (USDA) and now in private research has hard facts concerning the anti-fungal properties of this bark, which can be purchased in the United States.

TABEBUIA SPP. BIGNONIACEAE PAO D'ARCO

by: James A. Duke, Ph.D., USDA, Beltsville Research Center

USES: The timber of many species, though an "axe-breaker", is used. Sawdust of T. avellanedae is resistent to termites, perhaps due to deoxylapachol. Recently there has been a flurry of interest in "herbal tea" made from ipe roxo, lapacho, and/or pao d'arco.

FOLK MEDICINE: According to Hartwell (4), the tea of the bark is used in folk remedies for adenocarcinoma (pancreas), cancer of the esophagus, head, intestines, lung, prostate, and tongue, Hodgkin's disease, leukemia, and lupus 4. Reported to be alexiteric, analgesic, anodyne, antiodotal, diuretic, and fungicidal, Tabebuia species show up in folk remedies for boils, chlorosis, diarrhea, dysentery, enuresis, fever, pharyngitis, snakebite, syphilis, and wounds (32).

The pao d'arco and ipe roxo popularity stems to such species as T. Avellanadae, T. heptophylla, T. impetiginosa, and T. ipe. Many Latin American species are used in folk medicines. According to Morton (42), the leaf decoction of Tabebuia heterophylla is used in the Bahamas for gonorrhea, and toothache. Costa Ricans take the bark decoction of Tabebuia rosea for colds, fever, and headache; the flowers, leaves, and shoots for snakebite. Guatemalans give the bark decoction to dogs to protect them from rabies; Mexicans take the root decoction for anemia, the leaf-and-bark decoction for fever (42). Tabebuia serratifolia has been used traditionally for cancer in Colombia, the activity probably due to quinone.

..."Lapachol was listed recently by Perdue (1982) among the most important antitumor agents from plants. There are many folk uses reported in the popular press. Californians tell me in 1983 that they are drinking pao d'arco for fungal infections and applying the decoction (one spoon soaked in a quart of water overnight) locally to Candida. They report favorable results. Personally I would not hesitate to apply such a decoction or drink so dilute a tea. Xyloidone, as noted, is active against Candida."

CHEMISTRY:: ..."According to Prakash and Singh (Pharmazie 35(12): 813. 1980), the stembark of T. pentaphylla contains lapachol, nonacosane, dehydrotectol, and beta-sitosterol, the roots hexacosane, dehydrotectol, beta-sitosterol, and oleanolic acid. Some species contain xyloidone, which is active against Brucella and Candida. Much of the activity may be traced to the lapachol. Lapachol, active against gram positive and acid-fast bacteria, as well as fungi, was once of great interest to the NCI. According to Cancer Chemotherapy Reports, Part 2, Vol. 4, No. 4, Dec. 1978, lapachol has shown antimalarial activity in animals and is a known uncoupler of oxidative phosphorylation.

More recently, lapachol was found to have anti-cancer activity. Lapachol, a quinone filed in 1967, was dropped from NCI investigations because of therapeutic inactivity. Reported by Hartwell (4) from Stereospermum suaveolens, lapachol occurs in several species of Tabebuia....." ..."Brazilian species of Tabebuia, known as pao d'arco and lapacho have gotten big press sporadically over the last 50 years as cancer remedies. Thus Stereospermum and Tabebuia, classical sources of lapachol, both have folk histories as "cancer remedies." I have received unsolicited testimonials from "recovered patients" supposedly cured by pao d'arco. Recently I submitted an unvouchered sample of ipe roxo ("Tecoma curialis") to the NCI for screening. This is also labeled pao d'arco herbal tea. There are no cancer claims on the label but the pao d'arco has gotten enough press to generate a North American interest in lapachol, dropped by NCI because of "no therapeutic effect." Hartwell (4) notes that lapachol was carried into clinical trial because "of its high Walker 256 activity even when given orally." Lack of toxicity permitted large oral doses but sufficiently high blood levels could not be obtained to show a therapeutic effect. While lapachol was inactive against L1210 leukemia, the sodium salt of lapachol was active.

TOXICITY: At high oral doses, lapachol causes nausea, vomiting, and a reversible prolongation of the prothrombin time, the latter effect possibly due to lapachol's structural similarity to vitamin K.

The following "quote" got me in trouble. "American herbal medicine experts Dr. James Duke, of the National Institute of Health, and Dr. Norman Farnsworth of the University of Illnois, confirm Martin's claims 'Taheebo undoubtedly contains a substance found to be highly effective against cancers.' Farnsworth told GLOBE."

I quote from the GLOBE newspaper as it was printed (September 15, 1981, GLOBE). Shortly thereafter, Tabebuia was being promoted under the bold headlines, " "1,000-year-ld Inca cancer cure works." In the PR material the three words "Farnsworth told GLOBE" has been deleted. I imagine that Dr. Farnsworth was as badly represented by the quote as I was, but note how the omission of three little words make it look as though Duke and Farnsworth were being quoted, not Martin.

Perhaps similar quotes may be taken from this chapter, but neither I, the editors, CRC, NCI, or the USDA are endorsing any herbal remedy for cancer. I am merely compiling information on biological activity of some plants and plant-derived compounds. Even though some folk cancer plants do contain biologically active compounds with antitumor compounds, we do not endorse herbal medication.

Directions for preparation of Pau d'Arco Tea. One heaping or two level tablespoons of the bark in 4 to 5 cups of water. Let boil together over low heat for 15 minutes. (Avoid using aluminum pots; glass, enamel, or stainless steel pots are preferred). Serve hot or cold throughout the day, preferably 4 times on an empty stomach (an hour before meals).

La Pacho Tree

The La Pacho Tree grows in Brazil and Pac D'Arco tea comes from this tree. Dr. Huemer recommends this tea for persons who have a Candida infection. I quote from "Let's Live Magazine, September 1983 page 64.

"I did hear of one promising new treatment for Candida infections. It is tea made from the inner bark of the LaPacho tree that grows in Brazil. The tree itself is uncommonly resistant to fungus. The tea is said to be effective orally and on epithelial surfaces..."

Dr.R. Huemer, M.D. is a graduate of UCLA School of Medicine and has his private practice in Westlake Village, California. In addition to being the author of many research and scientific articles, Dr. Huemer has been a guest on various radio and television shows. He is the current President of the Orthomolecular Medical Society, and is also a member of the American Aging Association, the International Academy of Preventive Medicine, the American Association for the Advancement of Science, the New York Academy of Sciences, and the National Foundation for Nutritional Research. He is Associate Editor of the Journal of the International Academy of Preventive Medicine and on the editorial board of Mechanism of Ageing and Development.

NATURALLY OCCURING ANTICARCINOGEN QUINONES

The Survival Factor In Neoplastic And Viral Diseases p. 296
book by: Wm. F. Koch, Ph.D., M.D. -Vanderkloot Press, Detroit, Mi., 1961

While searching in Nature for plants that present chromophore groups of the order we have proven to be anticarcinogenic ....three were found in Australia and Africa and two in Brazil. ....The Brazilian pigment has not been identified as to structure except by ourselves since we find it to be both the para and ortho forms of a naphtoquinone in isomerism in two different trees. Here they can be extracted from the inner bark, and are named the Pau Arco Amarilo and Roxo for the paraquinone and ortho quinone forms respectively. Both are proven to be curative in cancer and other diseases.

AUSTRALIAN TEA TREE OIL- Australian Tea Tree Oil is distilled from the leaves of Melaleuca alternifolia, a tree species indigenous of the north coast of New South Wales, Australia. Tea Tree Oil possesses powerful germicidal, fungicidal and antiseptic properties, and is non-toxic and non-irritating to normal tissue. These characteristics have lead to widespread acceptance and use in first-aid, dental and surgical practice in Australia. The properties of Tea Tree Oil have been known since the pioneering work of Penfold & Morrison early in the century and has been well documented in the popular and scientific literature.

American College of Obstetricians & Gynecologists, Edwardo F. Pena, M.D., Vol. 19, No. 6, June 1962- MELALEUCA ALTERNIFOLIA OIL

(Summary) Australian Melaleuca Alternifolia Oil in suitable dilutions was found to be highly effective in treatment of trichomonal vaginitis, moniliasis, cervicitis and chronic endocervicitis.

TO ORDER: Oil of Melaleuca, Inc., 2222 Teton Plaza, Idaho Falls, Idaho 83401 1 (800) 624-2825) in Idaho. Toll Free all other states 1 (800) 523-4513

(Continued)

ANTIBIOTICS AND ITS ROLE IN SYSTEMATIC CANDIDIASIS

THE CONNECTION BETWEEN ANTIBIOTICS, THE THYMUS AND CANDIDA

Maxwell G. Shepherd: Candidiasis: An Infectious Disease of Increasing Importance. New Zealand Dental Journal 78:89, July 1982

Since the introduction of antibiotics and with the use of corticosteroids and immunosuppressive agents, there has been an increase in the prevalence of both superficial and systematic candidiasis. An indication of the prevalence of fungal infections in the community can be gleaned from the amount spent on anti-fungal agents. In 1979, the wholesale value of anti-fungal drugs in the USA was $104 million; this compares with the $220 million spent on penicillins.

NOTE: IF YOUR ARE ON ANTIBIOTICS HAVE YOUR DOCTOR GIVE YOU VITAMIN C

Robert Cathcart, M.D.: Method of Determining Proper Doses of Vitamin C for the Treatment of Disease by Titrating to Bowel Tolerance- Journal of Orthomolecular Psychiatry: V. 10 No. 2 1982

Dr. Cathcart's experience in utilizing vitamin C in large doses has extended over a 9 year period and has involved over 9000 patients. The purpose of this paper is to describe a method which maximizes the effectiveness of ascorbic acid taken orally for various diseases and stress processes.

Candida Albicans-Candida infections occur less frequently in patients being treated with antibiotics if bowel tolerance doses of ascorbic acid are simultaneously used. Ascorbic acid seems to have little effect on established candida infections. It may be found that appropriate antifungal agents will penetrate tissues saturated in ascorbate better.

NATURAL ANTIBIOTIC IN WHEAT SEEDS

Vol. 42, No. 8--PLANT DISEASE REPORTER--Aug. 15, 1958-Peter Ark, Professor of Plant Pathology, University of California, Berkeley, California

Abstract Seeds of both barley and wheat contain an antibiotic principle active against Gram-positive bacterial and fungi when tested in vitro. ....An antibiotic principle active against all tested Gram-positive organisms was detected in various degrees of strength from both wheat and barley seeds.

Discussion: The existence of antibiotics in higher plants has been known to scientists for some time. ...Grummer and Tokin emphasize naturally-occurring antibiotics in higher plants as contributing factors of natural immunity in plants....

*NATURAL ANTIBIOTIC FOR CANDIDA IN THE FORM OF 'GARLIC'

Vol. 43, No. 2--PLANT DISEASE REPORTER--Feb. 15, 1959
CONTROL OF CERTAIN DISEASES OF PLANTS WITH ANTIBIOTICS FROM GARLIC (ALLIUM SATIVUM L.) by Peter A. Ark, Professor of Plant Pathology, University of California, Berkeley, California

Antibiotic Action of Garlic in Vitro

From the experimental tests it is evident that garlic contains a volatile fraction that is quite toxic to both the bacteria and the fungi. ...." rusts and facultative fungi were strongly affected by the garlic extracts."

Summary and Conclusion [1]Garlic juice and aqueous and organic solvent extracts of garlic exhibit antibacterial and antifungal properties in vitro and on leaves and fruit.

NATURAL ANTIBIOTIC FOR CANDIDA - SOAKED WHEAT SEED WATER

A natural antibiotic that can be used on a daily basis for Candida is "Rejuvelac" (soaked wheat seed in water). To make Rejuvelac use 3 cups spring water to 1 cup soft spring wheat (organic). Let stand first time 48 hours in room temperature. Pour soak water out and refill again with 3 cups spring water. Let stand second time 24 hours. Pour soak water into jar and use as fermented drink. Use same seeds once again with 3 cups water and pour off second time in 24 hours. Cover jar loosely, allowing air to enter. Rejuvelac contains many B vitamins, besides being a natural antibiotic. *Dr. Peter Ark, Professor Emeritus of the Department of Plant Pathology, University of California Berkeley, published papers in the '40's and '50's on the inhibitory effect of soaked wheat seed water to fungi. (Use organic seeds and rinse before you soak.)
*Use organic garlic only. All other garlic is being irradiated by FDA.

THE EFFECTIVENESS OF S.G.P. ON DENTAL PATIENTS WITH MERCURY RESTORATIONS -A PILOT STUDY by Samuel J. Wong, Jr., D.D.S., and David A. H. Zhu, M.D.

Since garlic grows in many parts of the world and is nontoxic by nature, it has been used for food as well as medicine for thousands of years. Upon recent studies, scientists discovered that garlic emits mitogenic radiation which may stimulate cell growth and rejuvenates body function.

By experimental studies S.G.P. (Special Garlic Preparation) may protect destruction of erythrocytes polluted by heavy metals, such as mercury.

Conclusion: The administration of Special Garlic Preparation (S.G.P.) may promote the elimination of toxic materials in the body. This research shows the effectiveness of S.G.P. in increasing the elimination of mercury via hair.

*SAUERKRAUT FOR LACTIC ACID

"Lactic acid is extremely important in providing a media for beneficial bacterial growth in the body, having a counteracting effect upon putrefaction in the colon." "Civilized" Diseases and Their Circumvention, by Max Garten, N.D., D.C.

Recipe:

One head of red/green cabbage
Wash cabbage leaves (save outer 3 cabbage leaves)
Juice remaining cabbage in Champion or Acne Juicer
Place the pulp of the juiced cabbage into
an earthenware or crock pot
Add 1 T. of kelp and stir
(thyme, dill, carrots or beets can be added for variety)
Pour cabbage juice into pot and push cabbage pulp down
until entire pulp is covered with the juice.
Cover top with remaining cabbage leaves.
Place plate on top
Weight down with heavy rock or gallon jug of water, etc.
Leave at room temperature for 3-5 days
Remove cloth, any foam or mildew, plate and weight
Store saurkraut in glass jar in refrigerator.

Sauerkraut Inhibits Candida
(See excerpt from Journal below)

Cabbage Juice= Vitamin U
Ulcers treated with Vitamin U rich extracts heal 3 to 6 times faster than those patients treated by conventional bland diets. (Healing takes place in 7 to 10 days instead of 37 to 42 days)

CABBAGE JUICE FOR PEPTIC ULCER AND CANDIDA

VITAMIN U CONCENTRATE THERAPY OF PEPTIC ULCER (Excerpt)
THE AMERICAN JOURNAL OF GASTROENTEROLOGY March 1954
Garnett Cheney, M.D. San Francisco, California

(This work was supported by a "grant-in-aid" by Merck & Co., Inc., Rahway, N.J. Inc., Rahway, N.J.)

"In October, 1952, the author reported the results of fresh cabbage juice in the treatment of 100 patients with peptic ulcer. These results indicated that cabbage juice contained an unidentified antipeptic ulcer dietary factor which promoted more rapid healing of peptic ulcers than has commonly occurred in employing the more conventional methods of therapy. In this series of cases, each patient received 1 liter of fresh cabbage juice daily, and no drugs were prescribed except symptomatically. It was stressed that heating or processing of the antiulcer factor, which has been termed Vitamin U, tended to destroy it.

A total of 102 patients were included in the present study. One hundred of these patients had a definite clinical diagnosis of peptic ulcer....

The peptic ulcers were located in the* esophagus in 4 cases; the stomach in 21 cases; the duodenum in 73 cases; and the jejunum in 2 cases.

The Vitamin U preperation which was administered to each patient was usually between 50 to 60 c.c. in volume, and each dose represented the equivalent of 1 liter of freshly pressed raw cabbage juice which had been concentrated by cold processing. In a few instances, the concentrate represented 2 liters of cabbage juice instead of one. Consequently, this form of concentrate was administered in a dose of 25 to 30 c.c. daily.

....It should be noted that pain relief in this series has not been produced by any form of medication, and it is the time at which the spontaneous appearance of pain actually ceases. ....Pain ceased in this group of 90 patients between the first and eleventh days. All but 8 of these were pain-free the first week. ....The average time of pain relief was 4.24 days.

TABLE 1 - SHOWS HEALING TIME OF ESOPHAGEAL ULCER

Vitamin U Concentrate Therapy in 4 Cases of Esophageal Ulcer

Case No..	Age & Sex	Duration		Peptic Ulcer Location	(By X-ray) Diam. In Cms.	Vitamin U Merck No.	Therapy Month	Patient Activity	Day of Pain Relief	Ulcer Crater Healing Time	Remarks
		Total Illness	Present Attack								
16	69M	4 yrs.	3 mos.	Posterior Wall	2.0	52R-3761	Oct.	Ambulatory	10th	10 days	Onset after partial gastrectomy
33	63M	7 yrs.	4 mos.	Anterior Wall	1.0	52R-3669	Oct.	At work	3rd	9 days	Also Meckels Peptic Ulcer
40	65F	2+yrs.	2 yrs.	Posterior Wall	1.0	51R-6827	Nov.	Ambulatory	2nd	10 days	Esophagoscopic verification
100	41F	3 yrs.	4 mos.	No Crater	-	53R-2514	May	Hospital	4th	-	Esophagoscopy- severe peptic esophagitis

Chaney-Vitamin U Concentrate Therapy of Peptic Ulcer

The therapeutic results of Vitamin U therapy of peptic ulcer which have been presented in this report indicate that this disease is fundamentally a disorder of nutrition. ....It has been postulated that Vitamin U, or some fraction or derivative thereof, increases the resistance of the mucosal lining of the esophagus, stomach and intestine to the erosive and ulcerating action of gastric juice which is high in acid content and rich in pepsin."

*See Mortality Weekly Report (9/24/82) next page regarding Esophagitis due to Candidiasis

---

UPDATE ON ACQUIRED IMMUNE DEFICIENCY SYNDROME (AIDS)-UNITED STATES (1)

MORBIDITY AND MORTALITY WEEKLY REPORT
September 24, 1982/Vol 31/No. 37

CURRENT TRENDS

Between June 1, 1981, and September 15, 1982, Center for Disease Control received reports of 593 cases of acquired immune deficiency syndrome (AIDS). Death occurred in 243 cases (41%).

Editorial Note: CDC defines a case of AIDS as a disease, at least moderately predictive of a defect in cell-mediated immunity, occurring in a person with no known cause for diminished resistance to that disease. Such diseases include KS, PCP, and serious 001.* Diagnoses are considered to fit the case definition only if based on sufficiently reliable methods (generally histology or culture). However, this case definition may not include the full spectrum of AIDS manifestations, which may range from absence of symptoms (despite laboratory evidence of immune deficiency) to non-specific symptoms (e.g., fever weight loss, generalized, persistent lymphadenopathy) (4) to specific diseases that are insufficiently predictive of cellular immuno-deficiency to be included in incidence monitoring (e.g., tuberculosis, oral candidiasis, herpes zoster) to malignant neoplasms that cause, as well as result from, immunodeficiency (5) Conversely, some patients who are considered AIDS cases on the basis of diseases only moderately predictive of cellular immuno-deficiency may not actually be immunodeficient and may not be part of the current epidemic. Absence of a reliable, inexpensive, widely available test for AIDS, however, may make the working case definition the best currently available for incidence monitoring.

Two points in this update deserve emphasis. First, the eventual case-mortality rate of AIDS, a few years after diagnosis, may be far greater than the 41% overall case-mortality rate noted above. Second, the reported incidence of AIDS has continued to increase rapidly. Only a small percentage of cases have none of the identified risk factors (male homosexuality, intravenous drug abuse, Haitian origin, and perhaps hemophilia A).

*these infections include pneumonia, meningitis, or encephalitis due to one or more of the following aspergillosis, candidiasis, cryptococcosis, cytomegalovirus, nocardiosis, strongyloidosis, toxoplasmosis, zygomycosis, or atypical mycobacteriosis (species other than tuberculosis or lepra); esophagitis due to candidiasis, or herpes simplex virus; multifocal leukoencephalopathy;..........

(1) Morbidity & Mortality Weekly Report-Sept. 24, 1982/Vol.31/No.37

in the footnote of the Editorial Note

In the Editors Note, CDC defines a case of AIDS as a disease, at least occurring in a person with no known cause for diminished resistance to that disease. Such diseases include KS, PCP, and serious OOI.* which refers to the foot note stating,*"These infections include pneumonia, meningitis, or encephalitis due to one or more of the following: ....."esophagitis due to candidiasis".......

The dictionary describes esophagitis as meaning inflammation of the esophagus.

Candidiasis causes inflammation in the esophagus area which in turn effects the Thymus gland (which is in the same area as esophagus) in its maturing of the T cells which are released to fight disease. Editor.

NEWSLETTER: Lawrence A. Plumlee, M.D. ENVIRONMENT HEALTH ASSOCIATION
12110 Webbs Chapel Road, Suite 305E, Dallas, Texas (703) 534-8354

Excerpt - "Dr. Patricia Lucas has hypothesized that the major cause of our immune disorders is due to defects in the gastrointestinal mucosa due to Candida."

VITAMIN C IN THE TREATMENT OF ACQUIRED IMMUNE DEFICIENCY SYNDROME (AIDS)
Robert F. Cathcart, III, 58 N. El Camino Real, #119, San Mateo, Ca. 94401
Medical Hypotheses 14: 423-433, 1984

Abstract-My previous experience with the utilization of ascorbic acid in the treatment of viral diseases led me to hypothesize that ascorbate would be of value in the treatment of AIDS (acquired immune deficiency syndrome). Preliminary clinical evidence is that massive doses of ascorbate (50-200 grams per 24 hours) can suppress the symptoms of the disease and can markedly reduce the tendency for secondary infections. In combination with usual treatments for the secondary infections, large doses of ascorbate will often produce a clinical remission which shows every evidence of being prolonged if treatment is continued. This clinical remission is achieved despite continuing laboratory evidence of helper T-cell suppression. There may be a complete or partial destruction of the helper T-cells during an initial infection that does not necessitate a continuing toxicity from some source to maintain a permanent or prolonged helper T-cell suppression. However, it is possible ascorbate may prevent that destruction if used adequately during that prodrome period. Emphasis is put upon the recognition and treatment of the frequent intestinal parasites. Food and chemical sensitivities occur frequently in the AID syndrome. A topical C-paste has been found very effective in the treatment of herpel simplex and, to a lesser extent, in the treatment of some Kaposi's lesions. Increasingly, clinical research on other methods of treating AIDS is being "contaminated by patients taking ascorbate.

USE OF CHLOROPHYLL (wheatgrass juice-grown from hard-red winter wheat) IN THE MOUTH FOR DEGENERATIVE DISEASE AND FUNGI (Candida)

COMFREY AND CHLOROPHYLL by Vincent Licata, Nutritionist

"Dr. Homer Junkin, of the Paris Hospital, Paris, Illinois, electrified the dental profession with the announcement that he had succeeded in controlling Vincent's Angina* (trench mouth) and advanced phyorrhea through the intensive use of the Green Liquid Chlorophyll. His method of application was to inject chlorophyll into the gums and the disease appeared to be cleared up in less than thirty days. "The gums tightened up entirely," Dr. Homer D. Junkin Commented, "and have remained clean since."

Two of Dr. Gurshkin's Temple University Colleagues in this investigation of chlorophyll, Doctors Redpath and Davis, were ear, nose and throat specialists. These doctors treated over 1,000 patients ranging from young children to elderly persons. They were suffering a wide variety of ailments from head colds, acute catarrhal inflamation and hay fever to acute sinus infections.

Dr. Gurskin, in commenting on his associates experience with chlorophyll writes, "It is interesting to note that there is not a single case recorded in which either improvement or cure has not taken place."

A recent report is that of two Pennsylvania doctors, Langley and Morgan, which tells of their experience with this substance and 40 patients suffering with skin diseases of eleven different types.

One of the most gratifying results of treatment with chlorophyll, say the doctors, was its ability to relieve itching and burning, and they state that this relief was almost immediate. But the physiological effect on the infected skin was as dramatic as the relief from itching and burning. 88 percent of these patients were "Clinically Cured."

CHLOROPHYLL, NATURE'S "GREEN MAGIC" by Theodore M. Rudolph Ph.D.

Why Chlorophyll is Useful Because anaerobic bacterial, a disease-producing micro-organism living within many human bodies, cannot live in the presence of oxygen or oxygen-producing agents such as Chlorophyll, the health protecting influence of this miracle compound is best described in the words of an eminent Temple University scientist: "It is entirely possible that bacterial being of vegetable origin, yet possessing no Chlorophyll ordinarily, undergo some biological change in the presence of this substance. Thus we must assume that some constructive effect is produced when Chlorophyll comes in contact with body tissues, whether normal or diseased, and Chlorophyll appears to exercise a normalizing influence as pertains to natural powers. In concluding his remarks, the

---

*Editor's Comment- Since one of the places Candida lives is the mouth & throat area, it would seem plausible that the taking in of Chlorophyll (wheatgrass/rejuvelac) would retard the growth of Candida in the mouth and throat area (thymus).

university scientist adds, "Chlorophyll has to a certain degree, an indirect action on bacteria as noted in anaerobic infections. ....'Chlorophyll, possessing the property of breaking down poisonous carbon dioxide, releases free oxygen, thus inhibiting or reducing the action of anaerobic bacteria.'

---

* WHEATGRASS JUICE-GIFT OF NATURE by Betsy Russell-Manning

Wheatgrass juice contains high amounts of CHLOROPHYLL. Chlorophyll resembles the molecules of human red blood cells and produces an unfavorable environment for bacterial growth, rather than by any direct action upon the bacteria themselves. (Grow your own wheatgrass with organic hard-red winter wheat!)

Dr. Chiu-Nan Lai, Ph.D[1] of the University of Texas System Cancer Center, Department of Biology, Houston, Texas has determined through using the Ames Bacterial Mutagenicity Test that CHLOROPHYLL is the active factor in wheat sprout extract which inhibits the metabolic activation of carcinogens.

Wheatgrass is a complete food animals have been observed to choose during periods of illness, a diet consisting almost exclusively of green vegetation. Wheatgrass is a survival food and can be lived on exclusively.

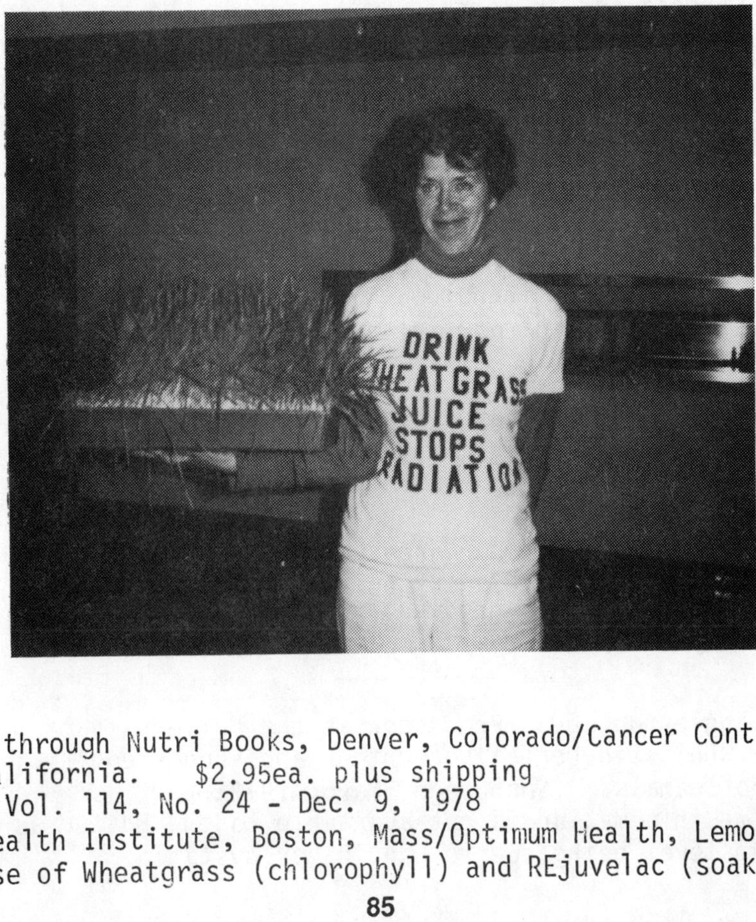

*booklet-Order through Nutri Books, Denver, Colorado/Cancer Control Society Los Angeles, California. $2.95ea. plus shipping
1Science News, Vol. 114, No. 24 - Dec. 9, 1978
2Hippocrates Health Institute, Boston, Mass/Optimum Health, Lemon Grove, Calif. also teaches use of Wheatgrass (chlorophyll) and REjuvelac (soaked seed water).

To order hard-red winter wheat (wheat berry) write Arrowhead Mills, Inc. Box 2059, Hereford, Texas 79045. These seeds are grown organically with no pesticides or chemicals.

To order a juicer to juice the wheat grass : Kevin Manning, 2504 Cross Hill Road, Louisville, Kentucky 40206. (Send money order "U.S. Postal" or Certified check only)

Manual/hand juicer $ 82.00 + $10.00 U.P.S.
Electric Juicer $295.00 + $7.00 New York; $7.00 N.Y. to Chicago
$13.50 from Chicago to West Coast

THE SPECTRO SCAN (Evaluations for Mg/CA/K/P) (Candida, High Potassium Levels & Heavy Metal Toxicity)

Dr. Burton Silver, Ph.D. invented the Spectro-Scan (High-Tech Computer based X-ray analysis), which is able to read the Intracellular Nutritional Mineral Analysis of the body. In other words, evaluations for Magnesium/Calcium Ratios--Phosphorus/Magnesium Ratios--Potassium/Calcium Ratios are read by this machine, along with other nutritional information of the body; (i.e., the ability to pick up HEAVY METAL TOXICITY)

Persons with Candida and/or persons with Candida who are taking Nystatin have an extremely high potassium level. According to Dr. Silver these patients have a potassium peak that goes right off the end of the scale. Dr. Silver said at this point he doesn't know if the high level of potassium is coming from the Candida or Nystatin.[2]

This test is non-invasive, safe, painless and fast. Since cells and tissues of the oral cavity reflect overall nutritional status, sub-lingual smears are conveniently obtained by briskly scraping the mucus-membrane on the floor of the mouth, close to the frenulum. This is the ONLY test for rapid tissue mineral ratios revealing intracellular levels of MG/CA/K/P.

This test is easily and quickly performed by health care assistants or doctor. The specimen is then mailed to Dr. Silver's San Bruno, California office where the machine makes its analysis. The results are then returned rapidly to the health professional by mail.

To find the Professional in your area using the Spectro-Scan write or call: SPECTRO-SCAN, INC. - 841 W. San Bruno Ave. - Suite No. 10 - San Bruno, California 94066 - Tel: (415) 872/0482 or (800) 874/4804 or (800) 874-4808

---

1 Dr. David Eggleston, DDS, Professor at the University of Southern California addressed the Wholistic Dental Convention and suggested 'Kyolic' (garlic) for irrigating root canals. (San Diego, March 1983)

2 At this time information is not available to the Editor as to the cause of the high potassium level being due to Candida or Nystatin.

CAPRISTATIN EXCELLENT FOR "CANDIDA"

CAPRISTATIN ACID is a NUTRIENT taken in tablet form in a resinous base which goes directly to the large intestine where it is released. It INHIBITS THE GROWTH OF ALL MONILIAS AND ESPECIALLY CANDIDA.

"ORI THRUSH" for Oral Candidiasis. It comes in a liquid form for gargling.

"ORI THRUSH" Concentrate also comes in liquid form for topical Candida (which appears sometimes as a skin infestation in the fingernails or toenails and as Eczema. The concentrate can also be used as a douche.

* A San Francisco M.D. uses these products on his Candida patients and has had excellent results.

The product can be purchased through:

Cardiovascular Research
1061 "B" Shary Circle
Concord, California 94518

(415) 827-2636

*This physician used Capristatin Acid in place of Nystatin (which is a drug).

MAXIDOLOPHIS SUPER POWERFUL ACIDOLOPHILUS

Maxidolophis contains billions of organisms.
Maxidolophis helps strengthen the intestinal tract.
Maxidolophis helps strengthen the immune system.
Maxidolophis inhibits disease causing yeast and fungus.

Maxidolophis can be purchased in San Francisco: New West Health Food Store
970 Market Street
San Francisco, Calif.
(415) 775-7760

Or through Manufacturer: Ethical Nutrients
1121 East Colorado
Glendale, California 91205
(818) 243-1700

CANDIDA CLEAR

Helps restore the body's nutritionally weakened immune system to its proper function.
Helps prevent chronic growth of the yeast Candida albicans, which may produce toxins that may result in diarrhea, constipation, gastritis, kidney and bladder infections, fatigue, yeast vaginitis, skin rashes, plus various mental, emotional conditions.
Aids in restoring normal colon ecology and maintains the delicate balance of intestinal flora.

Candida Clear contains garlic, vitamin A (in the form of Beta Carotene, caprylic Acid.)

Candida Clear is most effective when the diet is altered to eliminate all yeast-containing foods.

Puregar	500MG
Caprylic Acid	70MG
Vitamin A (Beta Carotene)	10,000IU
Selenium (I-Selenmethionine)	100MG
Taheebo	100MB

Julie Estrada (415 392-8555)
c/o BioNet, Inc.
517 Washington St., Suite 201
San Francisco, Ca. 94111
$13.60 + $1.10 shipping

Editor's Note: Candida Clear is recommended by Dr. Emanuel Cheraskin, M.D., D.D.S. Dr. Cheraskin is on the staff at the University of Alabama.

CANTROL

Nature's Way Cantrol (Candida Control Pack) is a complete nutritional approach for the control of Candida albicans. Each Cantrol pack contains a combination of natural ingredients that helps to control Candida. These ingredients come in portion-controlled packages for added convenience and freshness. Cantrol's high potency formula helps keep yeast colonies from overpopulating in the intestines where they grow. One major ingredient in Cantrol is Primadophilus brand acidophilus, contained in unique enterosoluble capsules. This allows it to pass through the stomach and be released in the intestines for maximum benefit.

Additional ingredients such as Nature's Way anti-oxidant, linseed oil and vitamin E are included in the Cantrol portion-controlled pack for nutritional support. We have also included a free booklet, "Dietary Guidelines and Program Overview" which provides dietary suggestions along with complete information on the Cantrol program

Cantrol may be purchased in health food stores everywhere. If Cantrol is unavailable in your area, write Nature's Way, 10 Mountain Springs Parkway, Springville, Utah 84663, or call toll-free 1-800-453-9000

BODY TODY

Natural Minerals For the Body. Body Toddy is a natural blend of a group of 60 major minerals and trace minerals extracted from a natural deposit of plant origin. Body Toddy is not a medicine or drug or stimulant. Body Toddy is pure mineral.
Price: $ 32 fl. oz., $21.00 To Order: Rockland Int'l 12215 E. Skelly Drive. Tulsa, Oklahoma 74128 (918 664-1390) or write Ron Stenner 2841 Soscol Ave. Napa, Ca.

CANDIDA CONTROL

One of today's foremost nutritional authorities has made a revolutionary breakthrough in expanding the frontier of natural healing.

Dr. A.S. Wheelwright is an internationally renowned Herbal Nutritionist with a Ph.D. in Chemistry. Compelled by an intense desire to find answers to man's greatest health concerns, Wheelwright has traveled the globe studying intensively with Chinese, European, South American and American Indian herbalists, healers and health experts. He has spent over 30 years in the laboratory researching and testing how specific herbs activate each vitamin and mineral. He has tested his findings with over 64,000 people. Through this wealth of experience, Dr. Wheelwright has discovered the secret to scientifically formulating high energy nutritional products. These assist the body to revitalize rapidly and naturally.

As a result, Dr. Wheelwright has now introduced a new line of products known as Systemic Formulas. These products work very specifically to provide the nutritional building blocks to support and rebuild body systems. They function in two ways. One is to stimulate the cells into activity to promote cleansing. The other is to relax the cells which encourages building and control of infection. Medical authorities have found Systemic Formulas to be powerful, yet gentle and safe in their action.

The following for Candida Control: Tai Ra Chi - Anti-Viro (ViVi) - Corrector

Tai Ra Chi contains: A concentrate of Pau de Arco herb from Peru with Ceriece from Jamaica and Cynita from South America. Preserved and extracted in 10% Spirits and 10% Vegetable Glycerine.

ViVi Anti-Viro contains: Taheebo, Lomatium Dissecutim Oil, in a base of 6x leptotoenia, lactose and natural herbal oils.
(ViVi utilized the rare and costly Shosone Sacred Oil from the herb- Lomatium Dissectim, long considered a powerful anti-viral (the only known herb in nature with anti-viral properties) by the Nez Pierce and Shosone medicine men. These Indians took a preparation of this oil to Dr. Krebs (of Laetrile fame) in San Francisco during the Flu Epidemic of 1918. It is said they were responsible for saving 40,000 lives. ViVi is broad spectrum for viruses and also has anti-fungal properties

#4 Corrector contains: Extracts of Basil Wintergreen, Spearmint, Grapefruit Rind, Wild Carrot. In an Herbal base.

Days 1 - 14. Begin with 1 drop Tai Ra Chi under tongue 1x/day. Gradually increase to 12 drops a day (6 drops in the morning, six in the evening.) Also treat drinking water (spring water) with 1 drop / 12 oz. Let it sit for several hours before using.

Days 15 - 30. Continue with Tai Ra Chi. Begin with 1 ViVi 1x/day between meals. Increase to 2 per day on day 18, one in the morning, one in the afternoon. Use Spearmint tea as a beverage (not peppermint).

Days 30 - 45. Continue with Tai Ra Chi; ViVi will end. Begin 1 Corrector #4 between meals. Gradually increase to 4/day, two in the morning, two in the afternoon. Note: Large or coarse-mannered people may need to use 6/day and in rare cases up to 8/day for the last few days. Continue with Spearmint tea.
Maintenance. Use 1 Corrector #4 each 3 days.

*Excellent Products-Editor

To Order these Products:

Write to: Systemic Formulas of California
P.O. Box 782
San Mateo, California 94401

Susan Kuss, Nutritionist
Tim Kuss-Distributor
(415) 349-5144

IMU-GEN

TO ORDER: SCIMETRIC, INC.
Route 1, Box 33A
Brandt, S. D. 57218
(605) 832-3191

IMMUNITY - THE CURE FOR ALL DISEASES

Have you ever wondered why one or two people in a household of four or five come down with colds, flu or other more serious illnesses and do not 'pass-on' their infirmities to the others? The answer is very simple. Those with weaker immune systems are very susceptible to bacterial infections and thus are unable to produce antibodies fast enough to fight off the rapidly growing organisms.

From the moment of birth, newborn babies nourished by colostrum (otherise known as the first days of mother's milk), receive their first protection against nature. After the first few days of birth, the thymus gland then takes over this protective role and continues to supply us with immune factors, known as "T-cells." By the time we reach our teens, this gland begins to shrink and our capacity of immunity begins to recede.

As our resistance diminishes, so does our ability to fight back when illness strikes. Production of antibodies to ward off harmful bacteria becomes a relatively slow process, requiring days or weeks. Obviously then, the invading bacteria escalates in number without sufficient white cells to fend off the attackers.

How does IMU-GEN work?

People constantly combat multitudes of disease-causing organisms present in their environment. Bacteria, viruses and other microbes frequently penetrate the skin or mucous membranes which is the signal for the initiation of our bodies' natural immune response. When this happens, two types of responses occur: one is humoral immunity, which leads to the production of antibodies, and the other is known as cell mediated immunity, known as CMI. Both types of immunity are concerned with the lymphocyte (a type of white blood cell). Lymphocytes all look similar, but there are two very important types. In healthy bodies an infection stimulates "B" lymphocytes into becoming numerous antibody producing plasma cells, which protect by attaching to the invader to protect the body. The other, "T" lymphocytes becomes activated and directly or indirectly kill the invading microbes.

The natural production of antibodies or the activation of "T" cells may take several days and in severe illnesses may not develop enough immune factors to overcome the invaders. If, however, the person possesses pre-formed antibodies or activated "T" cells, the invaders, from a broad spectrum of infections or inflammations, may be quickly destroyed and normal health is maintained.

Because IMU-GEN protects the body against bacterial invaders, it is often used in the prevention of and therapy prescribed for Candida , or yeast infections, and appears highly qualified to encourage the body's resistance to the yeast cells.

SEROYAL, INC.

A COMPLETE DIAGNOSTIC AND THERAPY PROGRAM CALLED THE "CANDIDA SYSTEM"

Some of the physicians and Ph.D's who helped in formulating these products are: H. Hagglund, M.D.; Jeff Bland, Ph.D., Dr. Guilford, Ph.D., Stan Bauman, Ph.D.

Serodex (formerly known as Candex) A Homeopathic dilution formulated to help improve the body's immunity in the treatment of diagnosed Candida albicans.

Some of the products new on the market will be: Serostatin, Serodophilus, Heavy Metal Detox, Immuno Forte, Hyper-Intestional Cleanser, etc.

These are just a few of the products Seroyal has developed. This complete line will take the patient through blood test analysis for Candida to aiding the patient in ridding his/herself of this fungus.

All products are sold to those only in the Health Care Profession. Ask your physician or health care professional to order these products for you.

Address: Seroyal, Inc., P.O. Box 6500, Concord, California 94524 (415) 676 7201

HERBS AN ENDANGERED SPECIES?

It would appear that herbs are indeed becoming an endangered species in Canada. The Bureau of Non-Prescription Drugs, assailed over-the-counter sales of garlic as "dangerous to public safety." The Agency has ordered the removal of all garlic preparations from health food stores. According to news releases the agency is studying all vitamin, mineral, plant and food supplements for "potential danger." Along with garlic, amino acids, (building blocks of the body), Propolis, Royal Jelly, Ginseng, Aloe Vera, Wheat-Germ oil, Cayenne, Horse Chestnut, have all been prohibited from health food stores. They are now being classified as "New Drugs", because they appear in tablet or capsule form.

World Research News
December 1985
15300 Ventura Blvd. Suite 405
Sherman Oaks, California 91403

Editor's Note: Please write your congressman/woman and state "You are being forewarned not to try to pass any bill like this here in the United States."

Note: The above research Organization will do extensive research on any material you the client requests. There is a fee involved. This research outlet has just opened and is run very well.

HERBS FOR CANDIDA

KROEGER HERB PRODUCTS

CANDIDA ALBICANS is a fungus. However, unlike plants, they require oxygen and have a nucleus in their cells. They contain no chlorophyll and cannot make their own food (scavengers).

Candida seems to prefer people as hosts. It seems to multiply best in those of us who:

- are prone to eating poor diets
- are taking drugs-including steroid type chemicals and hormone altering drugs like the birth control pill
- have broken down our immune system from stress and/or
- have not replenished our intestinal flora after anti-biotics.

Candida's favorite places to growth are the mucous surfaces of the gastro-intestinal and genitourinary tracts. Its toxins readily move through the bloodstream to all parts of the body producing such symptoms as:

- sensitivity to molds
- gastritis
- distention & bloating
- constipation
- diarrhea
- gas colitis
- headaches
- depression
- lethargy
- hyperactivity
- acme
- yeast vaginitis
- menstrual irregularities
- cramping
- kidney & bladder infections
- cystitis
- allergic symptoms like hay fever, sinusitis
- earaches
- hives
- food allergies
- chemical sensitivities
- fatigue
- cold hands & feet
- joint pains which travel from joint to joint
- numbness
- loss of libido

Candida Albicans can even be the culprit in endometriosis.

WHAT TO DO?

- Avoid all yeast products
- Reduce your intake of refined carbohydrates and alcohol
- Avoid brewers yeast, raw mushrooms, chocolate, sweets, dairy products, nuts and nut butters.

Take Hanna's Specialty Herb formula KANTITA. It has proved immensely helpful in the fight against CANDIDA ALBICANS-the fungus among us.

INGREDIENTS: Condurango Bark
Yellow Dock
Red Clover Tops
(eat with a little yogurt)

Suggested Retail Price: $8.00 per bottle (75 capsules)
When ordering by mail, please enclose 75¢ per bottle for postage and handling

(continued)

KROEGER HERB PRODUCTS CONTINUED

HERB	OTHER HELPFUL SUPPLEMENTS	DESCRIPTION	INGREDIENTS
CHEM-X 2 twice/daily between meals	A,B-Complex, Aloe Vera	Transmutes chemical deposits, Helpful for fatigue from exposure to chemical pollutants, smoke, and aromatic hydrocarbons.	Black Tea, Condurango Bark, Red Clover, Yellowdock, Paprika, Chaparell, Spikenard

Herbal Anti-Booze

All physicians as well as laymen agree. "A drinking problem is a sickness." Yes, it is! It is the old enemy CANDIDA ALBICANS, encased in the liver and pancreas.

Whenever, by accident or by disturbed friendly bacteria in the intestines, Candida albicans overgrows, it may reach the liver and pancreas and be encased therein. People become addicted to alcohol. They may end up with the disease called ALCOHOLISM.

HERBAL ANTI-BOOZE will break this encased fungus disease. HERBAL ANTI-BOOZE is safe, time proven and very effective.

To order all of the above products: KROEGER HERB PRODUCTS
1122 Pearl St.
Boulder, Colorado 80302

Echinacea: Research conducted mainly in Germany over the past ten years reveals that Echinacea possesses most of its acclaimed medicinal properties and may be highly effective for the treatment of viral infections and the stimulation of the immune system. Research published in the United States in 1972 demonstrated antitumor activity of a lipid soluble component from Echinacea. Recent findings suggest that the active principle of Echinacea stimulates the immune system by binding to carbohydrate receptors on the cell surfaces of T-lymphocytes which in turn induces their nonspecific transformation, production of interferon, and the secretion of other lymphokines. The antiviral activity of Echinacea preparations appears to be directly related to the release of interferon by T-cells and other undifferentiated parenchymal cells.

See Wacker, A., and Hilbig, W., Planta Medica 33, 89-102 (1978), etc.

Feverfew: Candida die-off gives Candida patients headaches

Feverfew is an herb that grows wild. According to Paul Lee, Ph.D. former professor at the University of California, Santa Cruz, "Feverfew

"They have confirmed it completely. Ninety percent of those who suffered from migranes, from headaches, are cured. The longer you take it the more effective it becomes. Arthritis comes next because it is also an inflammatory disease and feverfew reduces inflammation.

Write to Paul Lee, Ph.D., Box 409, Santa Cruz, Ca. 95061 and he will send you some. You also may be able to get it in the Health food Stores.
This is an excerpt from Let's Live, July 1986.
titled: Your Headache is Over: Interview with Paul Lee, Ph.D., by Maureen Salaman

HOMEOPATHIC REMEDIES FOR STRENGTHENING THE IMMUNE SYSTEM

Mercurius Sol., Arsenicum Album, Thuja, Lachesis, Carcinosin.

Write Homeopathic Educational Service, 2124 Kittredge Street, Berkeley, California 94704, (415) 653-9270 (M-F 2-6 p.m. P.C.T.) *

Write to the above address for a homeopathic self-care medicine kit! (one for the beginner, one for travelling, and the third one as a comprehensive kit.

Write to the above address for a homeopathic catalog. Be sure to enclose a sase (business size)

*The National Center for Homeopathy is a nonprofit membership organization established for the purpose of promoting homeopathy through education, publication, research, and membership services. Write: National Center for Homeopathy, 1500 Massachusetts Avenue, N.W., Washington, D.C. 20005. (202) 223-6182.

EFFECT OF ORALLY CONSUMED ALOE VERA JUICE ON GASTROINTESTINAL FUNCTION IN NORMAL HUMANS; by Jeffrey Bland, Ph.D., Linus Pauling Institute of Science and Medicine, Palo Alto, California

...the effect of Aloe Vera juice supplementation appeared to be that of altering colonic biota. Those subjects that had heavy overgrowth of fecal bacteria and some yeast infection, were found to have improved fecal colonization and decreased yeast after the Aloe Vera Juice supplementation.

The function of Aloe Vera juice in promoting proper gastrointestinal function, based upon the information from this preliminary study, may be to regulate gastrointestinal pH while improving gastrointestinal motility, increasing stool specific gravity, and reducing populations of certain fecal microorganisms, including yeast.

To Order:

Dr. Donald Barber, D.D.S.
6010 Main Street
Williamsville, N.Y. 14221
(716) 632-7310

Aloe Vera Juice
Forever Living Products
$14.95 qt. (add $1.50 shipping)
$179.40 case

$OXYC_3$ is an oxidative drug, as the name implies. Nascent oxygen released with the use of this drug permeates membranes and directly kills candida. It is quite powerful and the effect is immediate.

American Biologics Hospital-Attn: Mike Culbert
Dr. Wolfram Kuhnau, M.D.
Phone No.
619-429-8200
800-227-4458

Stateside Address:
1180 Walnut Ave.
Chula Vista, Ca. 92011

CANDIDA BALANCING - HUMAN ECOLOGY BALANCING SCIENCE

The Candida balance is a very individual balance or correctional method. It will reset all the electromagnetic switches, including acupuncture meridians, particularly two energy systems that I have recently discovered to be affected by Candida and more particularly the toxin it secretes- "Acetaldehyde", (100 times more toxic then its little brother Formaldehyde. These two toxins affect the brain hemesphere integration and heart hemisphere integration. Loss of brain hemisphere integration results in dyslexia, spaciness, poor balance and weakens the nervous and immune systems.

Loss of hemesphere integration results in cold hands and cold feet, a pale look and poor circulation. Both brain and heart integration can now be accomplished by a simple exercise in minutes. Procedures for balancing all the meridians and energies that have been off-set by Candida can now be corrected in an individual manner in approximately an hour. The body will then be able to heal itself if nutrition and other ecological methods are followed, (e.g. removing mercury and other poisons from the body, TMJ alignment, etc.)

Steven Rochlitz, M.A.
Wholistic Health Consultant
Nutritional and Environmental Analysis
P.O. Box 1134
Setauket, New York 11733
(516) 689-9776

EDITOR'S NOTE: Rochlitz has been teaching this method all over the world and practitioners as well as lay people are finding amazing results. Mr. Rochlitz became environmentally ill (a universal reactor) when he was studying for a Ph.D. in Physics; thus stopping to heal himself. Mr. Rochlitz's will be publishing his new book this fall, titled, ALLERGIES AND CANDIDA- with an Energy Balancing Answer (With Brain and Heart Integration).

Townsend Newsletter for physicians just recently devoted an entire issue to Mr. Rochlitz's method of energy balancing.

POT-POURRI OF REMEDIES FOR ENHANCING THE IMMUNE SYSTEM

Cranberry Juice- Contains A,C.B complex, potassium, manganese, iron and calcium
Gooseberries- A natural laxative, good for digestion. (Mix with banana in blender add water)
Bromelin- Good for digestion
Thyroxin- Ideal way of fighting depression and mood swings.

GENTIAN VIOLET - quoted from the 27th Edition of the United States Dispensatory, 1973

Gentian violet is an antibacterial, antifungal and anthelmintic dye. It inhibits the growth of the causative agent of Vincent's angina, as well as growth of many molds, as Monilia, Torula, Epidermophyton and Trichophyton. Sutton (J.A.M.A.,110 1733, 1938) recommended such use in impetigo, furunculosis, secondarily infected dermatoses, and dermatomycoses. ....Gentian violet is often helpful in controlling pruritus ani and vulvae because it clears up secondary infections. Although aqueous solutions stain skin and clothing, the stains may be removed by washing. Topical application of a 1 percent solution is effective in the treatment of infections due to Candida albicans, as in thrush. Gorrell (Clin. Med., 302, 1945) used a 1 percent aqueous solution in treating leukorrhea when molds or yeast were present in the discharge. ....Gentian violet is active against (pinworm)

Locally gentian violet is nontoxic. When taken orally it may cause nausea, vomiting, diarrhea, and lassitude.

Dose. -The usual dose of gentian violet is 60 mg., given orally, 3 times daily, before meals, for 8 to 10 days in the treatment of pinworm infestations, and for 30 days in the treatment of liver fluke infestations.

For topical application a solution containing 1 percent of gentian violet and 10 percent of alcohol in purified water is used.

Several physicians mentioned Gentian Violet in their lecture at the 1985 Candida conference in San Francisco. Please check with your physician for use of Gentian violet.

TESTING FOR CANDIDA

In recent months, research for establishing a procedure for detecting the presence of Candida has resulted in 3 tests now being used with good results reported:

California Allergy Laboratories Hemogenetics Division has developed its "Light" test to measure the immune response of patients to Candida Albicans. For more information contact:

California Allergy Laboratories
101 South San Mateo Drive, Suite 315
San Mateo, Ca. 94401
(415) 342-8323

Immunodiagnostic Laboratories has developed a testing procedure for identifying Candida antibody levels in the patient. For information contact:

Edward E. Winger, M.D.
Pathologist
Immunodiagnostic Laboratories
400- 29th St.
Oakland, Ca. 94609
(415) 839-6477

Osler Welch Laboratory
2929 Summit
Oakland, California
Tel: (415) 835-8293

DUTCH PRIDE-BIO-"10"

It is always good news when a product appears on the scene that shows solid evidence of being effective against Candida albicans. Added good news is that efficacious amounts of this newly available preparation is many times removed from any toxic or untoward side-effects resulting from its use.

BIO-"10" has been under investigation in the United States for 15 years, and the following opinions of competent professionals reflect the promise that is inherent in the many testimonials that have been received attesting to its efficacy.

UNIVERSITY OF CALIFORNIA, DAVIS; Daniel Tuse', Ph.D. (Doctoral Candidate-at time of study)

"E-100 (BIO-"10") was 12% more inhibitory to the growth of Saccharomyces sp. in liquid culture that Amphotericin B, and 16% more inhibitory to C. albicans than its widely used counterpart. Agar diffusion studies showed that E-100 (BIO-"10") was 2 1/2 times more potent than Am-B at the lowest dose tested for Saccharomyces sp.and over 3 times more potent than Am.B for C.albicans."

UNIVERSITY OF CALIFORNIA, DAVIS; S. Anderson Peoples, M.D., Professor of Pharmacology (Emeritus)

"...where utilized in vivo, it (BIO-"10") combines with the natural bodily functions and immune responses to become an effective medication with virtually no toxic or side effects."

STANFORD UNIVERSITY (1984); James D. Berg, Ph.D., Medical Microbiology-Env. Eng.

"The third potential mechanism for E-100 (BIO-"10") involves utilization of chlorite by cells, particularly leukocytes, as a substrate to increase the efficiency of a group of enzymes known as peroxidases...there are two interesting outcomes of chlorite utilization by these enzymes. The first is that the immune system may be directly enhanced by the increased rate of oxidation of foreign material by the leukocytes. The second result is an increased ability by all metabolically active cells to scavenge free radicals."

James R. Privitera, M.D., Covina, California

"In the almost seven years I have been using BIO-"10" in my practice...I have dispensed it to several hundred patients with not one report of any ill or untoward effect. At this time I have seen it work in a variety of ways...I know that BIO-"10" has a significant contribution to make to the field of medicine, and I'll be happy to cooperate in any way I can to bring it about."

Thus, there is strong evidence to indicate that BIO-"10" can act as a supplement to the body's immune system and, apparently, its use as a dietary aid can raise the efficiency of the body's resistance to better combat infections, toxic agents, and other dysfunctions. This information is for educational purposes only, and is not meant to prescribe treatment for any particular disorder or disease.
For further information as to availability, price and possible distributorships, please contact: Ms. Ember Safford, Dutch Pride Products, P.O. Box 1651, Cottonwood, Arizona, 86326. Tel. (602) 634-7066

VITAMIN "O" - THE OXYGEN NUTRIENT

A complex carbohydrate is a high oxygen food. Complex carbohydrates are vegetables, whole grains, seeds, and nuts. (Fruits are too high in simple sugars to be classified as complex carbohydrates.) ...fats are oxygen robbers. Protein is composed of 20 to 50 percent oxygen. ...It is obvious that complex carbohydrates have the most oxygen. ....Oxygen provides the spark of life. Nutrients provide the fuel for burning. The correct fuel/oxygen mixture is required for the best of health.

An acidic condition, caused by the accumulation of acidic by-products, occurs in poorly oxygenated cells. Soft drinks, caffeine, and red meats are among the substances that cause systemic (whole body) acidity.

Common yeast infections (Candida albicans) occur frequently in an oxygen-poor body. Because of the low oxygen environment, the Candida albicans generates a substance that is responsible for cellular damage. This disrupts intestional absorptive processes and impairs the function of lymphocytes and red blood cells thereby reducing immune defenses.

Dr. Levine describes the role of oxygen as it relates to human electrical energy: "Like the electrical circuits in your home, your body is also electrical. Oxygen forms the positive terminal of your cellular battery. Energy from fresh natural foods provides the current...

Vitamin "O" may be purchased through:
Nutri-Cology
400 Preda Street
San Leandro, Calif. 94577
(800) 545-9960

$15.95 pro-oxygen wafers +
$ 1.00 for additional literature, includ- postage and handling.

The above paragraphs are excerpted from an article in the July 1986 issue of Let's Live Magazine. Mrs. Kamen is author of "Osteoprosis: What It Is, How To Prevent It, How To Stop It".

Editor's Note: Vitamin "O" contains Siberian Ginseng which is extremely high in Organic Germanium. (Organic Germanium is believed to be a key active principal in many nature healing substances such as Aloe Vera, Ginseng, Garlic, Chlorella, etc.

NEW: AN ALTERNATIVE TO DRUGS IN THE TREATMENT OF CANDIDA

TO ORDER: Marsha Smith
8 Muriel Pl.
Fairfax, Ca. 94930
(415) 459-5013

*CANDASTATIN by Multiway

SPECIAL NUTRITIONAL SUPPORT IN YEAST MANAGEMENT

EACH 6 TABLETS SUPPLY:

Pancreatin..............180 mg
Calcium Ascorbate......2,250 mg
Vit. B-1.............. 60 mg
Vit. B-2................60 mg
Vit. B-6................60 mg
Biotin..................100 mg
Beta Carotene (Vit A) 18,000 I.U.
Vit. E (d-a-Tocopherol 300 I.U.
Zinc Chelate............18 mg
Selenium (Sodium Selenite.30 mg

L-Cysteine.............450mg
L-Typosine.............360mg
L-Glutamine............360mg
Betaine HCI............ 60mg
Thymus-Lymph-Spleen Complex.......360mg

*Contains NO preservatives, sugar, starch, salt, wheat, corn, soy, yeast or milk derivatives.

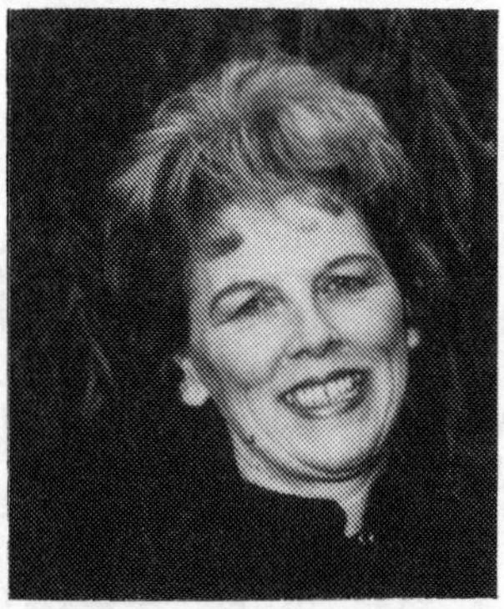

Dorothy Iversen

From Candida to Better Health

by
Dorothy Iversen
7185 Union Ave., Mayer, MN 55360

CANDIDIASIS?

I had never heard of the disease until last year. Unknowingly however, it was my miserable "companion" for at least 30 of my 52 years! Every bout with pneumonia or a flu would end with yet another antibiotic, leaving me with diarrhea, indigestion and allergic reactions. With each new sickness, I was progressively worse. I finally refused to see a doctor for my ailments, for they just did not know the damage their drugs were doing to my system. When three of my four babies developed "Thrush" shortly after birth, they still had not diagnosed the Candidiasis. (Thrush is a yeast infection that occurs in the mouth of babies. It is picked up from the mother as the baby comes through the birth canal.) In each case, the baby promptly was treated; they did nothing for me!

As a result of this yeast infection that came from so many antibiotics, my problems grew worse and worse. I developed a 25 year history of back problems that never got better. I did not know I was allergic to numerous foods that were irritating my intestines and weakening the muscles to my back...The CAUSE was not corrected, so the trouble progressed to my neck and arms. I lost most of my strength and was in pain much of the time. I never suspected a disease called Candidiasis and the related allergies were to blame! Suffering with severe fatigue and unexplained bouts of depression that I could not understand, I felt guilty that I was unable to control my "roller-coaster" emotions...Now, instead of visiting medical doctors trying to get help, I was making the rounds with chiropractors, hoping someone could help my painful back and the chronic diarrhea I had had for twelve years without relief.

In 1979 I developed three lumps on my left breast. The largest of the three was cancerous, and I treated with a naturopathic doctor who used only herbs and natural methods. My ability to digest or assimilate food was almost nil; as a result, my mineral level was extremely low as well. This doctor put me on a program, similar to the one used by Dr. William Kelley, which of course, is shunned by most uninformed medical people. Part of my program consisted of taking "pancreatic enzymes" around the clock. On a vegetarian diet, these enzymes (meant to digest meat), work to "digest" deficient and cancerous cells, throwing the toxic, cancerous material into the blood stream for elimination. I will not go into all the other parts of my cancer treatment here, but will say that after being on this program for about eight weeks, the two smaller lumps softened and disappeared, proving the program worked! These early signs were a great encouragement to continue, inspite of the pressure from friends who thought I should be going to a medical doctor for a possible mastectomy, (the popular treatment then), or even go in for chemotherapy which would have completely destroyed my already deficient immune system. It was during this time my faith was strengthened. GOD began to show me some incredible things in the Bible, "hidden from the wise and prudent, and revealed...unto babes" (Matt. 11:26) Surely that was me! Study had become incresingly difficult because of the Candida, however, I felt God's Spirit take over in areas where I needed help.

One day I was puzzled by a verse in Rev. 18:23 that says, "...all nations are deceived by her sorceries." I wanted to determine exactly what that verse meant, so I looked up the word "sorcery" and found that the Greek word is "PHARMEKIA". The English root word "pharmacy" deals with the dispensing of drugs, as well as magic, sorcery and witchcraft. "All nations have been deceived" by the administration of these drugs...No wonder I had gotten sicker each time I was given antibiotics. Jer. 46:11 confirmed what GOD had showed me, "...in vain shalt thou use many medicines, for thou shalt not be cured." How thankful I was that the Lord had sent me a health care professional who refused to use these drugs and used herbs instead! With great hope, I continued the program for about nine months when the largest cancerous lump softened and disappeared! The cancer was gone!

Although now free of the cancer, I still suffered other afflictions connected with the Candida. I was embarrassed that I was sick so often, picking up pneumonia, bronchitis, and every "bug" that came along, not to mention the chronic fatigue, diarrhea, back problems, menstrual and vaginal problems, chronic athlete's foot, and a similar fungal infection in my nostrils, and probably throughout my system. (We spent hundreds of dollars on athlete's foot remedies that worked only temporarily, and a much greater amount trying to relieve my painful back!)

Finally, five years after the cancer, a wonderfully alert chiropractor diagnosed the Candidiasis for the first time. I was put on a yeast-free, sugar-free, low carbohydrate diet, along with Caprystatin, a non-prescriptive medication. He pinpointed my allergies and I was wonderfully relieved of much of my back problems. After several months, however, my general condition was only slightly improved. In fact, the strict diet seemed to make everything worse...Upon hearing a lecture about all the wonderful results people were getting using **hydrogen peroxide,** and knowing it is a **natural** product found in mother's milk, in rain and snow, and in all fresh fruits and vegetables, etc., I decided to try it. I started by taking just three drops of 35% food grade hydrogen peroxide (h.p.) in a 6 oz. glass of apple juice or distilled water, always at least an hour after eating or drinking. This 100% natural product has the ability to seek out foreign bacteria, FUNGUS, even strep germs and will kill them without harming any surrounding tissue! I felt it was working so I increased the dosage until I was taking 25 drops each day. Nausea and a slight headache occurred, lasting about an hour. I was not alarmed when this happened, for I knew it was seeking out the fungus, and like the cancer treatment, the h.p. was killing toxic material, throwing it into my blood stream, causing the nausea before being eliminated.

After taking the maximum dosage of 25 drops once a day for a couple of weeks, I then increased to twice, and finally to three times a day. The total plan was over an eight week span, building up to three times a day at the maximum dosage, and then tapering off gradually to once a day. Because a large pocket of Candida remained in my prolapsed transverse colon, I went through the program again, this time using a natural intestinal cleanser to clean out this infecting pocket that was multiplying and distributing the Candida throughout my system. (Dr. Christopher's "Eight-In-One" worked best for me, though Sonne's Intestinal Cleanser works well. I mixed the product as directed and let the mixture sit for a couple of minutes to "gel" before adding the peroxide. Stir and drink.) Using the peroxide three times a day with the intestinal cleanser produced a beneficial "healing crisis". I felt as though I was coming down with a flu, then expelled some long, tough and fibrous fecal material. After this was passed, I began to feel better!

The hydrogen peroxide was clearly what had killed off the excess Candida albicans, although I feel other supplements have contributed to my rebuilding success...I take a good yeast-free multi-vitamin/mineral supplement called "Basic Preventive", (by Advanced Medical Nutrition, Inc.) To encourage hormone production and vaginal elasticity and health, I take "Fem-H" and "BB-T", both by Dr. Christopher under the NuPro label.) I use Orithrush douche and also take Vital-Dophilus to maintain a good flora in the vagina and intestines respectively, I also take Golden Seal, Kyolic Garlic, and Pau d'arco capsules, all anti-fungal agents. Depression and fatigue were constantly a problem, and the low carbohydrate diet made this worse, partly because of my extremely low blood sugar level. NuPro's "P-INS" have helped to rebuild my pancreas and keeps my blood sugar at a more normal level, also relieving the emotional dips and extreme fatigue. Amino acid capsules have helped improve mental alertness, memory, hormonal balance and emotional stability. Altogether, I have been treating the excess Candida for fifteen months, but have been on the h.p. for about 6 months and now take a daily "maintenance" dosage of 20 drops each night before retiring. (I also take 25 drops when coming down with a cold or flu. It is effective in killing the germs in about an hour's time if taken as soon as I begin to feel sick. I have also used it to treat my athlete's foot by soaking my feet in a 3% solution persistantly for 20 minutes daily, and continuing for at least 10 days after all symptoms disappeared.) The h.p. has given me wonderful new energy, and I require much less sleep each night!

I still do not eat yeast foods like bread or mushrooms, etc., but do eat fruit and carbohydrates now, along with limited dairy products, and limit my meat to poultry and fish. I eat plenty of steamed or raw vegetables and salads. Because of the allergies, I rotate my foods and do not eat any food more than once in a four-day period, preventing further allergic reactions to additional foods. I also take "Antronex" (Standard Process Labs), a natural anti-histamine that helps prevent reactions to allergies.

Because most Candida victims have used every avenue possible trying to get well, I will share some additional things that have helped me understand the problem better...Through my illnesses, I have been drawn to principles GOD gave us in the Bible that apply...

For explicit instructions on the efficient operation of any product, you would follow the "Manufacturer's Handbook", of course. Certainly GOD, **our Creator,** knows how **we** operate best! We must regard **His** instructions to be just as valid and necessary as any other book of instructions, if we are to regain individual and national health! MEN have been playing "god" long enough! Our "Instructor's Handbook" (the Bible), tells us to eat foods "whose seed is in itself", and can reproduce "after its kind". This includes green herbs, vegetables, grains, fruits, and nuts. (Gen 1:11, 29, 30).

In early Bible days, men lived nearly 900 years, eating this diet. However, because of immorality GOD sent Noah's Flood, and afterward shortened their life span to 90 years by telling them they could now eat meat for the first time. (Gen. 9:3) He promised HEALTH, however, by specifying which kinds of meat they should eat in Ex. 15:26 and Lev. 11.

HYBRID fruits and vegetables do not have that "seed" that can reproduce by themselves. They are man's creation, without regard to the Creator's instructions, and in the end, will not bring us health...

Likewise, yeast products and mushrooms do not have "seeds within themselves". They are reproduced by spores, are parasitic in nature, living off other organisms. Further, they are grown in the dark, thrive on rotting, decayed material or pure manure. (I notice trees that are dying, for example, often have a visible fungus growth on the trunks. This is just the natural life to death process, helping to speed up the decay of an already dying tree. Fungus never lives on a HEALTHY HOST!...) It is not surprising, therefore, that yeast-based antibiotics have caused so much harm, for they thrive on unhealthy, decaying material... in US! It is also quite significant that Unleavened bread was commanded for the feasts in the Bible.

("Leavening" or yeast is always symbolic of sin throughout the Bible.) Since those feast days are symbolic of future times, the wise will refrain from yeast-bearing foods and drugs...!

In tenderness and love, GOD confides to us in 3 John 2, "BELOVED, I wish **above all things,** that thou mayest prosper and **be in health,** even as thy soul prospereth"! Although our knowledge is still incomplete, we certainly are headed in the right direction when we let our Heavenly Father guide us to health He has promised, (and even that ETERNAL life), by following His instructions. Truly His Word, the Bible, "is a lamp unto our feet, and a light unto our path!" (Ps. 119:105)

Reprinted with permission
Health Consciousness, October 1985
Roy Kupsinel, M.D. Editor
P.O. Box 550
Oviedo, Fla. 32765-0550
(305) 365-6681

IX

THE USE OF HYDROGEN PEROXIDE, OZONE, LASER, HYPERBARIC OXYGEN FOR CANDIDA, ETC.

Dr. Sol Silverman, DDS and Professor of Oral Medicine at the University of California in San Francisco recommends hydrogen peroxide in saline solution as being a good control for Candida in the oral cavity. See Chapter III of this book for a review of this lecture by Dr. Silverman.

---

41 million Americans have serious arthritis, 20 million have herpes, 13 million have serious diabetes. This is 74 million or over one third of our population and we have only covered three diseases. At the beginning of this century we were one of the healthiest nations on this earth.

Some of the reasons we are not healthy are: our air, water and food are not what they were 75 to 100 years ago. We have polluted our air, we need additives for our water to make it safe to drink, and our food has lost its trace elements, long leached from our soils. We now must use supplements to help supply what has been lost. One of these supplements is oxygen.

Oxygen is the most abundant element on earth, it comprises 45.6% of the earth's crust and 20.95% of dry air. It is one of the most vital and necessary elements to support life. Oxygen is so vital to good health that hospitals have it installed in the patient's rooms. All rescue units ambulances and life support systems are equipped with it. Without oxygen you can live only a few minutes.

Oxygen taken internally, is capable of eliminating microorganisms in the human body to the extent that arthritis, cancer, ulcers, hives, and a total of 35 diseases could be eliminated or controlled.

Through the research efforts of Dr. Edward Carl Rosenow (1875-1966) author of 450 published medical papers and associated with the Mayo Clinic for over 60 years, a technique has been developed by which these microorganisms can be controlled. His basic tenet was that we live in an ocean of microorganisms, the body is like a world. In the world of the body are millions of microorganisms. Little creatures each seeking their own habitat, food and environment. Just as animals in our world live in different climates, eat different foods, multiply, prey on others, infect, go through metamorphosis, pollute streams, so these little microorganisms invade our bodies and seek out their proper habitats. These microorganisms do the following:

-attack cells and enter them, building cocoons around the stricken cell; thus cutting off the blood supply and causing the cell to lose its specific function, so that it can only live and multiply into cancerous tumors.
-cling to the lining in the nervous system and short-circuit some of the electronics in the central computer of the brain.
-give off calcium waste matter that cements bones together
-lodge in liver and kidneys, and with their bile form stones
-gnaw away at the joints (inflammatory arthritis)

One of the simplest sources of this healing oxygen is in hydrogen peroxide. Hydrogen peroxide traces back through to the origin of time. It gets into our rain and snow from the ozone layer high in the earth's atmosphere. Ozone (O_3) is free oxygen (O_2) plus an extra atom of oxygen. This extra atom of oxygen splits off very easily, and does so when it comes in contact with water. Water (H_2O) now becomes hydrogen peroxide (H_2O_2). Compared to chlorine, bacterial and viral disinfection with ozone is up to 5000 times more rapid. (McGraw-Hill Encyclopedia of Science & Technology 5th Edition, p. 728). This is why many cities in Europe use ozone and hydrogen peroxide in their drinking waters. Many brands of bottled water that you buy in this country have been ozonated for your protection. Hydrogen peroxide is found in our fresh fruits and vegetables; some from rain and some is manufactured in the photosynthesis process. (Gen. Biochemistry Furton & Simmonds, p. 338). If we were to eat fresh fruit and vegetables in their raw state we would get this healing oxygen into our bodies.

We tested human mother's milk and found it contains a good amount of natural hydrogen peroxide. Colostrum milk (first milk secreted after birth) has an even stronger hydrogen peroxide content. In testing natural spring waters, we found the spring water at Lourdes, France contained the strongest amount of hydrogen peroxide in its natural form.

In the past twenty years, there have been over 1,000 medical articles published on the qualities of hydrogen peroxide.

The FDA (Food & Drug Administration) in Federal Regulation Vol 46, Number 6, January 9, 1981 in effect gave the food industry a green light to use hydrogen peroxide in the "Aseptic" packaging process. The FDA has further ruled that hydrogen peroxide can be used in the processing of cheese and related cheese products (part 160), and as an antimicrobial agent in whey processing. They have also ruled it to be used in cleaning and healing mouth injuries. It is used in milk in 45 countries around the world. If one were to put a teaspoon of 3% hydrogen peroxide in a glass of fresh milk it would kill all the micro organisms. As a result the milk will not sour, even without refrigeration.

There are many peroxides available on the market, however many have stabilizers in them. The very best are Re-agent and Food Grade hydrogen peroxide. Peroxide is sold in drug stores and grocery stores as an antiseptic;

There is an abundance of healing oxygen in many of the raw foods we eat, however, we lack an adequate supply because of the way we process our food. Heat destroys or neutralizes hydrogen peroxide, lessening the benefits to our body. This is why the subject of drinking hydrogen peroxide; it will supplement this vital oxygen and help keep one well.

The above information is for educational purposes only, and is not meant to prescribe for any particular disorder or disease. Names and addresses and phone numbers of people who claim to have been helped by the use of the hydrogen peroxide program can be obtained by writing to Box 81, Union Rd., California, Ky. 41007 (606) 635-9297 or 6600 Trail Blvd. N., Naples, Fla. 33940 (813) 597-4111 - Fr.Richard Willhelm, B.S.

Fr. Willhelm studied under Dr. Robert Oppenheimer, Ph.D. at the University of California, Berkeley & Dr. Enrico Fermi, Ph.D. (Nobel Prize 1934) at the University of Washington.

USING 35% FOOD GRATE HYDROGEN PEROXIDE (H_2O_2)

Use the dosages listed in the chart with 5 ounces of distilled water, juice, or milk. DO NOT USE WITH FRESH PRESSED CARROT JUICE (there's an enzyme in the carrot juice that breaks H_2O_2 down into water and oxygen), CARBONATED DRINKS, OR ALCOHOLIC BEVERAGES. (When reaching higher dosages, use more water or juice as needed).

Take on an empty stomach, 1 hour before a meal, or an hour after a meal. If your stomach gets upset at any level, stay at that level, or go back one level. NOTE: Candida victims may need to start at 1 drop 3 times per day.

To Make 3% Solution (Using 35%):
Mix 1 oz. of 35% hydrogen peroxide into 11 oz. of distilled water. This makes 3/4 pint of 3% solution.

To Make 8% Solution (Using 35%):
Mix 4 parts of 35% hydrogen peroxide to 13 parts of distilled water.

To Make 12% Solution (Using 35%):
Mix 1 part 35% hydrogen peroxide to 2 parts of distilled water.

Possible Reactions to Hydrogen Peroxide:
Skin erruptions, nausea, sleepiness, unusual fatigue, diarrhea, colds (in head or chest), ear infections, boils, or any other method that the body uses to emit toxins from the body (the toxins have been rooted out by the use of hydrogen peroxide). This is the natural way for the body to cleanse and the natural cleansing will be of short duration, as you continue to maintain your program. Above all, even if you must decrease the dosage, continue the program, don't give up.

If you get a cleansing reaction, you may want to increase the dosage to hasten the cleansing. A cleansing is the effect on the body of bacteria dying off, or various forms of poisons being released through the eliminative organs of the body, i.e. skin, lungs, kidneys and bowels.

Remember: When hydrogen peroxide comes in contact with virus and streptococcus, it will liberate free oxygen (O_2). This may be happening in your stomach. If your stomach feels uneasy, it is only the hydrogen peroxide seeking out the virus and streptococcus to destroy.

CAUSTION: If you spill 35% hydrogen peroxide on your skin, immediately rinse under tap water. It will burn and turn the skin white. Avoid spillage.

DOSAGE SCHEDULE FOR 35% H_2O_2

1st day, use 9 drops (3 drops, 3 times/day)
2nd day, use 12 drops (4 drops, 3 times/day)
3rd day, use 15 drops (5 drops, 3 times/day)
4th day, use 18 drops (6 drops, 3 times/day)
5th day, use 21 drops (7 drops, 3 times/day)
6th day, use 24 drops (8 drops, 3 times/day)
7th day, use 27 drops (9 drops, 3 times/day)
8th day, use 30 drops (10 drops, 3 times/day)
9th day, use 36 drops (12 drops, 3 times/day)

10th day, use 42 drops (14 drops, 3 times/day)
11th day, use 48 drops (16 drops, 3 times/day)
12th day, use 54 drops (18 drops, 3 times/day)
13th day, use 60 drops (20 drops, 3 times/day)
14th day, use 66 drops (22 drops, 3 times/day)
15th day, use 72 drops (24 drops, 3 times/day)
16th day, use 75 drops (25 drops, 3 times/day)

For more serious complaints stay at 25 drops, 3 times per day for 1-3 weeks. Next graduate down to 25 drops, 2 times per day until the problem is taken care of. This may take from 1-6 months. Don't give up.

When free of complaints, you may taper off by taking:

25 drops once every other day, 4 times.
25 drops once every third day for 2 weeks.
25 drops once every fourth day for 3 weeks.

A good maintenance would be 5-15 drops per week, depending on the amount of cooked and processed foods you are eating.

THE DROP REFERRED TO IS UNDILUTED 35% HYDROGEN PEROXIDE.

Note: Candida victims may need to start at a dosage of 2 drops, 3 times per day and work up.

Information furnished by ECHO
BOX 126
Delano, Mn. 55328

Subscription Rate: $10.00 - 6 issues - Write to the above address
Echo is an educational organization whose purpose is the research of Hydrogen Peroxide.

Hydrogen Peroxide Used in Hot Tub- From Echo Newsletter

35% Hydrogen Peroxide is being used at a racquet club in its hot tub spa. It is reported that the spa water is yeast free, virus free, doesn't froth or maintain any amount of foam, no odor, and is a lovely blue. This method of purification has been practiced for over two years.

NOTE: If a person is on medication, the physician may suggest treating the medication as a food, thereby taking the peroxide one hour before or one hour after taking the medicine.

Remember

Deep breathing of fresh air, along with exercise is very important, Hydrogen Peroxide need not be kept in refrigerator.

ADDITIONAL USES FOR HYDROGEN PEROXIDE
(information furnished by ECHO NEWSLETTER)

Vegetable Soak: (In place of Clorox)
Add 1/4 cup 3% H_2O_2 to a sink full of cold water. Soak light vegetables (lettuce, etc.) 20 minutes, thicker skinned vegetables (like cucumbers) for 30 minutes. Drain and dry (they keep longer too!).

If time is a problem, you can spray the vegetables with straight 3% H_2O_2, let stand for a couple of minutes, rinse and dry.

To Freshen Kitchen: Keep a spray bottle of 3% (straight) in the kitchen. Use it to wipe off counter tops and appliances. It disinfects and gives the kitchen a fresh smell. Works great inside the refrigerator! (P.S. works on formica desk tops too).

Washing/Laundry: Add 8 ounces of 3% to your wash in place of bleaches with fumes!

Marinate: Place chicken or beef in a casserole (avoid use of aluminum pans), and cover with 3% hydrogen peroxide. It may take several pints depending on amount of meat/chicken. Place, loosely covered in refrigerator overnight. The next day, rinse and cook.

In the Dishwasher: Add 2 oz. of 3% hydrogen peroxide to your regular washing formula. Your glasses will really sparkle!

Sprouting Seeds: Add 1 ounce 3% hydrogen peroxide to 1 pint of water and soak the seeds overnight. Add the same amount of hydrogen peroxide each time you rinse the seeds. Some people have reported 3/4" sprouts in 24 hours!

Plants: Put 1 oz. 3% Hydrogen Peroxide in 1 quart of water. Water or mist plants with this solution.

Put 8 ounces white sugar, and 4-8 ounces 3% hydrogen peroxide in 1 gallon of water. Use this as an insecticide spray.

Humidifiers/Steamers: Use 1 pint 3% H_2O_2 to 1 gallon of water. (Helps keep them clean too!)

In the Bathroom: Keep a spray bottle of 3% hydrogen peroxide in the shower. Spray your body after washing to replace the acid mantle on your skin that soap removes.

Spray toilet paper with 3% hydrogen peroxide before wiping.

Use 3% on a cotton ball as a facial freshener after washing.

Add 1/2-1 pint 35% hydrogen peroxide to a full bathtub for a detoxifying bath. (Note: try not to use this after 6-7:00 p.m. - the increased absorbed oxygen may keep you awake!)

Athlete's Foot: Soak feet nightly in 3% hydrogen peroxide.

Mouthwash: Use 3% hydrogen peroxide. Add a dash of liquid chlorophyll for flavoring if desired. "Peroxol" is a commercial brand presently sold. It is 1 1/2% hydrogen peroxide with flavoring to mask the taste.

Toothpaste: Use baking soda - add enough 3% hydrogen peroxide to make a paste. Or, just dip your brush in 3% hydrogen peroxide and brush. (There is a new commerical brand out called PerioGene, it is a hydrogen peroxide gel).

Douche: Equal parts of 3% hydrogen peroxide and water is the maximum dosage. Start with more water, and gradually increase the amount of 3% you add.

Enema: 6 Tablespoons 3% hydrogen peroxide to a quart of water is the maximum dosage. Start with 3 tablespoons and gradually increase the amount.

Colonic: 1 pint 3% hydrogen peroxide to five gallons of water is the maximum dosage. Start with 1/2 pint and gradually increase the dosage.

WHERE TO PURCHASE HYDROGEN PEROXIDE (35% Food Grade)

Jackie Easterbrook	A.J. MacDonald
8063 Clares Drive	719 North Loma Drive
Sarasota, Florida 33580	Lodi, California 95240
(813) 355-9163	(209) 368-8681

For further literature on Hydrogen Peroxide write or call:
Elizabeth Muelhaupt, c/o Rainbow Associates, 7148 Meridian Road, S.E., Olympia, Washington 98503. (206) 456-0916

ECHO NEWSLETTER: (Excerpts) September/October 1984
Volume 1, Number 1

CHLORINE IN DRINKING WATER OR HYDROGEN PEROXIDE?

Business Week Magazine, 5-7-84, Page 118.
Ozone: The water purifier that could edge out chlorine.
Ozone has the ability to destroy bacteria 5,000 times faster than chlorine. The first two cities in the U.S. to use this process are Casper, Wyoming, and Potsdam, New York. Los Angeles, California is building a $120 million plant that will be the largest in the world in the U.S. at a Cincinnati, Ohio based corporation. Canada and Switzerland are also building these machines.

CALIFORNIA SUPER MARKETS AND HYDROGEN PEROXIDE

Some super markets in California are misting their fresh fruits and vegetables with H2O2. They are finding this increases the shelf life. Could this be the answer to the nitrites used by restaurants to keep their greens fresh longer?

Newsletter Address: ECHO
P.O. BOX 126
Delano, Minn. 55328

CANCER RESEARCH OF VIRGINIA LIVINGSTON, M.D.

The following paper on the Cancer Research of Virginia Livingston, M.D. presents her findings of microorganisms as being one of the causes of cancer and other degenerative diseases. This summary will help the reader see more clearly how hydrogen peroxide once taken internally will flood the body, releasing oxygen and thus destroying these microorganisms, yeasts and fungi which live without oxygen.

OXYGEN TRANSFERRING AND HYDROGEN TRANSFERRING ENZYMES IN THE PREVENTION OF CANCER

The Prime Cause and Prevention of Cancer
Revised lecture at the meeting of the Nobel-Laureates on June 30, 1966
at Lindau, Lake Constance, Germany
by Otto Warburg

"The prime cause of cancer is the replacement of the respiration of oxygen in normal body cells by a fermentation of sugar. All normal body cells meet their energy needs by respiration of oxygen, whereas cancer cells meet their energy needs in great part by fermentation. All normal body cells are thus obligate aerobes, whereas all cancer cells are partial anaerobes. From the standpoint of the physics and chemistry of life this difference between normal and cancer cells is so great that one can scarcely picture a greater difference. Oxygen gas, the donor of energy in plants and animals is dethroned in the cancer cells and replaced by an energy yielding reaction of the lowest living forms, namely, a fermentation of glucose.

The key to the cancer problem is accordingly the energetics of life... ...the oxygen transferring and hydrogen transferring enzymes were discovered and chemically isolated. ...The fermentation of cancer cells was discovered decades ago; but only in recent years has it been demonstrated that cancer cells can actually grow in the body almost with only the energy of fermentation. Only today can one submit, with respect to cancer, all the experiments demanded by Pasteur and Koch as proof of the prime cause of a disease. If it is true that the replacement of oxygen-respiration by fermentation is the prime cause of cancer, then all cancer cells without exception must ferment, and no normal growing cell ought to exist that ferments in the body."

Dr. Warburg won the Nobel Prize in Medicine in 1931 for his discovery of the oxygen transferring enzyme of cell respiration and was voted a second Nobel Prize in 1944 for his discovery of the active groups of the hydrogen transferring enzymes.

The following articles are summarized from the medical journals showing the wide use of Hydrogen Peroxide for the body.

a) Simple Painless Treatment of Warts

b) Killing of Blood-Stage Murine Malaria Parasites by Hydrogen Peroxide

c) Influenzal Pneumonia: The Intravenous Injection of Hydrogen Peroxide

d) Removal of Cholesterol and other lipids from experimental animals and human atheromatous arteries by dilute hydrogen peroxide

e) Catalase as a protective shield

f) Hydrogen Peroxide mediated Killing of Bacteria

g) Generation of H2O2 in Biomembranes

h) Peroxide Enemas in Obstipation

i) Hydrogen Peroxide release from Human Blood Platelets

j) Cell Division in Normal and Transformed Cells: The Possible Role of Superoxide and Hydrogen Peroxide

k) Iowa Conference on Hydrogen Peroxide

l) The Effects of Hydrogen Peroxide on the Ehrlich Carcinoma in Laboratory Mice: St. Thomas Institute, Cincinnati, Hoio, Nov. 15, 1982

m) Oxygen Intermediates are Required for Interferon Activation of NK Cells

n) Knighton, et al, Oxygen for Prevention of Wound Infection

o) General Biochemistry

p) Could Oxygen be a New Wonder Cure?

q) Stroud's Digest on the Diseases of Birds

r) Bacteria May Help Prevent Infections

TRANSLATION FROM THE GERMAN CUMULATED INDEX MEDICUS 1962

SIMPLE PAINLESS TREATMENT OF WARTS

English Translation by:
Elke Olson

CUMULATED INDEX MEDICUS 1962
Hydrogen Peroxide Therapy
Manok M: (On a Simple and Painless Treatment of Warts)
Hautarzt 12:425 Sept. 1961 Germany

An easy and painless treatment of Warts: There is still not a lone method of wart treatment which as everyone wishes, is painless; doesn't leave scars; doesn't render one unable to work and doesn't harm later on. The non-uniform therapeutic methods mirror itself in a lot of steps of mechanical, physical or chemical types, because none are meeting the above qualifications.

Either the methods are too bloody and painful, or they are unsuitable as they leave damage behind. Besides one has to expect residue if there aren't disfiguring scars left behind.

In this short and preliminary communication we don't intend to talk about all the therapeutic methods available, but only our own.

We thought to use an old disinfectant 30% H_2O_2 (Hydrogen Peroxide).

The now therapeutic results justify this preliminary report. It seems that by this really easy and painless means, the wart can be removed. The technic itself is very easy. One needs a sharp spoon, but not to remove the wart, rather to open the surface. One doesn't need to get to the root which would cause it to bleed. Because of this way it is painless. But it is necessary to have the medication go into the wart. With an eyedropper drop 1 drop of 30% H_2O_2 onto the opened surface and let it dry. After 2 or 3 days scrape off the dried layer and add another drop of H_2O_2. How many times depends on the size of the wart. For middle sized warts it'll take usually 4 to 5 applications. Larger ones will take longer. With Verrucae Planae Juveniles the most it will take is 2 applications to have it disappear without a trace. Of special importance is, that the Plantar Wart, which is otherwise hard to remove, can be treated successfully that way. The pain stops mostly after the 1st or 2nd application, so the patient shouldn't have any trouble walking.

After the application the patient will feel at most a prickly sensation, which will last a few minutes. After that it could itch, which also disappears after a short time.

So far we have treated 30 patients this way with good results. This treatment takes a little longer but is painless and not bloody.

It is important to realize that the wart will disappear without leaving any kind of residue. One will not be able to see where the wart was.

A try with Papillomata Acuminata failed completely it seems though, that after removing with Podophyllin the residue can be prevented by moistening the area with H_2O_2.

That it isn't a suggestive influence shows in a one-sided treatment. The untreated warts were not influenced. The treated ones disappeared.

Anyway we will be testing the worth of this method in the hope that corresponding to the existing experience it will prove itself.

Summary: A preliminary communication of a painless and not bloody treatment of warts with H_2O_2 (Hydrogen Peroxide).

Killing of blood-stage murine malaria parasites by hydrogen peroxide
Hazel M. Dockrell and John H.L. Playfair; Immunology Department, Middlesex Hospital Medical School, London W1P 9PG, England
Infection and Immunity, Jan. 1983. p. 456-459

"Both nonlethal Plasmodium yoelii and lethal Plasmodium berghei were killed in vitro by hydrogen peroxide at concentrations as low as 10^{-5} M. Higher concentrations were required in the presence of added normal erythrocytes. Injection of hydrogen peroxide in vivo significantly reduced P. yoelli parasitemia.... "

Influenzal pneumonia: The intravenous injection of hydrogen peroxide
T.H. Oliver: The Lancet, Feb. 21, 1920 p. 432

"In view of the possibility of a further outbreak of influenza accompanied by broncho-pneumonia, another method of combating the extreme toxaemia and anoxaemia appears to be worthy of record, more particularly so as the clinical importance of the latter has recently been discussed by Professor J.S. Haldane. It is noteworthy that in his paper he lays especial emphasis on the primary need of oxygen in solution in the blood."

Effects on Patients.
The first case was an Indian with broncho-pneumonia of influenzal origin and intensely toxaemic. He had been delirious for two days previously, and was selected as being the worst case in the ward and to all appearances moribund. Two ounces of a ten-volume solution of H_2O_2 were diluted with 8 ounces of normal saline... ....The change in the mental condition was remarkable, the patient, who previously had had to be tied in bed owing to delirium, was within six hours of the injection sitting up and asking for food; he slept well the next night and from that time improved in every way, eventually being invalided to India as a walking case three weeks later."

CONCLUSIONS: From our experience we conclude that-

1. H_2O_2 can be given intravenously without gas embolism being produced.
2. The anoxaemia is often markedly benefited.
3. The toxaemia appears to be overcome in many cases.
4. The mortality (48 per cent) compares very favorably with the 80 per cent in similar cases not so treated, and more so when it is remembered that we only treated the most severe and apparently hopeless.

REFERENCES ON HYDROGEN PEROXIDE

Removal of cholesterol and other lipids from experimental animals and human atheromatous arteries by dilute hydrogen peroxide
James W. Finney, M.A., Bruce E. Jay, B.S., George J. Race, M.D., Harold C. Urschel, M.D., John T. Mallams, M.D., and George A. Balla, M.D., F.I.C.A.
From the Charles A. Sammons Research Division, Baylor University Medical Center, Dallas, Texas. Work supported in part by A.C.S. Grant No. T-284A, The Moody Foundation, Dallas Heart Fund, U.S.P.H.S. Grants No. CA 07127-02 and CA 07127-02S1, and USPHS Grant No. DE 21.

"From these studies the following points have been made: hydrogen peroxide is broken down very rapidly when introduced into the blood stream in both rabbits and humans; in dilute solutions, intravascular hydrogen peroxide has no unacceptable deleterious effect on formed blood elements, and the breakdown of hydrogen peroxide by biological fluids results in the supersaturation of these fluids with oxygen. The magnitude of the supersaturation is equivalent to several atmospheres of oxygen."

Catalase as a protective shield: Guest Author: Peter A. Ward, M.D. is Professor and Chairman of the Department of Pathology and Interim Dean of the University of Michigan School of Medicine. Dr. Ward has published many key papers in the field of immunology and has achieved international eminence as a leading authority in the field of complement research.

...."acute respiratory distress syndrome ("shock lung"), or ARDS, is an ideal candidate for treatment with catalase..."

"This article presents a novel and intriguing approach to treating certain important inflammatory disorders such as arthritis, shocklung, systemic lupus erythematosus, glomerulonephiritis, and myocardial infraction. It is based on the observation that polymorphonuclear (PMN) leukocytes, which are prominent cells in the inflammatory reactions, flood the tissues with hydrogen peroxide (H_2O_2). Whereas, hydrogen peroxide is beneficial when it kills bacteria ingested by the PMN leukocytes, it is harmful when it kills normal cells in the lungs, kidneys, joints, or heart. Since hydrogen peroxide can be inactivated by catalase (which converts it to harmless water and oxygen) catalase has been tested experimentally to prevent inflammatory reactions of the lung and heart and the results have been favorable.

TABLE 2

Human Pathological Conditions That May Be Amenable To Treatment with Catalase

1. Immune complex diseases (systematic lupus erythematosus, immune complex vasculitis, or glomerulonephritis. Goodpasture's disease involving kidney and/or lung, cold and warm autoimmune hemolytic anemias).
2. Rheumatoid arthritis.
3. Acute respiratory distress syndrome ("shock lung").

Hydrogen peroxide mediated killing of bacteria: Dennis P. Clifford and John E. Repine: Webb-Waring Lung Institute and the Pulmonary Divisions of the Departments of Medicine and Pediatrics, University of Colorado Health Sciences Center, 4200 East Ninth Avenue, Denver, Co. 80262. Molecular and Cellular Biochemistry 49, 143-149(1982)

"Polymorphonuclear leukocytes (PMN) or neutrophils have multiple systems available for killing ingested bacteria. Nearly each of these incorporates H_2O_2 indicating the essential nature of this reactive oxygen intermediate for microbicidal activity. ..."These mechanisms appear important since deficiencies of H_2O_2 production, myeloperoxidase or lactoferrin frequently increases their owner's susceptibility to infection."

Generation of H_2O_2 in biomembranes: T. Ramasarma: Biochimica et Biophysica Acta, 694 (1982) 69-93 Elsevier Biomedical Press; Department of Biochemistry Indian Institute of Science, Bangalore 560 012 (India)

"Knowlege of the generation of H_2O_2 in cellular oxidations has existed for many years. It has been assumed that H_2O_2 is toxic to cells and the presence of catalase is indicative of a detoxication mechanism. Other radicals of oxygen were recently recognized to be more potent destructive agents of biological material than H_2O_2 in some cellular oxidation processes leading to several important metabolites. Thus, the generation of H_2O_2 in cellular processes seems to be purposeful and H_2O_2 can not be dismissed as a mere undesirable byproduct. ....The capacity for generation of H_2O_2 is now found to be widespread in a variety of organisms and in the organelles of the cells."

Peroxide enemas in obstipation: (Correspondence published in the South Africa Medical Journal) SA Mediese Tydskrif Deel 63 8 Januarie 1983

"To the Editor: A patient with longstanding absolute constipation was recently referred to our District Sister for manual removal of faeces. This practice is unpleasant for both nurse and patient, besides being unnecessary Since it does not seem to be widely known, I wish to mention my method of disimpaction using a peroxide enema.

A solution is made of 30 ml hydrogen peroxide with 600 ml cool tap water and a funnel and catheter are used to run this solution through the anus by gravity only. The solution of peroxide bubbles on contact with the faeces and fragments it. The loose detritus is washed out and gradually the entire mass breaks down.

This procedure should be performed with the patient on a bedpan and the surroundings well protected, because the plug of inspissated faeces usually holds back a large amount of liquid faeces and when it is dissolved the liquid floods out.

This method was originally devised to treat elderly patients with obstipation who had undergone cataract operation and in whom straining at stool could have had tragic results. In particularly obstinate cases the strength of the solution may be slightly increased, bearing in mind the sensitivity of the rectal mucosa. J.H. Marks (Heideveld Day Hospital-Heideveld Cape Town)

Iowa Conference on Hydrogen Peroxide
Week of September 12, 1983
Winifred Wirth
Cincinnati, Ohio

Recently Iowa considered the effects of H_2O_2 on immature animals not bearing the Ehrlich carcinoma. Mice used were Swiss from the King Laboratories... At 5 weeks of age animals normally weigh 25 grams, and at 7-8 weeks of age, 32 grams. Administration of H_2O_2 began at the 5-weeks age and continued thereafter.... Beneficial effects include growth to a much larger size and an almost doubled life span. The implication for humans is indeed exciting.

Normal cells produce their own H_2O_2....

In retrospect, the cancer problem is perhaps a minor aspect of the H_2O_2 investigation. Heart disease, arthritis, ageing, etc. should perhaps take priority, since the control of these greatly affects the usual "cancer age."

The sad, but obvious truths, as experienced with the advent of Penicillin, even if H_2O_2 is eventually the answer to the cancer problem and the above-mentioned degenerative diseases, are these facts substantiating the one-way street aspect of H_2O_2--

(1) It is impossible to get a patent on it.

(2) It would be opposted by drug and pharmaceutical companies who are essentially commercial ventures.

(3) Physicians would ban together in opposition to its use--it is simply too inexpensive and available.

The Effects of Hydrogen Peroxide on the Ehrlich Carcinoma in Laboratory Mice: St. Thomas Institute, Cincinnati, Ohio; Nov. 15, 1982

In 4 out of 8 experiments involving 197 mice, and to a lesser extent in a fifth experiment, the oral administration of hydrogen peroxide in a fifth experiment, the oral administration of hydrogen peroxide by stomach tube, or perhaps better in the drinking water, was effective in the treatment of mice bearing the Ehrlich carcinoma as judged by mortality and delay in palpable tumor incidence.

Oxygen Intermediates are Required for Interferon Activation of NK Cells
Helfand, Stephen L: Journal of Interferon Research Vo. 3, Number 2, 1983, pp. 143-151

...The results suggest then that IFN may stimulate the production of low amounts of H_2O_2 and possibly other oxygen intermediates (OH) which are a necessary event early in the pathway of IFN activation of human NK cells.

...We present evidence here which is compatible with the suggestion that H_2O_2 and possibly other oxygen intermediates, may also play a role in the IFN-mediated augmentation of cytolytic function in another effector cell type, the human natural killer (NK) cell.

...These results raise the possibility that the chemiluminescence response generated by IFN may be due to the liberation of H_2O_2, OH, and possibly other oxygen intermediates.

Knighton, et al, Oxygen for Prevention of Wound Infection
Arch Surg. 119:199-204, 1984

....Animal studies from UCSF have demonstrated enhancement of host defenses in the prevention of wound infection involving certain bacteria. Knighton, et al, liken prophylactic use of increased inhaled oxygen to the use of prophylactic antibiotics.

The use of oxygen to enhance host defenses in the prevention of wound infection at the time of surgery may be a preventive as well as treatment modality in the near future, if animal studies are borne out in humans. Oxygen therapy appears to be as effective as antibiotic prophylaxis.

General Biochemistry
Fruton & Simmonds: Published by Wiley & Sons, New York
P 338-339

It will have been noted that in the direct oxidation of a reduced flavin by O_2 one of the products is H_2O_2. This property of flavins assumed some interest when it was discovered that Penicillium notatum contained a yellow protein (notatin) which, in the presence of D-glucose, appeared to be an antibacterial agent. The subsequent identification of notatin and glucose oxidase explained the mode of antibacterial action, since the oxidation of glucose by O_2 in the presence of notatin results in the formation of bactericidal amounts of H_2O_2. ...Other flavoproteins (e.g., xanthine oxidase) that catalyze the formation of H_2O_2 have also been shown to act as antibacterial agents.

SPECIAL TREATMENT GIVES HOPE FOR THOSE WITH CANCER AND MULTIPLE SCLEROSIS.

Could Oxygen be a New Wonder Cure?
by Karen Davis: Women's World. (The Woman's Weekly) July 31, 1984
177 North Dean Street, P.O. Box 6700, Englewood, N.J. 07631

In South Africa studies have shown that oxygen may help fight cancer. Tumor cells that are low in oxygen can survive radiation treatment. Placing cancer patients in pressurized chambers is thought to force more oxygen into tumor cells and help radiation destroy cancer....

The hottest debate concerns multiple sclerosis. A study reported that 12 of 17 patients receiving oxygen therapy showed objective improvement of symptoms.

....some MS patients who get HBO therapy at private clinics insist it helps them. ...Oxygen therapy is now being taken much more seriously. It is being tested for use in preventing paralysis in head and spinal injuries, in speeding bone healing and in treating colitis, meningitis, sickle-cell anemia and pelvic inflammatory disease. And specialists are backing up all claims with sound research. "The medical community will then be more willing to accept HBO, and it will become available to patients everywhere," says Dr. Davis.

Book: Stroud's Digest on the Diseases of Birds
L.G. Marcus & R. Stroud - 1943
Minneapolis, Minn.

Robert Stroud used sodium perborate and hydrogen peroxide to cure birds. (sodium perborate in water gives you hydrogen peroxide)

The book is an alphabetically arranged compendium consisting of a complete report of the researches of the author and a digest of the extant knowledge of this subject, written from the point of view of the practical canary breeder.

Bacteria May Help Prevent Infections
Associated Press May 29, 1984
Minneapolis Star and Tribune

Doctors can ward off serious infections in newborns by giving them harmless bacteria that compete against dangerous microbes, according to a Columbia University researcher.

Dr. Katherine Sprunt said Monday that she had used bacteria normally found in the throat to establish a healthy balance between microbes and prevent the runaway growth of harmful bacteria.

Inside the body there is a kind of microscopic botanical garden where growths helpful and harmful compete for a niche in which to live.

Our natural bacterial flora appear to be good for us, said Sprunt. Disturbing the status quo is potentially bad for us, and key constituents of our flora can be used to help us.

She described the procedure at the annual meeting of the American Association for the Advancement of Science.

If all goes well babies will develop this beneficial internal mix of bacteria within the first week of life. And in the throat, one form predominates -a harmless microbe called alphahemolytic streptococci.

The problem occurs when something else gets a head start and becomes the most common bacteria, spreading throughout the body and causing serious infections, such as meningitis or pneumonia.

This abnormal colonization - as doctors call it - seems to occur in about 8 percent of newborns who spend their first days in intensive care units. But it is more common in babies whose natural bacteria have been thrown out of kilter by antibiotics. Half of these youngsters are at risk of developing serious infections.

In an effort to head off the problem, doctors gave 44 babies a single dose of a form of alpha-hemolytic streptococci, called strain 215, that was taken from a normal youngster. The bacteria grew and became the dominant variety in the throats of 31 infants, and none developed serious infections.

Several of the treatment failures apparently occurred because the babies were taking antibiotics. When these were eliminated from the final statistics, the good bacteria versus bad bacteria strategy worked 89 percent of the time.

Once the transplanted bacterium took root, it was able to withstand onslaughts of penicillin and seemed to last indefinitely.

Just how the good bacteria squeeze out the bad ones is not clear, although some speculate that they may release a germ-killing chemical, such as hydrogen peroxide.

EDITOR'S NOTE: TWO OTHER WAYS IN WHICH TO ENHANCE THE IMMUNE SYSTEM

HYPERBARIC OXYGEN AND OZONE

(See following pages)

WHAT IS OZONE?

Ozone is an oxygen compound which also occurs in nature. Approximate 30 kilometers above the earth's surface, a layer of ozone is found, called the oxonosphere; it guarantees that the damaging parts of high-energy UV (ultraviolet radiation coming from the sun are filtered out before they reach us.

Many countries around the world use ozone in their water purification system, i.e., Russia, Belgium, German, France.

Editor's Note: The following information on medical ozone has little in common with the above information.

OZONE THERAPY

In addition to its ability to kill viruses, ozone is able to kill bacterial and fungi or yeasts. In selected patients with the Candida albicans syndrome, it can be useful both in aiding the iradication of the yeast but also in enhancing one's immune system.

It appears that ozone therapy holds much promise as an adjunctive therapy for a variety of illnesses. Applications of medical ozone available are as follows: Intraarterial application, Intestinal insufflation, Intramuscular application, major and minor autohemotherapy, ozonized water, Intraarticular injection, External application.

Health professionals administering ozone therapy in the United States.

West Coast

Dr. Eddie Barr, M.D.
930 Town and Country Village
San Jose, California 95128
(408) 247-7521

East Coast

Dr. M.J. Packovich, M.D.
Karin W. Kovalicky, R.N.
Medical Nutrition Center
585 Winters Avenue
Paramus, New Jersey 07652
(201) 967-5081

For names and addresses of other practitioners in the United States using ozone please contact the U.S. Representative Terrance McGrath, c/o Medizone Suite 3R, 240 Central Park South, New York, New York 10019 (212) 977-8951 or 977-8952.

This therapy has been given approval for scientific research by the FDA 1985.

Some of the pioneering researchers in the medical field using ozone include:

Dr. Joachim Varro, M.D. (surgeon) Dusseldorf, Germany
Dr. Josef Issels, M.D., Director of Issels Cancer Clinic,
Bad Wiessee, Germany
Dr. Ottokar F.V. Rokitansky, M.D.
Austrian Medical Assn. for Ozone Therapy
Vienna, Austria

Dr. Joachim Varro, M.D.
Fr. Richard Willhelm,
and Editor in Naples, Florida
1986

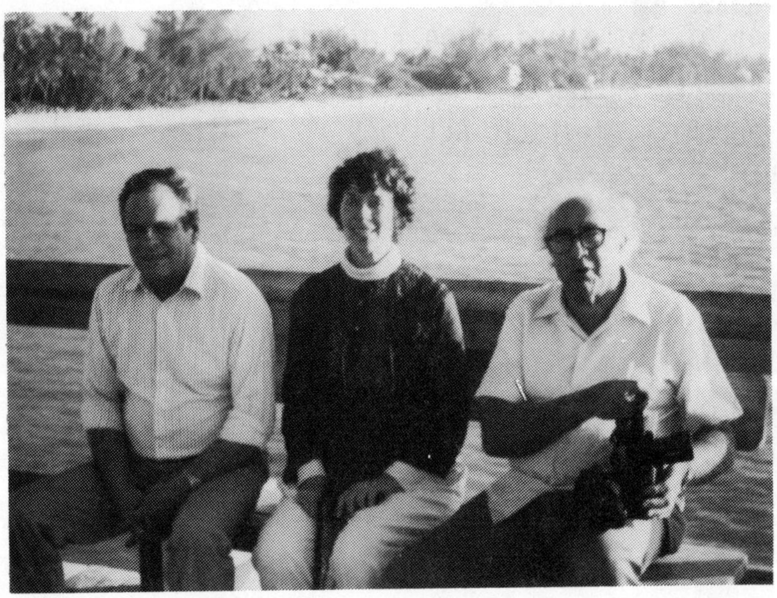

OZONE IN THE DENTAL PRACTICE
A lecture by Dr. Fritz Kramer, DDS, M.D.
Nurmeberg, Germany

It is possible to use ozone with excellent success in the dental practice just as in the medical practice.

The reasons are:

1. Ozone is a powerful disinfectant
2. Ozone has a hemostatic effect, particularly in the case of oozing hemorrhages.
3. Ozone has a good cleansing effect, this being of great advantage when cleaning out wounds in soft and bone tissue
4. Ozone improves the local supply of oxygen to the wound thus causing an improvement in the healing of the parts affected, and
5. Ozone locally increases tissue temperature in the area of the wound, which markedly improves metabolic processes.

Now with the development of the Hydrozotom machine, dentists are offered reliable, functional equipment which makes ozone therapy a practical reality.

THERAPY WITH OZONIZED WATER

Rinsing or bathing of the oral cavity with ozonized water is indicated in the following condition:

gingivitis
parodontosis
thrush (oral monoliosis)
stomatitis

THE MECHANISMS OF HYPERBARIC OXYGEN
AND INDICATIONS FOR ITS USE 1983
by Richard A. Neubauer, M.D.
(Hyperbaric Physician)

Endocrine Effects:
1. Stimulation of thymus and adrenal glands

Alteration of Immune mechanisms
Bactericidal and Bacteriostatic Activity
- Anaeorobic
- Aerobic
- Bacteriodes

Anti-fungal Effect
1. Mucormycosis
2. Actinomycosis

Ocean Medical Center
4001 Ocean Drive
Lauderdale-by the Sea, Fla. 33308
Tel: (305) 776-5800

Laser Beam

Dynatronics, Inc.
Mr. Denny Rippy,
Vice President
270 W. Crossroads Square
Salt Lake City, Utah 84115
(800) 874-6251

Dynatron 11-20 (Laser)
Price: $4875.00 + $20.00 shipping

Double Blind Studies done in the following areas: Canker Sores (all infections of the mouth respond); Wound Healing; Pain Control Studies; Rheumotoid Arthritis; Sensory Nerve Conduction

This laser is in the final stages of approval by the FDA for individually trained medical practitioners

EDITOR'S NOTE: It has been reported that laser stimulates the immune system, which would in turn be beneficial to the Candida patient.

X

THE USE OF HYDROGEN PEROXIDE IN DENTISTRY FOR GUM DISEASE

VIEWPOINT - KEYES TECHNIQUE (ADA News) December 14, 1981 (Excerpts)

My personal experiences in dentistry have been as a researcher, an academician with primary responsibility for teaching periodontial to dental students at the University of North Carolina, and as a periodontist in fulltime private practice for the past 17 years.

Unlike Dr. Gottsegen and his colleagues, my observations of the Keyes programs and techniques are based on considerable personal experience with and direct clinical application of the Keyes' treatment regimes....

Certainly, there are no radical nor unproved procedures in the total Keyes' treatment regimes, no therapies that put patients at risk. The worst that could happen under Dr. Keyes' conservative treatment programs would be that this treatment might not be fully effective. I have found it is, though, and only then decided to comment....

According to the most recently published epidemiologic studies, periodontal disease in the US is rampant and of epidemic proportions, despite the establishment-promoted and accepted surgical therapies and treatment prevalent today.... Periodontia's therapeutic failures are due to several factors:

- surgery simply is not a very rational approach to the treatment of infectious disease;
- surgery is rapidly becoming a treatment modality that only a minority of the citizenry can afford;
- the pain accompanying and occurring as a consequency of periodontal surgery generates a groundswell of patient agonizing and complaining that is contagious, attention-getting....and that frightens millions of periodontal patients who need treatment away from the periodontist's office and into the oral surgeon's office.
- surgery is an ineffective way to destroy bacteria and their byproducts, which are the primary and initiating causes of periodontal pathology....

I have used the Keyes' programs for more than a year on 350 to 400 patients. I can honestly report better treatment results than I have experienced in 25 previous years of periodontal practice when I used all of the sophisticated periodontal surgery modalities available to the profession.

Every dentist or periodontist I know that has fairly and objectively tried Dr. Keyes' nonsurgical, conservative treatment programs seems to agree with my own enthusiastic commentary, which fairly shouts..."It really does work-magnificently!"

The only negative factor that I have been able to observe in the Keyes' programs is that these programs are far less income-producing than their surgical counterparts. But the benefits accruing to the patient from Keyes'...therapies are overwhelmingly beneficial. If success in treatment is personally rewarding to the therapist, then there are great compensations.

Paul M. Cummings, Jr., DDS, MSD
Wilmington, North Carolina

USA-TODAY
HEALTH- Karen S. Peterson
JULY 19, 1984 -Gum Disease: Experts Disagree on Best Treatment

When Dr. Jerry Gardner's gums were swollen, he was referred to a specialist-a periodontist, who treats diseases of tissues and bones supporting the teeth.

I was told I'd need all my upper teeth pulled, say Gardner, a gastroenterologist with the National Institutes of Health in Bethesda, Maryland. So I tried Dr. Paul Keyes. That was six years ago and so far I haven't lost a tooth. And that's with no surgery.

Treatment of gum disease is one of the hottest controversies in dentistry. At the center is Dr. Paul Keyes, a former laboratory investigator with the National Institute of Dental Research for 27 years, who plans to publish a six-year study this fall in the Journal of the American Dental Association.

About 32 million Americans suffer from gum disease, an infection that over a period of years attacks tissues holding the teeth. Gums commonly bleed, swell and cause bad breath. In 10 percent to 15 percent of cases, damage can be severe, eventually causing tooth loss.

There is no known cure. Some periodontists use surgery to pare down the pockets of infection and expose the bacteria to treatment. But even after surgery, the disease can recur.

Keyes believes his technique can save patients from oral surgery. Critics call his method simplistic and unscientific.

...one study is under way specifically testing Keyes' entire treatment. By December, the Department of Periodontics at the University of Minnesota, Minneapolis, will publish the results of its three year, 300-patient study.

With the Keyes method, infectious bacteria from the patient's mouth are first diagnosed with a special microscope.

Then the teeth are deep-cleaned above and below the gums to remove bacteria. Tender gums are irrigated with a bacteria-killing solution.

Next come the instructions that raise the hackles of periodontists. Patients are taught to rub a mixture, usually of baking soda and hydrogen peroxide, into their gums. That is followed by drenching the gums in a salt solution.

...Delores Dinapoli of Westchester County, N.Y., went to a Keyes advocate, Dr. Daniel Zonan. Two years ago I went to a butcher who cut up one-fourth of my mouth. I looked like a chipmunk. Another periodontist suggested still more surgery, but I couldn't face it. After treatment with Dr. Zonan, my gums don't bleed or taste of pus. I have no pain or swelling.

Keyes' technique is less expensive for the patient, less traumatic, less painful and stressful, says Dr. Paul Cummings of Wilmington, North Carolina. Cummings has taught gum surgery. Now he is a convert to Keyes' method. "We have had at least some success with 98 percent of about 1,500 patients using the Keyes approach."

SPARE THE SCALPEL
AND SAVE THE
GUMS

By Judith Randal
Sunday, January 21, 1979
THE WASHINGTON POST

....Using an instrument called a periodontal probe, he had found that deep pockets had formed near almost every tooth. In these enlarged spaces at the gum margins, the toxins of chronic infection had already undermined the support of several teeth.

Extensive surgery was advised to remove or shave down these pockets so that I could do a more effective job of home care. I was told to have one already wobbly tooth extracted, to get my gums and the rest of of my teeth into the best shape possible, and to return for the surgery in about a year. It would take six months to complete and would cost $2,500 or more....

There matters might have rested had I not done some reading suggesting that there is no conclusive evidence that people who have gum surgery, even repeatedly, keep their teeth any longer than people who do not. From a call to the National Institute of Dental Research (a part of the National Institutes of Health), I learned of an experimental alternative program there and, after obtaining a referral from a physician friend, became a patient of the NIDR's Dr. Paul H. Keyes.

Keyes is perhaps best known in dental circles for animal experiments he performed with Dr. Robert Fitzgerald demonstrating conclusively what had long been suspected but never proved: that bacteria cause tooth decay. He also deals with periodontal disease as fundamentally a problem of infection. For this reason his office is equipped with a $2,000 instrument few other dental offices have-a microscope linked to a camera and small television screen that fit neatly on a countertop.

As he took sample scraping from my mouth and displayed them for me on the screen, hundreds of thousands of rod-shaped and corkscrew-shaped bacteria danced before my eyes like nothing so much as a blazing brushfire, while more slowly moving pus cells ominously reminded me that pyorrhea means "discharge of pus." With the microscope Keyes can tell at once - and so can the patient - whether the scaling he does and the self-care he prescribes are having the desired effect of extinguishing these fires. Without it, both patient and dentist would be in the dark.

Keys showed me how to wet baking soda with just enough hydrogen peroxide to make it into a paste and how to massage it into my gums first with a toothpick placed in a special holder (or with a rubber tip) and then with an electric toothbrush. I was to do this once a day on both sides of my gums.

For many patients this, followed by use of a Water Pik, empties the germs from those bacterial pockets for as long as the patient sticks to the routine, or at least reduces the germs to the point where the destruction does not progress. Keys chose baking soda and hydrogen peroxide for the job not only because they are harmless and inexpensive, but also because baking soda shrivels the germs and hydrogen peroxide introduces oxygen into the mouth. The more oxygen there is in their environment, the less likely these bacteria are to survive.

More often than not, the payoff from this treatment is gratifyingly fast. Generally, it is only a few weeks before bad breath disappears, gums no longer bleed when probed, and loose teeth begin to tighten up. However, the microscope may disclose persistent underlying infection, and this calls for the introduction of a strong table salt solution-epsom salts if the patient has high blood pressure and must avoid sodium-into the Water Pik.

....Of the 75 or so people with severe gum disease treated by the NIDR in the last three years, some had sought to avoid surgery and others had had it at least once, only to have it fail. Most whose mouths were not already in hopeless condition have retained all or nearly all their teeth.

Much the same has been true of the patients of the few other dentists who have invested in a microscope like Keyes and tried his techniques. One of these continues to do gum surgery, but much more sparingly than before. His billing for such surgery dropped from $30,000 in 1974 to just $800 last year, and even those patients on whom he operates are taught the NIDR regimen.

....only about 2,500 of the nation's dentists have had the advanced training in gum surgery that qualifies them as periodontists, whereas an estimated 32 million Americans have pyorrhea so severe that they are in imminent danger of losing their teeth. The sheer arithmetic of the situation-a caseload of over 12,000 patients per periodontists-speaks loudly for an alternative approach that professionals with less training can administer and supervise.

Fewer than half those 32 million are thought to be actually under treatment now and, according to current estimates, 90 million more Americans have gum disease in its earlier stages, which has also been shown to be responsive to the Keyes regimen.

Note: Dr. Keyes has retired from the National Instutites of Health and heads his own research foundation, "International Dental Health Foundation" 11800 Sunrise Valley Dr. Suite 832, Reston, Virginia 22091 (703) 476-6110

The reader may call or write to Dr. Keyes for a dentist who practices his concepts.

EFFECT OF HYDROGEN PEROXIDE ON DEVELOPING PLAQUE AND GINGIVITIS IN MAN
Journal of Clinical Periodontology: 1979:6: 115-130
Jan Wennstrom and Jan Lindhe
Department of Periodontology, Faculty of Odontology,
University of Gothenburg, Gothenburg, Sweden

"The results demonstrated that a mouthwash which released hydrogen peroxide effectively prevented the colonization of filaments, fusiforms, motile and curved rods as well as spirochetes in developing plaque. The mouthwash which was used as the only oral hygiene measure during a 2-week period furthermore markedly reduced the amount of plaque formed and significantly retarded gingivitis development. It is suggested that H_2O_2 released by mouthwashes during rinsing may prevent or retard the colonization and multiplication of anaerobic bacteria."

DENTAL RECORD Sept. 1886

The Archives of Dentistry

"Hints of the Use of Peroxide of Hydrogen" is the subject of an editorial article. Perhaps the most valuable use of it is in purifying the roots of teeth in which the pulps have died and decomposed. To illustrate, we will give our experience with two central incisors in the same mouth. The two teeth had been filled at quite an early age, perhaps fifteen years, the patient, a lady, being about twenty-five when we filled the teeth.

Applied the rubber dam, removed all the decay without reaching the pulp chamber, the teeth being void of sensibility and having that peculiar appearance belonging to a tooth having a dead pulp; proceeded excavating, until the pulp chamber was penetrated, found the chamber filled with a soft, offensive mass. Applied on cotton, peroxide of hydrogen, after removing all the putrid mass that we could with a broach; continued to apply H_2O_2 until there ceased to be any bubbles, applied iodoform, dried the cavity, filled the canals with gutta-percha and the tooth with gold. That was in September, 1884. The tooth has given no trouble since.

On the following day treated the other incisor, but found the pulp canal filled with pus when opened. The same happy result followed as in the case of its fellow of the opposite side.

Since that time have pursued the same practice in a number of similar cases. Deem it good practice to wipe out all cavities with H_2O_2 just previous to filling.

A simple test is to take a few drops in the mouth; it will form bubbles if it is good. ....the dentist should always procure it in the original bottle, and in hot weather keep it in a dark, cool place, well corked."

SALT, SODA & HYDROGEN PEROXIDE.... (Excerpts)

...IS IT ENOUGH?

Florida Dental Journal Summer, 1981/Vol. 52, No.2: Paul H. Keyes, D.D.S.

The merits of monitored and modulated therapy (MMT) in the management of the bacterial complexes associated with destructive periodontitis can be attained only by the systematic exclusion of alternative hypotheses. The value of MMT cannot be assessed from descriptions of it in the lay press nor by biased discussions in professional journals.

Almost all members of the dental profession have been working with the hypothesis that odontolysis (dental caries) and destructive periodontitis are not the consequences of transmissible or infectious bacterial diseases. Obviously with this postulation clinicians need not employ therapies directed toward specific bacterial targets. I hasten to add, if this hypothesis be correct, the biological and ecological conditions in the oral cavity would be unique in all of nature; and the relationship of bacteria to oral disease would be different from all of the findings of Pasteur, Koch and other microbiologists who have studied the relationships of bacteria to disease in other parts of the body.

If physicians who treat bacterial infections need to use a rationale that embraces: 1) the identification of bacterial targets, 2) the application of drugs having the potential to inactivate identified pathogens, and 3) the appropriate tests to determine if the microbial factors have been eliminated in addition to abatement of clinical symptoms; then why do so many dentists feel they can take bacterial control for granted? Something must be amiss for so many patients to experience progressive deterioration of their dentitions despite their best efforts and those of clinicians!

...Between 1910 and 1941, the dental profession should have listened to one of the pioneers in periodontics, Thomas B. Hartzell, Many times during this interval Hartzell tried to tell his colleagues (periodontists in particular) that if bacteria did not colonize tooth surfaces and invade the teeth themselves or the crevices surrounding them, we would not have carious lesions and destructive periodontitis. He also tried to tell them how to combat the consequences of "germ life on teeth".

For 20 years there has been mounting evidence that only specific microorganisms have a high odontopathic and periodontopathic potential. On the basis of these findings we should proceed with the conservative view that we are dealing with: 1) specific bacteriopathogens, 2) transmission of pathogens from person to person, and 3) the possibility of diagnosing, treating and monitoring specific microorganisms or microbiological complexes. From microscopic examinations of bacterial aggregations removed from healthy subjects and persons with creviculoradicular infections we have found five differences between the specimens in 1) types of microorganisms, 2) number (ipso facto), 3) cellular organizations, 4) dynamic behavior, and 5) pyogenic potential, (J. Dent. Res. 59(a):387, 1980).

These findings are consistent with many of Hartzell's observations and consequently our therapeutic program follows his recommendations of: 1) education of patients in the role bacteria play as cofactors in pathogenesis of periodontal lesions, 2) careful professional debridement of radicular surfaces with antiseptics, and 3) training of patients in the use of antibacterial home-care procedures. We use various agents as adjuvants...... hydrogen peroxide...water irrigators...toothbrushes...

Obviously this program cannot be handled without monitored and modulated therapy (MMT). ....If a patient is not in good control, i.e., has high counts of white blood cells and bacteria not found in healthy subjects, we adjust, modify or modulate the therapy to bring the best control possible.

It is my personal conviction, and also that of a growing number of general dentists and periodontists who are now using MMT, that success in the management of dentobacterial disease is enhanced by reducing uncertainty about the level of bacterial control patients attain from the various therapeutic measures employed.

It should be obvious that therapeutic programs can vary widely. There are no panaceas. And every measure has its limitations! Microscopic evaluations help to disclose those limitations. As matters now stand, both clinicians and patients may go through motions with good intentions. But neither really know whether he has been successful until after an interval of several years, there has been no gross clinical evidence of progressive disease. Furthermore, when clinical evidence of deterioration becomes apparent, what are we going to offer the patient? More of the same? I for one am saying, "No!" And so are many colleagues who do not believe that clinical appearances are satisfactory indicators of microbiological conditions. From my perspective, clinicians who treat creviculoradicular infections without MMT are open to criticism. If adequate microbiological control cannot be attained after use of appropriate therapeutic alternatives, the clinician and patient should know it early in the treatment program. Then both, knowing that no reasonable effort was spared to control the bacterial problem, can accept the outcome with equanimity."

XI

NUTRITIONAL COUNSELING FOR CANDIDA, RECIPES & FOOD IRRADIATION

Dr. Bruce Pacetti, D.D.S. - Cytotoxic Food Tests and Balanced Body Chemistry
c/o Dr. Ed. Bonomo, D.D.S.
2301 Rama Road
Charlotte, No. Carolina
(704) 535-2833

After twelve years of practicing reconstructive dentistry, personal health challenges led him to nutrition. He studied with Melvin Page, D.D.S., researching Dr. Page's unique approach to body chemistry evaluation and its relation to oral disease. Dr. Pacetti also began studying the research of Drs. Weston A. Price and Francis M. Pottenger, Jr. and became a board member of the Price-Pottenger Nutrition Foundation.

Pacetti has specialized in body chemistry analysis, TMJ/cranial work and nutrition. He lectures extensively around the world on the Cody chemistry principles and the Price-Pottenger materials.

Dr. Pacetti has lately devoted his energies to reinterpreting cytotoxic test results for the most effective utilization of these valuable clinical evaluations. Some of the most exciting results are now being seen in the correlation of the cytotoxic food sensitivity test, the phagoutic index test, the comprehensive stool test and T & B lymphocyte activity.

Dr. Helyn Luechauer, D.D.S. - Balancing Body Chemistry
3169 Barbara Court — Nutrition
Los Angeles, California
(213) 876-6440

Esther Thaler, C.M.T. - Nutrition Counselor
c/o Int'l Health Institute — Live Cellular Analysis
(Under D. Wm. Kelly, D.D.S.)
1901 Avenue of the Stars-Suite 1774
Los Angeles, California 90067
(213) 552 2677

Suzanne Peoples, M.D. - Candida
c/o Life Care Center, Inc. — Acupuncture
76 E. McNab Road — Chelation Therapy
Pompano Beach, Florida 33060 — Food Allergy Program
(305) 786-0370 — Nutritional Counseling
Orthomolecular Counseling
SOMA Neuro-Muscular Integration

S. S. Bursuk, N.D. - Bionutritional Analysis of Blood Chemistry
(Consulting Health Educator to dentists, physicians, etc.)
56 Woodmont Road
Melville, New York 11747
(516) 491 0550

Protocols for kinesiological & vertebral adjustments & protocols for verifying which organs & glands are in dysfunction
Optimum Nutritional Intake
Supplementation with vitamins, minerals, herbs, enzymes
Importance and role of exercise

FOOD IRRADIATION AND CANDIDA

"By the end of this decade, if all goes according to plan, nearly half the food Americans eat will have been treated with doses of ionizing radiation, the deadly by-product of nuclear reactors. Since early 1984 the Food and Drug Administration has been working - quietly, with little public input and virtually no organized opposition - to approve guidelines that would allow food distributors to irradiate foods. The regulations would allow for the exposure to radiation of foodstuffs ranging from lettuce and tomatoes to beef, liver, seafood and grain, beginning as soon as September 1985.

To this day, both the Pentagon and the DOE refuse to release the results of their research into long and short-term effects of eating irradiated food. As the product of a military research program, they say, such information is classified in the interest of national security.

....According to Dr. John Gofman, the author of a respected book on radiation and human health, efforts to reliably determine the long-term safety of irradiated foods would require a survey of some 200,000 people administered over a period of 50 or more years.

However, one indication of the problems irradiated food may cause was provided by the results of AID research conducted in southern India in the 1970's. The study, published in the February 1975 American Journal of Clinical Nutrition reported that irradiated food may be linked to leukemia, or blood cancer. In the study, all ten children fed irradiated food developed blood abnormalities associated with leukemia. A control group fed non-irradiated food showed no such abnormalities.

Gofman's is not the only voice expressing concern about the possible health effects of food irradiation. In a 1984 report on 12 sets of experiments involving irradiated chicken meat, the U.S. Department of Agriculture warned that two of the department's studies "had some possible adverse findings which will require careful consideration before the process can be declared safe." Mice that had eaten the irradiated chicken meat in one study showed an increase in testicular tumors, cancer and kidney disease. Another study found a radiation-related increase in deaths among the offspring of flies fed the chicken.

The Environmental Protection Agency, also in a 1984 report, stated that "irradiation of grains and vegetables stimulated the production of toxins some 1,000 times more deadly than EDBs." (EDB, Ethylene DiBromide, was widely used as a pesticide until it was linked to cancer and banned from use last year.)

Critics of the process say the gamma rays destroy some of the nutritional value of foods by breaking down vitamins A,C,E and especially B. But more frightening they say, are the possible by-products of irradiation and the potential impacts on microorganism that feed on the irradiated food.

"When radiation hits food," explained Jeff Reinhart, a biochemist who is a co-founder of the Coalition to Stop Food Irradiation, "molecules are changed, and vitamins are changed. Some of the by-products that are produced are highly toxic."

Bay Guardian
Feb. 27th 1985

Jeff Reinhart sums up the irradiation of food with the "3 Ds", Depletion, De-activation, and Destruction of nutrients!

The irradiation of foods will stress the immune system further, adding to the total body load of toxic chemicals.

Just how much will it harm our foods? According to Reinhart it will vary. In other words, it will depend on the type of food, how much it is irradiated and for how long. There are variables involved.

The irradiation of food will increase the inflammatory reaction which has already been amplified by Candida. In other words, one will become more ill after ingesting irradiated food.

"The only way to ensure that the food you buy has never been irridated will be to choose your products with care. Irradiation prevents vegetables from sprouting: any vegetable that has visible signs of life will be free of nuclear contamination. However, a potato that sits on a shelf for two weeks without so much as sprouting an eye has probably been irradiated, biochemist Jeff Reinhart told the Bay Guardian. Lettuce that doesn't wilt, bananas that don't turn brown and bread that never turns moldy all may be exhibiting signs of food irradiation.

Reinhart says, perhaps the safest way to avoid irradiated food is to shop at farmers' markets-where the produce comes direct from the farm - and at stores that sell only organic food."

Bay Guardian
Feb. 27th, 1985

It would take about 10 generations of rats and approximately 20 months total to equate the effect of irradiation of food on these rodents to the human. Yet, this simple test has not been done. I ask you the reader why this test has not been done and in the same breath why has the Department of Energy refused to give us the results of tests on the irradiation of foods, (simply stating it would not be in the best interests of National Security) Again, I ask you the reader, what kind of nonsense is this, when our very lives are at stake? - Editor

*For Further Information on the
COALITION TO STOP THE IRRADIATION OF FOODS
P.O. Box 59-0488
San Francisco, California 94159
Tel: (415) 56N-CSFI

*The Coalition to Stop the Irradiation of Foods is a Non-Profit Organization and Donations are gladly accepted.

Other sources to become involved to stop food irradiation: Health and Energy Inst. Washington, D.C. 20006 (202)543-1070; National Health Federation, 5001 Seminary Rd., Alexandria, Va. 22311 (703) 379-0589. Vermont Alliance to Protect Our Food; Vergennes, Vt., (802) 877-3289

CLOROX BATH FOR CLEANING FRUITS AND VEGETABLES

For cleaning fruits and vegetables against chemical and pesticide poisoning. Dr. Hazel Parcells gives the following instructions for cleaning foods with Clorox for highly chemically allergic patients.

The Clorox treatment will remove from the foods insecticides, preservatives, colorings, metal salts, bacteria and fungi.

Pre-Clean Foods: Separate the foods to be treated into the groups, keeping each food group separate throughout the procedure.

Vegetables: Leafy vegetables (such as spinach, lettuce), root vegetables (such as carrots, potatoes,), heavy skinned fiber vegetables.

Fruits: Thin-skinned berries and thin-skinned fruits (such as peaches, apricots, plums, etc.), heavy-skinned fruits (such as apples, all citrus fruits, bananas and pears).

Eggs: Eggs are at the top of the list of allergy-causing foods. This may be due to the pesticide sprays used around the pens and nests. The egg shell is porous and can absorb these poisons very quickly. Salmonella bacteria may also be present in the egg, as they are often found in the fowl.

Meats: (Poultry, fish, beef, lamb, pork.) Meat, poultry and fish are often preserved or processed with antibiotics, nitrites, nitrates or other unnatural preservatives. Beef tenderizers are commonly used. Frozen meat, turkey or chicken should first be defrosted.

For further information write to: Dr. Hazel Parcells, D.C., N.D., Ph.D., 111 Cardenas Drive, Albuquerque, New Mexico

HYDROGEN PEROXIDE FOR FRUITS & VEGETABLES

For clean fruits and vegetables against chemical and pesticide poisoning. Hydrogen Peroxide is 5000 times more effective in killing bacteria than chlorine. Use 4oz. of Hydrogen Peroxide (3%) in a dish-pan full of water.

Use 1oz. of Hydrogen Peroxide (3%) to a gallon of water to water your plants,

If you use 35% Hydrogen Peroxide for cleaning vegetables and fruits, use 1oz. to a gallon of water.

HYDROGEN PEROXIDE FOR YOUR BATH

Use 2oz Hydrogen Peroxide (35%) in a bath full of warm water. Soak for 20 minutes. If you use 3% Hydrogen Peroxide pour in a quart to a tub full of water.

SOME THOUGHTS ON: MILK/SALT/SUGAR/SOFT DRINKS/COFFEE

HOMOGENIZED! by Dr. Kurt A. Oster

"We have all heard the dairy industry slogans: "Milk is a Natural"... "Milk is the Perfect Food"... "Everybody Needs Milk"... and we have all received the message from Mother, "Drink your milk, dear."

NOT SO! According to research by Dr. Oster, Chief of Cardiology, Emeritus at Bridgeport's Park City Hospital. He is also a current Fellow of the American College of Cardiology, and of the American College of Clinical Pharmacology.

Two heart attacks motivated Dr. Oster to research the process of the build-up of plaque in the arteries conducive to heart disease. Funding his own way, Dr. Oster traveled to remote areas of the world seeking evidence to justify his discovery of the effects of homogenized milk on the human body. From Dr. Oster's research it was concluded by "statistics around the world that the heart disease rate in a country is proportional to the consumption of homogenized milk.

To order: Marcia Smith, 8 Muriel Place, Fairfax, California Cost $2.00 plus $1.00 shipping, California residents add 6 1/2% sales tax.

SALT

Decreasing your salt intake doesn't have to mean decreasing the pleasures of living and eating. Nor does a sodium-controlled diet have to turn your life into a series of sacrifices and denials. Even small changes in the amount of sodium you consume may help decrease your risk of illness.

An alternative to salt: CORRECTED SALT. Metabolically balanced salt. Will not aggravate high blood pressure. Tastes exactly like salt and has no bitter aftertaste.

Corrected salt is prepared from ordinary salt with the addition of commonly available non-toxic mineral salts, which do not change the taste. This information is based on sound scientific reasoning.

To order: Multiway Distributor, Marsha SMith, 8 Muriel Pl., Fairfax, Ca. 94930 Cost: $14.50/25oz., $7.70/8oz., $8.75/250 individual packs. (415) 459-5013

SUGAR

THE SWEET KILLER IN YOUR CUPBOARD by Carlson Wade
Special report on sugar

Most processed and manufactured foods are hidden sources of sugar. You must read the labels! Take a look in your cupboard right now. Do you see sugar? Toss it out of the house. It is as dangerous and deadly as any poison.

Whether known as sugar, sucrose or dextrose, it is still an undesirable non-food that should be eliminated from your food program.

Some of the health-robbing consequences of sugar are now given to you: boosts blood pressure, causes scalp dandruff disorders, villain involved in diabetes, may cause heart trouble, causes mental problems, tooth decay, overweight.

An entire copy of this article (excerpt only printed here) may be purchased 100-$3.00. 50 copies $2.00.

Send your name and address and check to NFA, Atlanta, Texas 75551

COFFEE

What's the story on Coffee and Decaffeinated Coffee?
Source: Better Nutrition, June 1983

There's some new and rather disturbing evidence of the possible harm that coffee may be doing to people who drink large amounts of the steaming black beverage every day. It comes from the National Institute of Mental Health, where biologist Paul Marangos gave mice a daily dose of the amount of caffeine that would be in four to eight cups of coffee.

At the end of two weeks, he found a proliferation of certain brain compounds which seemed to suggest that the caffeine given to the mice acts as a chemical antagonist, blocking the normal action of an essential brain compound called adenosine. According to a report in Science News, February 12, 1983...
...The brain reacts by producing new sites for adenosine, ...which causes abnormal sedation (and a craving for caffeine) whenever the effects wear off. He also found a disturbance in brain receptors which are involved in controlling anxiety.

....drinkers are choosing to decaffeinate themselves, by switching to coffee from which practically all of the caffeine has been removed.

But there's a Catch 22 situation there, as well. An Australian scientist reported in the British Journal Nature, January 26, 1983, that there is yet another chemical compound in coffee which is also present in the decaffeinated kinds, but not in tea or cocoa, which blocks the activity of another brain substance called naloxone. The average cup of coffee contains five times the active dose which this scientist used in his experiments. So it seems that anyone drinking large amounts of even decaffeinated coffee may find certain nervous troubles because the brain substances that work as both painkillers and mood elevators have been blocked by this newly found compound in coffee.

SOFT DRINKS

In addition to the high sugar content which need not be specified, optional ingredients that also do not have to appear on the label include any one of 12 nutritive sweeteners, 8 acidifying agents, 32 buffering agents, 17 emulsifiers, 6 foaming agents and one anti-foaming agent. In all, the government permits some 679 artificial ingredients to be used in mass produced soft drinks, according to "Natural Fruit Sodas" Report, from Health Falley Natural Foods.

Among the more questionalbe additives are food colorings, and 90 percent of food colors, says ralph Nader's Health Research Group, are synthetic. Most are coal-tar derivatives, to boot. "U.S. Certified Color" does not mean certified for safety, but simply means that it has met government standards which allow a certain percentage of impurities to be present.

TESTING YOUR OWN pH to Monitor and Control Your Body Chemistry/Candida

Use Narrow Range pH paper for testing the alkaline or acidic condition of the body. Immediately upon awakening in the morning place the Narrow Range pH paper on the tongue, remove and read the range of numbers.

The pH of the body should be between 7.2 and 7.5. If it is under 7.2 you are acid and must eat more alkaline foods. (See chart below) If the reading on the paper is above 7.5 you are too alkaline and you must eat more acid foods. (See chart below)
The following chart excerpted from the book, Nature Has a Remedy by Dr. Bernard Jensen, BiWorld Publishers, P.O.Box 62, Provo, Utah 84601
This Acid-Alkaline Chart is reprinted with permission.

ACID-ALKALINE CHART

The following table of foods is from Ragnar Berg of Germany.

Foods preceded by the letters "AL" are alkaline forming **Foods preceded by the letters "AC" are acid forming**

Column No. 1 Nonstarch Foods		Column No. 2 Proteins and Fruits		Column No. 3 Starchy Foods	
AL Alfalfa	AL Artichokes	AC Beef	AC Buttermilk	AL Bananas	AC Barley
AL Asparagus	AL Beans (string)	AC Chicken	AC Clams	AC Beans (lima)	AC Beans (white)
AL Beans (wax)	AL Beets (whole)	AC Cotage cheese	AC Crab	AC Bread	AC Cereals
AL Beet leaves	AL Broccoli	AC Duck	AC Eggs	AC Chestnuts	AC Corn
AL Cabbage (white)	AL Cabbage (red)	AC Fish	AC Goose	AC Corn meal	AC Crackers
AL Carrots	AL Carrot tops	AL Honey (pure)	AC Jello	AC Grapefruit	AC Corn starch
AL Cauliflower	AL Celery knobs	AC Lamb	AC Lobster	AC Gluten flour	AC Lentils
AL Chickory	AL Cocunut	AC Mutton	AC Nuts	AC Macaroni	AC Maize
AL Corn	AL Cucumbers	AC Oyster	AC Pork	AC Millet rye	AC Oatmeal
AL Dandelions	AL Eggplant	AC Rabbit	AC Raw sugar	AC Peanuts	AC Peanut butter
AL Endive	AL Garlic	AC Turkey	AC Turtle	AC Peas (dried)	AC Potatoes (sweet)
AL Horseradish	AL Kale	AC Veal	AL All berries	AL Potatoes (white)	AL Pumpkin
AL Kohlrabi	AL Leek	AL Apples	AL Apricots	AC Rice (brown)	AC Rice (polished)
AL Lettuce	AL Mushrooms	AL Avocados	AL Cantaloupes	AC Roman meal	AC Rye flour
AL Okra	AL Olives (ripe)	AL Cranberries	AL Curants	AC Sauerkraut	AC Tapioca
AL Onions	AL Osterplant	AL Dates	AL Figs	AL Squash (hubbard)	
AL Parsley	AL Parsnips	AL Grapes	AL Grapefruit		
AL Peas (fresh)	AL Peppers (sweet)	AL Lemons	AL Limes		
AL Radishes	AL Rutabagas	AL Oranges	AL Peaches		
AL Savory	AL Sea lettuce	AL Pears	AL Persimmons		
AL Sorrel	AL Spinach	AL Pineapple	AL Plums		
AL Soybean (products)	AL Sprouts	AL Prunes	AL Raisins		
AL Summer squash	AL Swiss chard	AL Rhubarb	AL Tomatoes		
AL Turnips	AL Watercress				

Non-starchy foods mix with proteins, fruits or starches; and proteins and fruits do not mix well with starchy foods.

Non-starchy foods mix with proteins, fruits or starches; and proteins and fruits do not mix well with starchy foods.

Source for Narrow Range pH Paper: Clarkson Laboratories
350 Trousdale Drive, Chula Vista, California 92010, (619) 425-1932
Cost $25.00 (case of 10 packages of strips)

LICK THE SUGAR HABIT
by Nancy Appleton, Ph.D.

Editor's Note: Lick the Sugar Habit is a forceful attack on lifestyle and eating habits that can lead to degenerative diseases. Nancy tells how excess refined sugar is linked to arthritis, cancer, heart disease, diabetes, and other degenerative disease.

"A practical life plan for attaining and maintaining good health... There are four "arenas" in which we act and produce basic effects on our chemical balance.

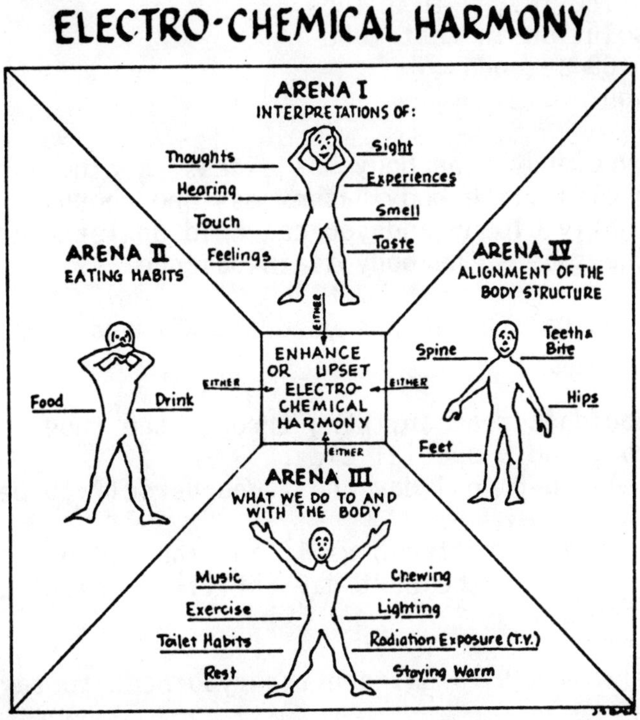

Arena I: The choices we make in interpreting what we and others do, think, and say. It is important to observe the language we use, and pay attention to the ways in which what we say, think, and do upset body chemistry.

Arena II: The choices we make in deciding what to eat. There are foods which upset the body chemistry, and foods which enhance it.

Arena III: Arena III deals with body mechanics and stimuli extrenal to the body. Body mechanics include chewing, toilet habits, and exercise. With good habits, you can help bring your body back into alignment.

Arena IV: The choices we make regarding alignment of the body structure. A body out of alignment, whether it be jaws, cranium, spine, hips or feet, will experience distress. Distress, in turn, upsets mineral relationships. Area IV is easy to deal with, if the other three arenas are in balance. A chiropractor makes an adjustment, and it will hold because there is good protein digestion and tissue integrity. If you are not functioning well in other arenas, and mineral relationships have been upset, tissue integrity will be compromised. A chiropractor may make an adjustment but it won't hold. The four arenas are interrelated; each must be balanced before health can be achieved."

Editor's Note: What I particularly like about Nancy's book is that she goes one step further and gives us a tool whereby we can actually monitor and balance our own body chemistry. See following instructions and address for kit.

The kit you will receive from Nancy will contain: 1 eye dropper, 1 test tube 1 tube containing solution and a booklet.

INSTRUCTIONS ON HOW TO USE THE TEST KIT

1) drop 10 drops of urine in the test tube
2) drop 10 drops of solution in test tube
3) shake up for 30 to 60 seconds
4) hold tube up to light
5) view it
6) if solution is very cloudy, the body has excess calcium
7) if solution is gin clear, the body has excess phosphorus
8) if solution is slightly cloudy and you can hold up lettering in back of tube and read through the tube - the body is in balance

Karen Stevens of Moraga, California has used the Kit and these are the results she found for herself:

(a) First day she couldn't read anything through the tube.
(b) She proceeded to go on a special diet.
(c) She tested herself in 3 to 4 day and found herself to be in balance and feeling better
(d) She then went off diet, tested herself and she had excess calcium.
(e) She tested herself again the next day (still off diet) and found she had excess phosphorus.

When you find your body is not in balance then you need to say on your special diet.

<u>Lick the Sugar Habit</u>, Choice Publishing Co. (1985) P.O. Box 3568, Santa Monica, California 90403-3568 Price $9.95 + $2.00 shipping

The test kit can be purchased through the same address. Price $15.00
Shipping $ 1.00
Calif. Sales Tx .97.

HOW TO REGULATE THE THYMUS AND FUNCTION OF THE T CELLS

The Nutritional Regulation of T Lymphocyte Function
969-985, 1979: D.F. Horrobin, M.S. Manku, M. Oka, R.O. Morgan, etc.
Clinical Research Institute of Montreal, 110 Pine Avenue West, Montreal
H2W 1R7, Canada: Medical Hypotheses 5 1975

Summary: Prostaglandin (PG E1) plays a major role in the regulation of the thymus development and T lymphocyte function and the evidence for this is reviewed. The production of PGE1 is dependent on nutritional factors with linoleic acid, gamma-linolenic acid, pyridoxine (B-6) zinc and Vitamin C playing key roles. Inadequate intake of any one of these will lead to inadequate PGE1 formation and defective T lymphocyte function. Megadose of any one are likely to be only minimally effective in the absence of adequate intakes of the others. By careful attention to diet it should be possible to activate T lymphocyte function in the large number of diseases including rheumatoid arthritis, various auto-immune diseases, multiple sclerosis, and cancer in which such function is defective.

FACTORS THAT MAY DEPRESS THE IMMUNE SYSTEM-"SUNLIGHT COULD SAVE YOUR LIFE"

"When enough ultraviolet light is received by the skin to produce a burning or reddening effect, increased levels of prostaglandins are produced in the skin. Prostaglandins are hormone-like substances that are produced from a certain essential unsaturated fat called linoleic acid.

Linoleic acid is found in polyunsaturated oils, especially corn oil. The more linoleic acid in the diet, the more there is in the tissues, and the greater is the production of prostaglandins. Prostaglandins are known to inhibit the immune system. Therefore, the more polyunsaturated fat in the diet, the more prostaglandins will form when the skin is reddened by the sun and the greater will the depressing effect on the immune system.

It is suggested that one way in which sunburning contributes to the formation of skin cancer is that it, in conjunction with a high polyunsaturated fat diet, depresses the immune system thereby leaving the body unable to check the growth of cancerous cells.

Polyunsaturated fat, itself, has been shown to inhibit the immune system. In fact, it does this so well that researchers are now using polyunsaturated fat in the diets of kidney transplant patients and those patients with skin grafts taken from other people, so the patients' bodies will not reject the foreign tissue.

Certain diseases may be caused by the body's becoming allergic to itself; that is, the immune system actually begins to destroy some of the body's cells. These diseases are called auto-immune diseases. Polyunsaturated fat has been used to inhibit the immune system in these diseases. It is apparent then that the inclusion of polyunsaturated fat in the diet directly inhibits the immune system even without an additional sunburning effect.

WHAT IS CAMP?

A very interesting substance found in almost all cells, including lymphocytes, is known as cyclic adenosine monophosphate. In medical circles this long name is shortened to cyclic AMP. However, for the convenience of our readers, we have chosen to abbreviate it even more, referring to this harmful substance from now on simply as "CAMP". If high levels of cyclic AMP build up in the lymphocytes, they become unable to function properly and will not be able to destroy cancer cells. CAMP may also depress other factors in the body's immune system.

There are may factors which may elevate the level of CAMP in the lymphocytes. An understanding of some of these factors is especially important to one who is interested in sunlight therapy.

Stress

Whenever a person is under stress or is emotionally upset, adrenalin is poured into the system from the adrenal gland. Adrenalin goes to the cells and stimulates the production of CAMP. The increased CAMP inhibits the ability of the immune system to destroy cancer cells. It is a well-known fact that cancer may follow an emotional upset or a period of severe stress.

The Cup

Coffee, tea, and chocolate contain stimulating substances known as caffeine, theophylline, and theobromine. These substances increase the amount of CAMP in the body cells because they block the destruction of CAMP which would normally take place. Increased CAMP depresses the ability of the lymphocytes to function, and is a stimulant to the nervous system. It is by increasing CAMP production in the cell, that coffee and tea are able to produce their stimulating effects. A decrease in gamma globulin has actually been found among coffee drinkers. There have been reports that coffee drinking is related to some types of cancer. The nicotine in cigarettes may also be a factor in lowered immunity, as smokers have been found to have decreased levels of gamma globulin.

Prostaglandins

In the chapter on cancer, prostaglandins were discussed as to their role in inhibiting the immune system. Prostaglandins (specifically prostaglandin E1 and E2) work by stimulating the cells to produce CAMP, thereby decreasing the lymphocytes' ability to destroy cancer cells.

As you recall from the chapter on cancer, if one eats freely of polyunsaturated fat, his body may be stimulated to produce excessive prostaglandins and these may inhibit his immune system.

.....the sun decreases levels of CAMP in the body and thereby increases the ability of the lymphocytes and immune system to function properly. This may be why sunlight is helpful in the treatment of tuberculosis and other diseases, including cancer...."

<u>SUNLIGHT COULD SAVE YOUR LIFE</u> by Zane Kime, M.D., Box 400, World Health Pub. Penryn, Ca.95663 Reprinted with Permission

JOURNAL SHOWS ALL PURPOSE (WHITE) WHEAT FLOUR FAILS TO BE COMPLETELY ABSORBED.

INCOMPLETE ABSORPTION OF THE CARBOHYDRATE IN ALL-PURPOSE WHEAT FLOUR
Isabel H. Anderson, B.S., Allen S. Levine, Ph.D., and Michael D. Levitt, M.D.
The New England Journal of Medicine, Vol 304, No. 15, April 9, 1981

Malasorption of the carbohydrate lactose is a common cause of flatulence, abdominal discomfort, and diarrhea in otherwise healthy persons. The possibility that such symptoms could result from malasorption of the other major dietary carbohydrates (surcrose or starch) has received little consideration since these carbohydrates are assumed to be completely absorbed in health.

We measured breath hydrogen to assess the absorption of the carbohydrate in white, all-purpose wheat flour. These studies demonstrate that nearly all normal subjects fail to absorb an appreciable portion of this form of starch, possibly because of an interaction between the starch and protein moieties of wheat flour.

Incomplete small-bowel absorption of carbohydrate provides the colonic bacteria with substrate for reactions that liberate hydrogen. A fraction of this hydrogen is then absorbed and excreted on the breath, providing a reliable indicator of carbohydrate malabsorption.

In this study, sizable increases in breath hydrogen were observed in 17 of 18 healthy subjects ingesting 100g of wheat starch in the form of macaroni or bread made from all-purpose white flour. ...Thus, wheat flour was incompletely absorbed in virtually all healthy subjects...

This study is from the Department of Medicine and the Department of Food Science and Nutrition of the Veterans Administration Medical Center and the University of Minnesota, Minneapolis, Minn. Address reprint requests to Dr. Levitt at the Veterans Administration Medical Center, 54th St., and 48th Ave. South Minneapolis, Mn. 55417

Supported by the Veterans Administration and the National Institutes of Health.

RECIPE BOOKS

The following recipe book is listed for the Candida patient.

California Clinic of Preventive Medicine Cookbook

2010 Jimmie Duarante Blvd.
Del Mar, California 92014
(619) 755-3340
(619) 275-4352

$9.00 + Shipping

The following four books are not specifically written for the Candida patient, but may be used, guided with the knowledge of what the Candida patient is permitted to have.

Evdie Mae's Natural Recipes — $3.95 + Shipping

Eydie Mae Hunsberger
Avery Publications
1978

The UnCook Book — $5.95 + Shipping

Elizabeth & Elton Baker
Drelwood Publications
1981

Communication Creativity
P.O. Box 213
Saguache, Colorado 81149

Introducing Macrobiotic Cooking — $9.95 + Shipping

Wendy Esko
Japan Publications
1979

Diet changes are required as time progresses; a macrobiotic counsellor in your area is suggested to meet these changes.

Fit For Life — $17.50 + Shipping

Harvey and Marilyn Diamond

Warner Communications Company 1985
666 Fifth Avenue-New York, New York 10103

The Candida Albicans Yeast-Free Cookbook — $9.95 + Shipping $2.05

Pat Connolly and Associates of the Price Pottinger Foundation

Price Pottenger Nutrition Foundation
P.O. Box 2614-La Mesa, Ca. 92041

The Candida Gourmet Cookbook
by the Candida Research & Information Foundation
31111 Palomares Road
Castro Valley, California 94552
(415) 582 2179

XII

SILVER (mercury) FILLINGS, THE IMMUNE SYSTEM & CANDIDA

YEAST INFECTIONS THRIVE BECAUSE THE IMMUNE SYSTEM HAS BEEN DEPRESSED BY MERCURY TOXICITY

"THE YEAST IS YET TO COME" by Carlton Fredericks, Ph.D. - Lets Live Magazine 1984 August (Excerpt)

"When systemic infection with candida is the ultimate cause of vaginal yeast infections, the approach has to be more comprehensive. The local therapies can be used, but the yeast colonies in the body obviously require attention. This calls for the low carbohydrate diet, accompanied by high dosage of biotin, supplements of lactobacillus which, in this instance, are taken by mouth, medication with garlic, and, in a significant percentage of the cases, an examination for mercury poisoning deriving from the amalgam used to fill teeth. Despite the reassurances of the dental societies, who seem more intent on protecting the profession from lawsuits than they are in shielding patients from the toxicity of mercury, there are yeast infections which thrive because the immune system has been depressed by mercury toxicity.

Reprinted with Permission by-
Dr. Carlton Fredericks, Ph.D.

IMMUNE SUPPRESSION PRODUCED BY MERCURY AND OTHER TOXIC METALS- From the Journals-

Koller, Loren, D.V.M., Ph.D.: Immunosuppression produced by lead, cadmium, and mercury. Am. J. Vet. Res., 34 (11):1457-1458, 1973.

There was marked immunosuppression in the rabbits given lead, cadmium and mercury in the drinking water. ....The significant aspect of the present study is that chronic exposure to lead, cadmium, or mercury produces immunosuppression to a viral agent.

Druet, P., Hirsch, F., et. al.: Immune Dysregulation and Auto-Immunity Induced by Toxic Agents

Several observations suggest that mercury acts, at least in part, by modifying T-B cell cooperation and induces a polyclonal activation. ....Data presented strongly suggest that Hg modifies immune homeostasis in BN rats and that, as a consequence of immune dysregulation, auto-antibodies are produced, some of which are of pathogenic significance. This dysregulation may result from an interaction of Hg with the cell membrane of lymphocytes. All these results indicate that toxic agents can induce abnormal lymphocyte interactions leading to auto-immunity as predicted by Allison.

Lawrence, David: Heavy Metal Modulation of Lymphocyte Activities. Toxicol. Appl..Pharmacol., 57:439-451, 1981

Heavy metals induce immunopotentiating or immunosuppressive effects which could result in immunopathologic effects on numerous tissues. Alteration of the immune responsiveness has been related to the toxicity of heavy metals. For example, mercury (Hg^{2+}), lead, cadmium, and cobalt have been reported to be immunosuppressive in vivo.

Eggleston, D., D.D.S.: Effect of Dental Amalgam and Nickel Alloys on T-lymphocytes: Preliminary Report. Journal of Prosthetic Dentistry: Vol. 51 Number 5, P. 617-623, May 1984

The purpose of this research project was to determine the effect of dental amalgam and nickel alloys on human T-lymphocytes.

.....Therefore, a malfunction or reduction in the number of T4-lymphocytes results in a depressed immune response to antigens. An extreme example of this is the autoimmune deficiency syndrome (AIDS), in which the incidence of Kaposi's sarcoma and infections with opportunistic microorganisms is relatively high because of a lack of helper T-lymphocytes.

....Immune homeostasis is dependent on a delicate balance of T4/T8 ratio at 1.8:1 to 2:1. A ratio below 1.8:1 or above 2:1 can predispose to autoimmune diseases such as systemic lupus erythematosus, hemolytic anemia, multiple sclerosis, severe atopic eczema, inflammatory bowel disease, and glomerulonephritis.

Preliminary data suggest that dental amalgam and dental nickel alloys can adversely affect the quantity of T-lymphocytes. ....Normal immune function depends on a proper quantity, quality and ratio of T-lymphocyte helper and suppressor subsets.

Page 151 refers to Dr. Eggleston's 1983 lecture before the Wholistic Dental Convention in San Diego whereby he states that autoimmune diseases, arthritis, Amyotrophic Lateral Schlerosis, Lupus Erythematosis, Multiple Sclerosis and some forms of cancer are auto-immune types of diseases.

JOURNAL OF ORTHOMOLECULAR PSYCHIATRY
3rd QUARTER 1983 Vol 12, NUMBER 3

Hanson, Mats: Amalgam-Hazards In Your Teeth

A person can be extremely sensitive to inhaled Hg (mercury) without showing + skin reaction (Stock, 1936). If the Hg comes to the skin from the circulation severe dermatitis can occur. Acrodynia-pink disease- was common when Hg-containing baby powders were used. Inner allergies of autoimmune type are not visible from the outside. They occur when proteins bind Hg (or other metals). The immune system will then not recognize the protein and react. Many manifestations of Hg poisoning have obvious immunological components. It is also known that autoimmune diseases can be elicited by mercury, i.e. myasthenia gravis (Kantarjian, 1961) and immune reactions towards kidney tissue are known (Kelchner et al., 1976). Since Hg can bind to thousands of different proteins and each individual has an unique immune system, the many and variable manifestations of mercury poisoning are not surprising. However, those described by Stock (1928) are the most common.

The majority of people might have sufficient resistance to Hg to have amalgam without becoming seriously ill. However, mercury kills cells which are not renewed, especially nerve cells. These cells are the ones we will need later in life as a reserve. No dentist can guarantee that the patient will not come to harm. It must also be pointed out that the other metals in amalgam are not harmless either. Tin poisoning from canned food is well known. Tin is partly transformed into organic compounds in the environment just like Hg and there is a distinct possibility that the same will happen in the human body. Organotin compounds are extremely toxic. Silver causes argyria, an irreversible grey discoloration of the skin. The possibility of "inner argyria" has not been investigated. Silver binds extremely strongly to proteins and is used in the most sensitive protein stain available and also to stain nerve cells.

We are exposed to an increasing load of toxic substances from the environment. The internal contribution from amalgam is the one which is easiest to avoid. The fact that amalgam has been used for over 100 years is no argument for harmlessness. The same can be said for asbestos and many other hazardous substances. The most surprising fact, however, is that dentists want to work with a material which constitutes a great risk to themselves, their personnel and patients.

Dr. Hanson is affiliated with University of Lund, Department of Zoophysiology, Helgonavagen, 3B, S.22362 Lund, Sweden Telephone: 046-10 93 54

Dr. Pleva is a 'Corrosion' Scientist and an expert on corrosion mechanisms. He is Manager-Corrosion Section, Steel Research, Uddeholm AB, Pb 703, S-68301 Hagfors 1, Sweden. Dr. Pleva himself experienced mercury poisoning until the removal of his own silver fillings. He relates his experiences in the following article published in JOURNAL OF ORTHOMOLECULAR PSYCHIATRY, VOL 12 NO. 3, 1983.

Pleva, Jaro, Ph.D.: Mercury Poisoning from Dental Amalgam

Conclusions: My own symptoms, the similarity with those of chronic mercury poisoning, their disappearance when the amalgam was removed, studies of corroded amalgam fillings, case reports and data in the literature show that all statements that silver amalgam is a stable alloy which cannot give symptoms of mercury, can be dismissed. Since the mercury content of old amalgam fillingsin all cases were lower than in fresh ones and could approach zero in some places, corrosion must have caused dissolution and evaporation of mercury and not enrichment in the fillings as sometimes has been claimed. Based on a knowledge of the complicated structure and corrosion properties of amalgam, the search for a stable amalgam must be considered unrealistic. Also a very limited corrosion might be unacceptable when the released metal is highly toxic.

For doctors, anxious not to harm their patients, there is today no reason to hesitate in their attitude towards amalgam. Very much indicates that too many people are exposed to great sufferings because some scientific areas have been neglected by the medical world. There are also reasons for a broad epidemiological study on the relation between civilization diseases and amalgam. As a first step the use of gold or other metals together with amalgam should be immediately stopped and existing contacts, including temporary ones, should be eliminated. ....All my observations, both as a patient and as a corrosion scientist, have reasonable explanations and can be supported by data from the scientific literature. ....Medical practitioners need to recognize the characteristic manifestations of mercury poisoning and it is also my hope that this report might help dentists to a better understanding of the hazards of amalgam and combinations of metals. Following are a list of Symptoms of the Amalgam Syndrome, some of which Dr. Pleva felt before he had his own silver fillings removed.

Irregular heartbeat
Strong pains in the left part of chest
Retinal bleeding
Dim vision
Inability to fix the gaze, uncontrollable eye mevements
A film over the eyes, dry eyes
A grey ring around the cornea
Red, irritated throat; inflammation in upper airways and pleurisy a year after the dental treatment
Difficulties in swallowing
Severe amnesia, anxiety, irritability; difficulty & even impossibility to control behavior; indecision
Loss of interest in life; tirdness; a feeling of being old
Resistance to intellectual work
Increases need for sleep
Vertigo
Headache (about once a week) often migrane-like
Facial paralysis
Painful pull at the lower jaw towards collar bone
Increased salivation, sour-metallic taste
Bleeding gums at toothbrushing
Joint pains, especially increasing 1981-2
Pains in lower back
Weakness of muscles, slow muscle action
Pressure, pains, "needles" in the liver
Asthmatic breathing troubles
Gastrointestinal irritation
"Needles" at lymph nodes under arms & in gro
Eczema

SILVER 'MERCURY' FILLINGS IN RELATION TO AIDS

On the following page Dr. Boericke refers to the gums becoming spongy, receding and bleeding easily when one has silver 'mercury' fillings. This in turn makes a perfect home for the fungi "Candida' to live. Which can turn in to 'oral Candidiasis' paralyzing the immune system (thymus) which matures the 'T' Cells to fight foreign invaders, and you then have what is known as AIDS. It has also been shown that the use of silver 'mercury' amalgam fillings causes what is known as 'amalgam tattoo' which is chronic inflammatory response to amalgam, (which would also make a good home for Candida). In Dr. Eggleston's lecture referred to earlier in this book it is shown that the 'T' Cell goes up and down depending on the insertion or removal of silver 'mercury' amalgam fillings.

HINTS FROM THE AMERICAN DENTAL ASSOCIATION

At one time the American Dental Association (ADA) recommended that scrap amalgam, the material left over after filling a tooth, should be handled like toxic waste: No one was to touch it. It must be stored under water in sealed containers, and disposed of only through local health departments.

WARNING: TO PEOPLE WHO WORK IN BUILDINGS THAT HOUSES DENTAL OFFICES

If the building has sealed windows and central ventilation, you may be exposed to mercury vapor. The air can be tested. If the mercury vapor exceeds OSHA limits, steps can be taken to reduce exposure.

OPERATIVE DENTISTRY, 1979, 4, 24-35
AMALGAM-YESTERDAY, TODAY, AND TOMORROW: Evan H. Greener

"In 1845, the American Society of Dental Surgeons passed a resolution "pronouncing the use of all amalgams as malpractice" and further demanded that each member sign a pledge not to use amalgams, use of which constituted expulsion from the society."

"Recent surveys have shown that, nationally, at least 10% of dental offices have mercury vapor in excess of "Threshold Limit Value"...."Last year, the result of a survey of 85 operatories in Seattle revealed 10-15% had ambient mercury over TLV, with signs of mercury poisoning in clinicians; and perhaps more frightening, 70% of the operatories had ambient mercury levels above 40% TLV. Recently, the British Broadcasting Corporation on prime time television reported similar statistics for England, so we must believe that the problem is universal."

METHY-MERCURY is the changing of inorganic mercury (which dentists use) by anorobic bacteria (bacteria that needs no oxygen in order to survive) in the gut of the human being and which is poisoning the entire system especially the nervous system. (See Chapter XV)

Silver 'Mercury' Fillings

Silver Mercury Filling consist of silver (65% minimum), tin (25% minimum), copper (6% maximum), zinc (2% maximum). This amalgam is then mixed with a 50-50 ratio with mercury. Silver mercury fillings can create toxicity throughout the body as the metal ions (or free metals) are released into the tissues, causing unrelated symptoms. Many remote dysfunctions of the body can be attributed to toxicity of dental metals.

Dentists used 200,000 pounds of mercury in 1980
Dentists will use 400,000 pounds of mercury in 1990.
Dentists will use 600,000 pounds of mercury by 2000.

In 1972 NIOSH (National Institute for Occupational Safety and Health) set the standard for TLV (Threshold Limit Value). The TLV in the Soviet Union is 1/5 the limit amount of mercury we allow in the United States. Most of Europe uses the Soviet Union's standard.

William Boericke, M.D., former professor of Materia Medica at the University of California, San Francisco stated, "Every organ and tissue of the body is more or less affected by mercury. It transforms healthy cells into decrepit, inflamed and necrotic wrecks, decomposes the blood, producing a profound anemia. This malignant force especially affects the lymphatic system with all its membranes and glands, as well as the internal organs, bones, etc. The mind is affected with loss of memory and weakened will power. In the mouth, salivary secretions are increased, gums become spongy, recede and bleed easily, crowns of teeth decay, teeth loosen, feel tender and elongate."

Metal poisoning has been increasing at an alarming rate since silver amalgam was first introduced in the United States in 1825. In a review of History of Medicine, these diseases were first recorded in America after, 'mercury' silver fillings were introduced in 1825:

Nephritis in 1827;
Hodgkin's disease in 1832
Leukemia in 1845
Addison's disease in 1849
Banti's disease in 1881
Gaucher's disease in 1882
Anorexia nervosa in 1888
Dercum's disease in 1892
Van Jaksch's anemia in 1890
Sickle cell anemia in 1910
Chronic monocytic leukemia in 1913

These diseases are of unknown origin, and yet they have common symptoms of heavy metal poisoning such as in the case of sickle cell anemia, leukemia, blood dyscrasia in children, and irregular osteoporosis of the calvarium that appears in Hodgkins disease.

THE CANCER CONNECTION BETWEEN DEVITALIZED TEETH AND MERCURY FILLINGS?

A chapter from the book, A Healing Crisis -The Whole Body Approach to Cancer Therapy, by Jack Tropp refers to the teeth as being the cause in many patients who develop cancer.

Dr. Josef Issels and 'Ganzheitstherapie' (whole body approach).

Dr. Issels gravitated on an oblique path toward the treatment of cancer. He received his first training as a surgeon and then decided on general practice so that he could get at the roots of illness. He became heavily involved in the pathology of chronic diseases because these cases represented the heaviest part of his patient load.

The aim of Dr. Josef Issel's basic therapy was to eliminate all causal factors such as dental and tonsilar foci, and fields of neural disturbance; abnormal intestinal flora, faulty diet, exogenous chemical and physical factors, and psychic stress.

Neural Therapy. Issels explains first that "the 'focus' is a chronic, abnormal, local change in the connective tissue, capable of producing the varied distant effects beyond its immediate surroundings, and therefore in constant conflict with local and general defense (Pischinger and Kellner). By this definition, even a fully-healed scar may sometimes act as a focus, spreading disease to distant parts of the body."

Dr. Issels concentrates, however, on what he considers to be the most lethal of these foci, namely, infected teeth and tonsils, indicating that "the removal of devitalized teeth and chronically diseased tonsils is one of the better-known aspects of my work...but I believe that if they are diseased, they cause the body's natural resistance to be lowered, thus acting as an important contributory factor to tumor development. In these cases, I insist on their removal.

"In addition, my experience shows a direct connection between dental and tonsillar foci and many of the illnesses responsible for early debilitation and untimely invalidizing."

"...The diagnosis and treatment of dental foci remains generally unsatisfactory. A survey conducted at my clinic found that, on admission, ninety-eight percent of the adult cancer patients had between two and ten dead teeth, each one a dangerous toxin producing 'factory'. Very often we are confronted with X-ray negative dead teeth, root remnants, and residual ostitis which had not been diagnosed and therefore had not been removed."

"Only total, thorough dental treatment will really succeed in giving the body's defense a chance. In addition to x-ray diagnosis, it is therefore necessary to use other diagnostic aids, such as infra-red techniques and tests, to estimate tooth vitality and periosteal resistance, and other electrometric methods."

Dr. Issels has studied this problem most intensively, and, in his challenging book Cancer: A Second Opinion, he discusses in impressive detail the scientific and medical data surrounding this problem, which led to his conclusions.

Issels considers that the toxic activity of odontogenic foci may be even "more perilous for the organism than their neural effects."

"...The identity and chemical structure of certain of the biogenic amines were mainly clarified in the 1950's by Schug-Koesters, Hiller, Gaebelein and others of the University of Munich. Following similar findings in America, the metabolic and exchange processes in solid dental structures were further investigated by the German researcher Spreter von Kreudenstein. He showed the drugs injected intravenously were, four to five hours later, discernible within the intradental capillary ducts of even devitalized teeth, and in a concentration only slightly lower than in the blood.

"That endodental exchange may also take place in the opposite direction has been reported by Artelstone (USA) and Djerassi (Bulgaria). If radio-iodine, I-131, is deposited in an evacuated pulp cavity which is then sealed off with a filling, the iodine will appear in the thyroid some twenty hours later, as can be demonstrated by taking a scintograph of the thyroid region. Similarly, dyes can be washed out of a sealed pulp cavity."

"All these findings prove conclusively that within solid dental structures, there may proceed an unimpeded substantial interchange in either direction. Consequently, odontogenic toxins, wherever they may have been produced are able to diffuse and circulate within the organism."

"...The close connection between teeth and tonsils was proven when it was observed that Indian ink injected into a sealed dental cavity appeared as spots on the tonsillar surface in about twenty to thirty minutes. These experiments showed that pathogenic substances from the jaw region, including toxins from devitalized teeth, are conducted to the lymphatic tonsillar ring, there to be detoxicated and excreted. Besides their 'natural' physiological load, the tonsils are thus additionally exposed to continuous attack by odontogenous toxins provoked by the devitalization of teeth."

Degeneration-Regeneration by Melvin E. Page, DDS -1949 Nutritional Development

Even in cases of injury to the body in general, healing ability may be related to dental conditions. A certain patient had, as he expressed it, never a sick day in his life until he was in an automobile accident. He spent the next three years and his life savings trying to get well. Eleven operations failed to close a fistula. Finally a new physician suggested that a dentist look at his mouth. After the removal of seven devitalized teeth, the fistula closed and the man became well.

CHELATE HEAVY METALS FROM THE BODY

CATACHELEX nutritionally supports circulation and has amino acids which have been shown to chelate HEAVY METALS. Catachelex also has proteolytic enzymes to insure the body's ability to digest protein, especially fibrin which is one of the main components of arterial plaque.

ADDRESS FOR CATACHELEX		PRICE
Mrs. Marcia Smith or -	Jerry Mittelman, DDS	\$69.00 (includes tape)
c/o Multi-Way	263 West End Ave. #2A	(+ Calif. tax)
8 Muriel Place	New York City, New York	\$ 2.00 (shipping outside
Fairfax, California 94930	10023	Calif.)
(415) 459-5013	(212) 874 4212	

BACKGROUND OF MULTIWAY. Dr. Dwight McKee, M.D. is one of the founders of Multi-Way and is the Director of Nutritional Research. McKee works in close contact with Dr. E. Revici, M.D. of New York. Dr. Revici is a native of Romania and had his own privately funded hospital in New York, where he had been able to help many patients suffering with A.I.D.S through his revolutionary and advanced methods of treatment.

Curriculum Vitae: D.L. McKee, M.D. (In part only)

B.A. 1970, Williams College: graduated cum laude, honors in chemistry, Phi Beta Kappa.

Case-Western Reserve University: studies in combined M.D. -Ph.D. program from 1970-1973. Completed first two years of medical school and did three years of graduate work and research in pharmacology. Research work focused on the role of cyclic AMP in the central nervous system, under the guidance of Dr. T.W. Rall, co-discoverer of the cyclic AMP. The discovery of cyclic AMP was awarded the Nobel Prize for medicine in 1972.

1976: Diplomat, National Board of Medical Examiners.

1977-1979: served as Medical Director of the Nutritional Academy, Des Plaines, Illinois. Taught bi-monthly, 3-day seminars to Doctors and Nutritionists on how to administer nutritional programs, based on a model of balancing the autonomic nervous system through nutrition. Served as medical editor of The Journal of the Nutritional Academy.

Member of American Medical Association.

HOW TO DETOXIFY MERCURY FROM THE TISSUES OF THE BODY

EDITOR'S NOTE: The following article from the April 1986 issue of Homeopathy Today refers to an article by an M.D. who suggests mercury main remain in the tissues (although mercury fillings are removed) with symptoms of mercury poisoning until it is removed from the tissues by homeopathic means. See following article.

<u>HOMEOPATHY TODAY Vol. 6, No. 4, April, 1986</u>: National Center for Homeopathy, 1500 Massachusetts Avenue N.W., Washington, D.C. 20005. (202) 223-6182

I have made some observations in regard to the bad effects of these mercurial fillings in the mouth, and have come to believe that the eliminative forces of the system are unable to cope with metallic poisons, unaided. A patient so affected, will carry mercurial symptoms all through life, unless they are treated with the indicated remedy. The removal of the cause is not sufficient to restore health. I have convinced myself of this by having the filling removed and putting them on placebo. The symptoms invariably continued until I prescribed a remedy based on the symptoms. -G.P. Waring, M.D., in discussion. IHA Transactions, 1906, pp. 148-9.

EDITOR'S NOTE: Dr. Roy Smudde, D.D.S. suggests that anyone environmentally ill to detoxify first with homeopathic remedies and then consider removing mercury fillings. He further suggests anyone who wants to remove the mercury fillings, but does not seem to have health related problems, that these patients start detoxifying the mercury maybe only two weeks before having the mercury removed.

Dr. Smudde feels the patient should remove mercury fillings from the body, (this is the ideal situation), however, if this is not possible because of environmental illness, homeopathic remedies would work very nicely for this patient. He suggests starting with homeopathic remedies six months before possible removal of mercury fillings for the environmentally ill.

The KEY TO SUCCESS in all of this, according to Dr. Smudde, is to keep the organs of elimination open in order to let the mercury travel to the outside of the body. In other words, detoxification of the body through all the avenues of cleansing. The organs of elimination are: Colon, Lungs, Kidneys, Skin and Mucous Membranes and Menstration in women.

ADDRESSES FOR HOMEOPATHY AND HOMEOPATHY KITS:

Homeopathic Educational Services (For Catalog send business envelope & SASE)
2124 Kittredge Street
Berkeley, Ca. 94704
(415) 653-9270 (M-F 2-6 p.m. P.C.T.)

For Mercury detoxification through homeopathy write to:

Roy Smudde, D.D.S.
11311 Camarillo, Suite 211
No. Hollywood, Calif. 91602
(213) 937-7373

SIDE EFFECTS OF METAL

HETEROGENEOUS ALLOYS: precious metal with CHROME, NICKEL & STEEL

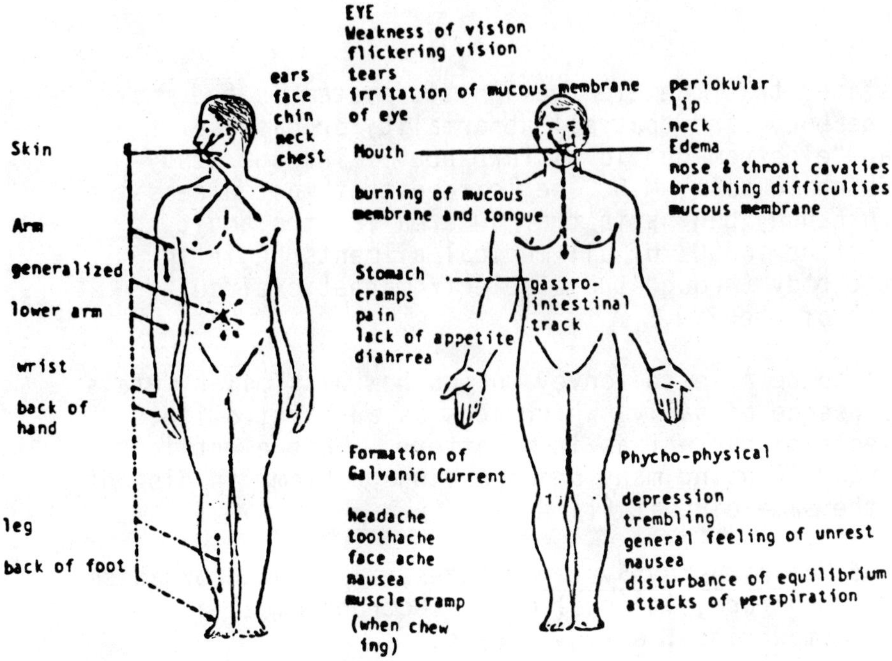

SIDE EFFECTS OF AMALGAM (edited by 24 authors)
(Healing Through Elimination)

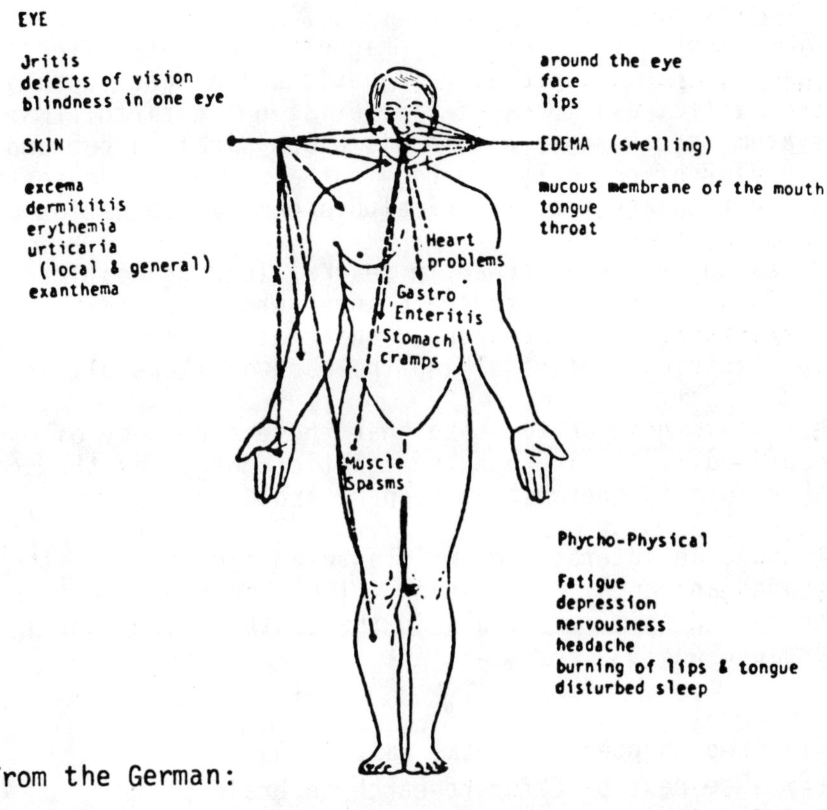

*Translated from the German:

Gasser, Von F.: Concerning foreign bodies in the mouth in research and practice. Schweizerische Monatsschrift Fuer Zahnheilkunde (SSO) 77(4): 307-323. April 1967

XIII

LECTURES ON THE ELECTROMAGNETIC BODY—MERCURY, NICKEL, "T" CELLS & AIDS

Dr. James Ouye, DDS states that the electromagnetic system is the most important system in the body, and that all abnormality or disease process starts with an "electromagnetic disturbance". Through studying the work of Dr. Reinhold Voll, M.D., he learned that most diseases (electromagnetic disturbance) begins in the jaw area for the adult. Dr. Voll has stated that up to 90% of all medical ailments begin in jaw area and affect the body through the bioelectromagnetic circuits related to that portion of the jaw.

In this chapter I hope to be able to convey to you how dissimilar metals in the mouth in the presence of saliva which acts as an electrolite, produces galvanic (electric) current as in a battery. This electricity is disturbing to the body, causing many unsuspecting problems in distant parts of the body on the same circuit.(1)

Jack Schwarz, author of Human Energy Systems states, "The human organism is not just a physical structure, it is also an electrochemical and electromagnetic organism made up of energy fields."

By measuring skin potentials, scientists have found that there are both alternating currents and direct currents coming from the body. Such currents arise from the migration of electrically charged particles, or ions, in the body tissues and fluids."

Albert Roy Davis, author of Magnetism and Its Effects on the Living System states, "Man is an electromagnetic animal and is subject to those forces that affect all forms of life existing on earth. Man's electromagnetic system is contained within his biophysical makeup and affects the total behavior of not only the body but also in many cases the changes in mental activities and the electrical biochemical operation of his system.

Research is now underway in several leading hospitals to show that man's brain is subject to severe changes when exposed to minor voltages and currents. (2) It has been found that the front of the skull is negative in electrical potential and the back of the skull is positive in nature."

Mr. Davis goes on to state that the entire body of man is a field of continually flowing electromagnetic energy and the space emissions of this form of energy have been recorded.

I found an interesting article in an old issue of the Dominion Dental Journal (Canadian Dental Association - 1902) on the effects of electric current through dissimilar metals in the mouth. (See Dental Galvanism Chapter-article No. 9)

(1) See Chapter on Dental Galvanism
(2) See next page for research on brain waves.

San Francisco Chronicle (Feb. 5, 1974) tells of a study to learn a person's thoughts through the use of a small computer that sorts electrical signals picked up by eight electrodes fastened like a crown around the scalp.

This clipping and the paragraph below show how we can manipulate the electromagnetic energy of humans and animals.

Other studies are being conducted at UC San Diego and in Spain whereby scientists are able to stimulate the brain of monkeys (through radio frequencies/electrical stimulation of the brain) and inhibit their movements or project or inhibit thought. -Editor.

Brain Waves May Tell What's On Your Mind

By Charles Petit

A study is underway at the Langley Porter Neuropsychiatric Institute here to learn if brain waves can reveal a person's natural aptitudes and intelligence — and possibly a person's thoughts.

Crucial to the study is the use of a small computer that sorts electrical signals picked up by eight electrodes fastened like a crown around the scalp.

With the computer, researchers can discover where in the brain various types of high frequency, low energy brain waves originate.

Scientists think that brain waves, instead of being non-functional side effects of cerebral electrical activity, may actually be carrying messages from one place in the brain to another.

Dr. Enoch Callaway, a psychiatrist, is directing the research with a grant from the Office of Naval Research.

The Navy's interest, he said, is mainly to see if computer analysis of brain waves could be useful in determining the aptitudes of new recruits.

Callaway described the project during this week's "merger celebration" marking the transfer of Langley Porter from the state Department of Health to the jurisdiction of the University of California Medical Center, its neighbor on Parnassus Heights for 30 years.

During an interview, the 50-year-old Callaway said it was 100 years ago that a German psychiatrist named Hans Berger first discovered brain waves. Berger hoped the rhythmic energies of the mind would reveal the secrets of extrasensory perception.

However, the use of the waves has been largely restricted to electroencephalograms that detect irregularities in brain waves — a means of diagnosing organic brain disease.

Considerable attention has also been paid lately to the conscious control of low-frequency brain waves, the most obvious example being "alpha wave bio-feedback" techniques.

However, Callaway's interest lies deeper in the brain where fleeting, high frequency waves of "electrical potential" flicker in curtains across the brain, often bypassing the neural pathways, usually thought to transmit the mind's internal messages.

Callaway is using computer techniques developed by a partner in the research, Peter Harris, a senior computer programmer.

Other things volunteers are asked to stare at flashing lights, or lights that change color, read a book, or stare at a picture, all while their brains are being monitored, said Harris.

By running tests repeatedly, the computer can pick out which electrical signals always accompany a specific stimulus.

So far Callaway and others in the field can distinguish between a person looking at a green light and one looking at a red light. They have also found that quickness of response is in some unexplained way related to IQ as measured with standard intelligence tests.

In addition, he has found that concrete, analytical thinking is accompanied by increased electrical activity in the left hemisphere of the brain, while intuitive and abstract thought brings the right hemisphere into dominance.

What it adds up to, said Callaway, is the possibility of charting areas of dominance in individual brains and correlating them with mental skills displayed by those individuals.

Further in the future is the possibility of monitoring the actual messages — if they exist — being transmitted across the brain. It may then be possible to use electronics to tell what a person is thinking, he said.

Callaway admitted that the Orwellian possibilities "are undeniable." Among the misuses possible, although far in the future, would be government thought control.

THE PHYSICAL PROPERTIES OF MERCURY IMPORTANT IN ELECTRONICS: Erwin F. Lowry: Sylvania Electric Products Inc., Salem, Mass. Annals of New York Academy of Science. April 1957
"....No other element possesses characteristics so peculiarly and eminently suited to the requirements of a variety of electronic devices."

SUGGESTED READING: (The following equally important!) Who Should Play God? & Algeny, both books by J. Rifkin. DAEDALUS (Journal of the American Academy of Arts & Sciences) Summer 1967 Deliberate Efforts to Control Human Behavior and Modify Personality by G. C. Quarton. Physical Control of the Mind by J. Delgato, M.D. Manipulation (Dangers and Benefits of Brain Research) by Erwin Lausch. All the aforementioned refer to 'Electrical Stimulation of the Brain'. See Bibliography for publishers and dates.

Electromagnetic Body

Most scientists believe in observable physics, however, there is also the virtual state (non-observable) of physics.

In physics there are two states in the human being:

No. 1. The Observable State. (This state has to do with what you can see, feel, hear, taste and touch).

No. 2. The Virtual State. (This state involves high frequency, the thought processes, out of body experiences, ESP, etc.)

In 1973 information began being disseminated about the electromagnetic system. We are a bio-electromagnetic and electrochemical system.

Our thoughts and our bodies are joined to the universe. Our energy goes out into space. We are dealing with electromagnetic frequencies that occur out in space. We are in contact with space and we are in contact with ourselves.

The very fact that we have electrons spinning around protons at a specific angle, produces an electromagnetic field. This is why we say the entire body is an electromagnetic system. This is why we say everything within the universe (plants, matter, air, our bodies) is electromagnetic and produces frequencies.

Every part of the human body is vibrating to different frequencies. There are many billions of different frequencies in our body. Different parts of one organ vibrates at different frequencies.

Dr. James Ouye, D.D.S.

The following material on the electromagnetic body, machines for measuring this energy,silver(mercury)fillings, T cells, etc. was given in three separate seminars. Following are excerpts from these seminars.

The first lecturer Dr. Roy Smudde, DDS practices in Los Angeles and uses electro-diagnosis (the Acupath and Dermatron machines and other wholistic modalities) to diagnose his patients. Dr. Smudde speaks on the electromagnetic energy field of the body and explains how the teeth, jaw joint and cranial mechanism control the rest of the body. He goes on to explain how certain dental materials can interfere with this energy field if one is allergic to these dental materials.

The second lecturer, Dr. Patrick Flannagan, Ph.D. is in private research in Tucson, Arizona at the Source of Innergy Laboratory. Dr. Flannagan is an inventor and author of the book, Pyramid Power, and has also done research for the U.S. Government. He has worked for the Navy on the "Man Dolphin-Communications Program". He worked at the Aberdeen Proving Grounds for the

Department of Unconventional Weapons, Warfare and Devices. Dr. Flannagan is now in private research where he has over 5 different systems for measuring the energy or vitality of the human body.

The third lecturer Dr. David Eggleston, DDS is Clinical Associate Professor, Department of Advanced Prosthodontics, University of Southern California. He is also in private practice in Newport Beach. Dr. Eggleston is doing private research on Silver(mercury) Fillings and how they effect the T cells and the immune system in the body.

Dr. Eggleston speaks on the Dermatron Machine for measuring the electromagnetic energy of the body, T Cells, Silver(mercury) Fillings and their relation to AIDS. He goes on to tell about new tests for measuring the T Cell level in the body, and how Nickel jewelry (earrings) can have an allergic effect on the body and answers questions from the audience.

Dr. Eggleston reports on Dr. Reinhold Voll M.D., of Germany who is the inventor of the Dermatron Machine and discoverer of additional energy circuits (meridians) in the body. For this and many more contributions to science Dr. Voll is a candidate for the Nobel Prize in Sweden for 1983, 1984. This is a new catagory for Alternative Medicine.

1983 July Cancer Control Convention
Doctors' Seminar
Speaker: Dr. Roy Smudde, DDS
on: Acupath & Dermatron Machines and How to Identify and Measure These Energies, Etc.

Holistic Dentistry takes into consideration the full range of the total body, but specifically anything in the mouth or that is used in the mouth. Many times the dental materials used in the mouth are potential allergens.

One of the abilities of the Acupath machine is to test and to be able to use the correct homeopathic remedy to neutralize energies which may be causing allergies. Electro-diagnosis is the actual electrical instrument we use to measure the acupuncture points of the body.

When I became interested in the Dermatron which is an instrument that measures acupuncture points, I also became acquainted with acupuncture, homeopathy and soon incorporated into my practice the concepts of cranioosteopathic methods. Thus I began dealing with the electromagnetic energies of the body.

The last 8 years I have been working in this area I have found that all diseases begin in the electromagnetic energy field and if you are able to photograph it with a Kirlian Camera, you can then find out what is going on and then at this time have an idea or opportunity to prevent it. If you wait until most of us were "trained" to wait, e.g., "if you waited until you had periodontal disease, root canal therapy, or whatever, it would be to late to prevent." If you wait until you have an ulcer, diverticulitis, or maybe cancer, it is again to late to prevent. You have already gotten it. So, the idea of electro-diagnosis is to determine what is going on in the electromagnetic field before the disease process has set in, whereby you have actual cell destruction.

Medical doctors today are using all kinds of tests for disease, i.e., EKG, EEG, Cat Scans, Blood Tests, Urinalysis. They are looking at a patient who either has a disease or doesn't have a disease. They have some trends they can look at. They see some things, some patterns happening and they can start predicting possibilities, saying, "You are going to have this or that". But it is still a little bit of guess work on their part.

What I would like to say is that we can prevent disease before this. This is the reason why I feel electro-diagnosis is the mainstream of preventative health diseases, in medicine and dentistry. Whatever you want to prevent, you can diagnose it and find it early before it gets to be a disease.

...One of the main reasons I am interested in dealing with allergies and any other pathology in the body, (because I feel I know after working in the field for 8 years) is that electro-diagnosis shows that the electro-magnetic energy field of the body is controlled and governed by the teeth, by the jaw joints and by the cranial mechanism and the rest of the structure. Structure to me means joints, muscles, teeth and so forth. We are talking about hard and soft tissues and we are talking about electromagnetic energy fields.

I am stating to you that diseases in the body begin in the electromagnetic field, Consequently, the bottom line is, if you are going to find out the causes of disease, you need to understand how to diagnose the electromagnetic field of the body.

1983 National Health Federation Convention
Speaker: Pat Flannagan, Ph.D.
Lecture: Electrical Energy Fields of the Body, Etc.

Dr. Harold Saxon Burr a professor of neurology at Yale University developed a devise he called an "L" Field Meter, or "Life Field Meter". The doctor discovered that the human body is surrounded by a complex electrical 'grid' structure and that if you can measure this 'grid' structure, you can actually evaluate the health of the body electronically. This was long before we had acupuncture instruments, acupuncture measuring equipment.

This was long before doctors were using the 'EAV' (Dermatron) machine from Germany, the 'Acuomatic', the 'Acuscope' and all these different electronic devices.

Dr. Burr was doing this 40 years ago. He was able to detect certain kinds of cancer with 99.8% accuracy, electronically, before cancer became physically observable in the body. He wrote over two hundred papers on this medical research and basically we use in our lab a 'Burr Electrometer' and variations of the Burr Electrometer to measure the vitality and energy of the human system.

In using this we can detect instantaneously the effects of stress, e.g., if you think a negative thought it will be indicated on the meter. This electrometer will detect the stressful effects of a negative thought. Kinesiology (muscle testing) will also detect the effects of a negative thought, however, it is not as accurate as an electrometer.

Thought can have an effect on the strength of the body. Energy follows thought. When you think negative thoughts you destroy all your energy systems. You cannot separate the physical from the mental. You cannot separate the observer from the observed. It's all integrated, it's all part of the complete whole. Our thoughts effect not only ourselves but other people.

All types of stress throws the electrical energy field out of balance first, and then eventually it throws the biochemistry system out of balance. Our environment is full of hidden stresses, i.e., the clothes you wear effect your vitality. Polyester clothing can drain your body more then anything else; simply because we wear clothes most of the time. Polyester sheets drain the body also. You wake up with less energy than you did the day before.

So, anything that is a continuous stress to your body will drain your vitality. This includes toxins, (environmental toxins such as lead poisoning), various toxins you find in the air, nitrates, nitrites in the foods, etc. These are forms of toxins that creates continuous stress in the body. The thought stress, emotional stress, hidden stresses, i.e., like electrical lights, TV stations, electrical stations, electrical fields, etc., drain your electromagnetic energy. (See book: How Safe Are Silver (mercury) Fillings?-Chapter VII "Environmental Factors that Disturb the body") Order through Cancer Control Society, Los Angeles. Ca. 90027, (213) 663-7801.

1983 Wholistic Dental Convention
Speaker: Dr. David Eggleston, DDS
Lecture: Electro-Acupuncture According to Voll (Dermatron), T Cells, Etc.

The Chinese concept that the body's energy flows along invisible channels called meridians has been unacceptable to the scientific western mind. The Chinese believed that the main cause of sickness is an imbalance of energy in the body. Some parts of the body becoming over supplied with energy while other parts have too little energy. This theory that disease is caused by an imbalance of energy is over 5,000 years old; since it was impossible to prove scientifically it was discarded by modern doctors as of no value.

Today, however Dr. Reinhold Voll, a physician in West Germany has helped change this discarded concept, after fighting all the way to the German Supreme Court to legitimize his research.

For the past 30 years Dr. Voll has been developing, along with his collegues, a system of electrical acupuncture (EAV) using the Dermatron machine. To understand the electrical acupuncture technique he has developed, we need a basic understanding of acupuncture, electronics and homeopathy.

Atoms are the basic structure of everything in the universe. Everything you see, feel and touch is made of atoms. An atom is made up of protons and electrons. The proton is the positive charged part of the atom. The electron is the negative charged part of the atom. The proton takes the central position as in a nucleus, with the electron spinning around it. Atoms put together form molecules, and molecules put together form substances, and all atoms have an electromagnetic field.

Before you have any disease process you must have a disturbed electromagnetic field. Many things can disturb this field. For instance, bad bacteria, fungus, virus's, poisons, inflammatory process, osteioitis, caused by poisons such as is found in pesticides, radiation and toxic dental materials. (I tie in the above 'fungus' with Candida-Editor)

William Tiller, past chairman of the Material Science Department of Stanford theorizes acupuncture works like an antenna system. "When you put an acupuncture needle into an acupuncture point, it's like raising the antenna on your car radio. You put the needle in, and it allows the body to give off excess electromagnetic energy, or if there is not enough energy it can pick up electromagnetic energy from the environment."

Acupuncture is one of the oldest therapeutic means to restore an energetic balance which has been disturbed by disease. The most important points for therapy are located at the beginnings or ends of meridians on the hands, feet and head. Dr. Voll has taken great interest in these points for more than 20 years.

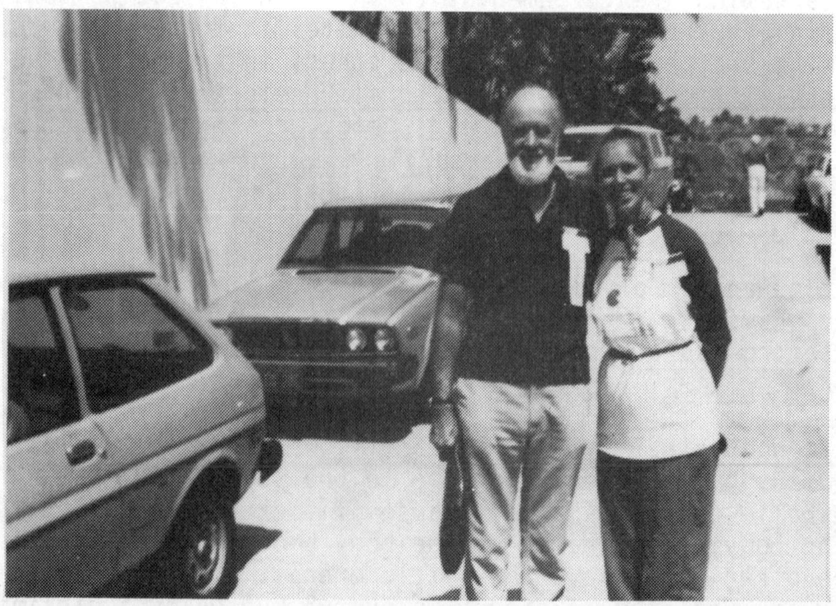

DR. WM. TILLER, Ph.D. of Stanford University, (a speaker at the 10th Mandala Holistic Health Conference) poses for photograph with Betsy.

San Diego
September 1984

Dr. Voll considering the above, felt indeed there was a relationship between pathology in the oral cavity and pathology elsewhere in the body. He then began studying the possibility of this relationship.

Dr. J. Thomsen, DDS and Dr. Voll mapped an electromagnetic connection between every tooth and the specific organs, muscles, and joints in the body. For an example, the front teeth (7,8,9 & 10) called incisors, are said to be connected meridian wise to the uro-genital system.

Benefits of "Electro-Acupuncture by Voll"

By 'EAV' measurements one can differentiate between acute, sub-acute and chronic inflammation; between initial, progressed or final degenerative processes in the body.

Every disease process begins by a change of the electrical potential, which can be identified by 'EAV' in its initial stages when the patient is still unaware of any sensations and when clinical conventional diagnosis cannot come forth with conspicuous results.

'EAV' can establish an immediate case report without prior access to the history of the patient, that is, based entirely on measurement readings. When location, severity of the disease, and the possible effects of the disturbance may be diagnosed in addition to latent initial diseases, and this coincides with findings from clinical exams; it can be taken as proof for the verification of acupuncture.

The 'EAV' method through the use of the Dermatron allows the dentist to determine chronic low level sensitivities to dental materials locally and systematically. This method also allows the dentist to measure the possible reaction to particular dental materials before they are placed into the oral cavity, and finally, this method allows the dentist to study the local and systemic effects of electrical current which has been produced by certain dissimilar and toxic metals.

The facet that has really interested me in this with dentistry, has been how we can implement this and how we can use it to further refine our dental skills in our dental diagnostic procedures. From using the Dermatron I've become somewhat aware that there is a possibility that certain dental materials may be harmful systemically. Before I got involved with the Dermatron and the electro-acupuncture, I was using amalgam and nickel based alloys rather extensively. ...Once you start using electro-acupuncture and start measuring some people, you won't use these materials. We saw major changes in electrical conductivity when we used these particular materials, mainly the nickel based alloys.

I would categorically state that no one should have nickel in their mouth.

Nickel has been used in dentistry for many years, with removable partial dentures. Removable partial dentures have up to 30% nickel. Many of them have no nickel at all. They are strictly chromium cobalt. Vitallium is a good example. There is no nickel in vitallium. Many of these chromium cobalt alloys have 5-10-15% nickel; it's a rare one that has up to 30. Those particular alloys have seemingly been well tolarated by patients. They have been used for many, many years. The newer based alloys have 60 to 80% nickel. Some of them have up to 1.8% beryllium. This is an entirely different situation with nickel at this percentage.

Laboratory animals that get nickel implanted into the body develop a high incidence of sarcomas and carcinomas and so forth. Those studies have been very well documented. There are similar metals which have been placed in as controls where no cancer developed, so it is definitely the nickel.

Nickel is used routinely by the national cancer centers to induce cancer in laboratory animals to study cancer. The nickel alloys they use are very similar to what we are putting in people's mouths. About 80% of the dental community is using nickel based alloys for porcelain fused to metal crowns.

The other factor that is involved here is the allergenic property of nickel. Nickel is the most allergenic metal known. There are more people allergic to nickel then all other metals combined. It's outright 9% of the female population and 9/10 of 1% of the male population. The theory is that the difference is because of jewelry. Nickel is also used in cosmetics. In the dyes for the coloring of the cosmetics; there are nickel oxides, and so forth.

So nickel is used in jewelry and nickel is used in cosmetics and that is why women have 10 times the incidence of nickel sensitivity as men. Men that pierce their ears have 33 times the incidence of nickel sensitivity as men that don't pierce their ears. That's in the ADA report (April 1982 Issue). We see this increase with women who pierce their ears; they have about 6 times the incidence of nickel sensitivity as women who don't pierce their ears.

In this ADA report it stated that the gold platinum in the nickel jewelry have gaps in it that you can see under a microscope. Just the infinitesimal amount of nickel that shows in the gaps of the gold plating is enough to sensitize a patient to nickel. That really blows your mind when you stop to think of the nickel we are putting in the mouth. Here you are talking about a fleeting contact of epithelia in a pierced earlobe on a gold plated nickel stud and the amount that is exposed on a microscopic level, and the exposure only lasts until the epithelium heals. Now we are talking about putting nickel in permanently in an area that has chronic inflammation and chronic irritation. It is imperative that the ADA run some research to determine if people with nickel restorations in their mouth have a higher incidence of nickel sensitivity than people that don't have nickel in their mouths.

The real problem is that when people are allergic to nickel they have a systemic reaction with no oral manifestation in most cases. So, I talk to dentists and they say I have been using nickel for 5 years and I don't see any problems in the mouth. The problem is not in the mouth. It occurs systemically. Joseph Moffa did some excellent research on this. He took ten patients with nickel sensitivity in all ten of them he put dental nickel alloys in their mouths and 8 of them had systemic reaction with no oral manifestation-8 out of 10. Moffa published this in the Journal of Dental Research and he further reported it in the Journal of Prosthetic Dentistry and then it was reported for a third time in the Journal of the American Dental Association. This is a classic study.

When you talk about 9% of females and 1% of males, you are talking about 12,000,000 people in the United States that shouldn't have nickel put in their mouth; that have a previous nickel sensitivity, let alone the number of people who are becoming nickel sensitive from the alloy that goes in the mouth. If 80% of those have a systemic manifestation, dentists are causing a major health problem....we are wiping out millions of people.

There is a dentist, a very close friend of mine, who practices in the Orange County area. He had one nickel crown placed on a lower molar and that night he broke out with a rash on his neck. That rash stayed there for a period of 6 months and finally I saw him and said, "Why don't we get rid of that nickel crown? After we had measured him, (Dermatron), He got up in the night at 2 o'clock in the morning and looked at his neck and that rash was gone.

It was interesting because in doing this research on nickel articles, I was reading Fisher's textbook on dermatology. His textbook is called Contact Dermatitis. It is a standard medical textbook and he lists in there that the most common systemic location from dermatitis from nickel allergy is on the neck. So, if someone is allergic to nickel and they put on a nickel bracelet they can break out with a rash on the neck. He also listed the thigh, the inner part of the thigh, and the neck as the two most common spots.

I do feel that people are being adversely affected by nickel and yet as dentists we just look in the mouth and the patient may slowly be developing some auto-immune problem, and that patient doesn't come back to your office. That patient goes to see a physician and then the physician will treat it symptomatically with cortisone and histamines and so forth.

Q. You mentioned nephritis as one of the things happening from nickel poisoning. Did you find a list of systemic problems which, if we heard the patient had we might suspect nickel or put us on our guard?

A. There was not a direct nickel toxicity that we can demonstrate.

The nickel seems to effect the auto-immune system. So, patients that have auto-immune diseases are the ones you should watch out for. Auto-immune diseases are arthritis, Amyotrophic Lateral Schlerosis (Lou Gehrig Disease)

Lupus-Erythematosis, Multiple Sclerosis and some forms of cancer. These are auto-immune types of diseases. We are looking for problems with the immune system. When we put something in the mouth that effects the immune system; we look for a problem that is an auto-immune problem.

"T" Cells

The state of the art in immunology now, on laboratory testing is with "T" cells. "T" cells are going to become more and more important. They really hit the journals because its the "T" cell problem with this virus that is passed between homosexuals; the A.I.D.S. problem (Acquired Immune Deficiency Syndrome) and "T" cells in someone with A.I.D.S., the "T-4" really drops down.

The "T" cells are a type of white blood cells. If you remember back from dental school, there are white blood cells made from bone marrow and there are white blood cells made from lymph nodes. The white bone cells that come from bone marrow would be the neutrophils, macrophages, basophils, macrophasias & eosinophils, these come from bone marrow. The ones that come from lymph nodes are the lymphocytes and of the lymphocytes, about 70% should be "T" cells. "T" cells mean that those white blood cells go through the thymus gland. Remember we were told the thymus gland was a vestigial organ; now it turns out to be an extremely valuable organ, because it mediates the "T" cells which have this tremendous effect on the immune system. I remember when kids had their thymus gland removed if they were chronically ill!

The "T" cells are white blood cells that are lymphocytes, that go through the thymus gland, and when they go through the thymus gland they become activated. They reach maturity. There are 10 types of "T" cells but only 2 types that are important. The "T-4" and the "T-8". The "T-4" cell is what is called the "T" helper cell. It's like the guy who walks through the forest and paints an 'X' on the trees that the logging crew has to come in and chop down. It's the one that identifies the cancer cells. It identifies the foreign bodies, it identifies the bacteria, *fungus, virus, etc.

The killer white blood cells, the macrophages, that engulf or phagocytize these foreign bodies, they don't know what to eat, unless that particle or organism has been labeled by a "T-4". In people with AIDS it wipes out their "T-4's". They have plenty of white blood cells to kill off bacteria and foreign bodies, but they are not labelled. So, these people are dying from the simplest forms of infection. They get a fungus or a staff or streph, and they die from it, because they don't have "T-4's" to go around and label the bad guys. So, the "T'4's" are the helper cells, they identify and they label the material that the other white blood cells (soldiers) come along and engulf.

The other "T" cell that is important is the "T-8". The "T-8" cell is the one that prevents the soldiers or killer white cells from becoming rogues (military police). The "T-8's" keep order in the soldiers' ranks in the macrophagia and neutrophils, etc. If you don't have enough "T-8's" your own white blood cells will run rampant and start attacking yourself, and that is the auto-immune diseases. If you don't have "T-8's" you have a problem in that your white blood cells may attack your joints, create arthritis or aggrevate it or may attack

*Candidiasis (Editor's Note)

myelin sheath and give you Multiple Sclerosis or attack collagen. Or you get a skin disease like lupus, scleraderma, or whatever.

LABORATORY TESTS FOR "T" CELLS

There are two laboratory tests you can get at this time by Smith-Kline. It is the best known and is the most highly regarded labs in the country. They can give you 2 tests. They can give you a test for total "T" cells They can also give you a "T-4", "T-8" ratio. You should have 1.5 to 2.2 (T'4's") for every "(T-8"). You should have 1.5 to 2.4 ("T-4's") for every % of ("T-8") you have.

People with AIDS have only .14'T" cells for every "T-8" they have. So, their "T-4's" are wiped out. The research we are doing in the office right now, is measuring "T" cells before, during and after we insert and remove amalgam and nickel based alloys. We are seeing the "T" cells just going crazy.

With most of the patients we are seeing, we are taking their amalgams out. We do it with consent. What we are doing with amalgam is we are measuring "T" cells baseline. We take the amalgam out, measure the blood, then we put the amalgam back in; remeasure the blood, then take it out again and put in gold or whatever and measure it again. With patients on the nickel, they are usually patients that come in with nickel. We measure the blood, then we take the nickel out and see if the "T" cell improves. Especially someone with a kidney disorder. (Referring to Case No. 1)* She had had this tremendous improvement the urologist said no one heals from (glomerulonephritis) at this stage. You get a +4 protein and creatine clearance that just doesn't heal. The way to confirm this, is to put the nickel back in. But it is hard to get the patient to accept that. So, it is really tough doing research and is not as simple as it sounds.

T CELLS AND 'SLIDES SHOWN'

Here is a patient that came in and really the number of amalgams present is not all that over-whelming. She had 2 class-1 amalgams, 1 class 2 amalgams upper and on the lower she had 3-class 1 amalgams. We measured this particular patient's total "T" cell level. Her total "T" cell level was at 47. The initial test you can get from Smith-Kline Lab. They have two tests; one will give you total "T" cell count and "T" cell % of lympocytes and the data I am going to give here is % of lympocytes that are "T" cells. You can also get a "T-4" to "T-8" ratio. That particular test has only been available the last few months. They use laser beam technology and monoclonal antibodies (which is the state of the art in immunology) to determine the "T-4"/"T-8" ratio.

I did some work with amalgams trying to find expressences of the work that Hal Huggins (dentist) has been doing and so forth. I tried to duplicate that and we could see some changes and some results, but it was nothing like what we are getting with "T" cells. (I have to talk to Hal about this-get him to do the "T" cell work as well). Because this is much more definitive and much more widely accepted in the medical community. "T" cells are used by physicians routinely on procedures. So they will accept that data.

*Not included here.

You have to wait 3 to 4 weeks before you will see a new balance of "T" cells from the variable that you have created. So, this particular patient was in her 20's, totally asymptomatic; on a woman's soccer team, good physical condition. She happens to be my dental assistant and she volunteered to go through this testing. Her "T" cell level was 47, which is extremely low. We took out the amalgams and prepared for gold inlays. We cleaned out every speck of amalgam. (I used TAB, we are finding less of a reaction to TAB then we are to other acrylic resins-made by Kerr). We seem to get less reaction with people who are chemically sensitive or have allergy problems. This material works very well. It is easily accessible through Kerr.

We made temporary restorations and placed those in the mouth. Then we waited 3 to 4 weeks with these temporary restorations. We re-took the blood test. Her "T" cell level went up to 73. I talked to the chief pathologist at Smith-Kline, Dr. Joe Patero and it just absolutely blew him away. They are working at Smith-Kline Laboratory in their pharmaceutical trying to get drugs to raise the "T" cell level. They haven't done anything like this! We got more of a "T" cell rise by taking out a few amalgams then they did by trying to raise it with drugs!

Q. What is the ideal "T" cell level?

A. The ideal "T" cell level is somewhere in the 70's. They say the average range is 50 to 80, but the closer to 80 the better and if you are depressed on your "T" cells then you have a higher percentage/chance of getting cancer, infectious diseases or auto-immune diseases, if your body can't identify the cancer cells it can't fight them.

A lot of the cancer research being done right now is to get the "T" cells up. Just from this preliminary data, I wouldn't want amalgam in anyone that is susceptible to cancer; has a family history of cancer or has already been diagnosed with cancer.

Q. How did you seat the temporary restorations?

A. I seated them with Kerr's Temp Bond Cement. We thought we might keep the "T" cells depressed if she was allergic to the temporary resins or the temporary cement. But fortunately she wasn't. Incidentally we checked her ahead of time with the Dermatron so we knew that she could handle the cement.

The first visit where we took out the amalgams, we made impressions, and the laboratory during this phase was making the gold inlay restorations. We bought her back into the chair and I just drilled some 'pits' into the temporaries and plugged them with amalgam. So, it didn't require any anesthetic. We just drilled some 'pot holes' into the temporaries and this incidentally was the first amalgam I had placed in three years.

The amount (amalgam) I put back in was somewhat less then what she had originally. I didn't put any in the upper jaw and these are somewhat smaller then the original ones and we put them in and just left them in for a month and rechecked the "T" cell level and it went back down to '55'. Now, again talking with the pathologist at Smith-Kline, the maximum they have been able to find on any control is 10% change from month to month. They have not identified a control yet that shifts more then 10%, so when she started at 47, if this was not a variable,(the maximum we could have seen in a change would have been up to 53), but it went up to '73' and by putting the amalgam back in, the maximum drop we could have expected was maybe down to '67' or so. The lab error was in the 10%.

They have done multiple blood drawing on the same patient at the same time and run it through separately. In other words, in the work on "T" cells, we don't have to run controls, because the controls have already been done. They know what the laboratory error is and they know what the standard deviation is on the control from month to month. That has been done on a large number of people.

They are using the "T" cell test to determine the immuno-suppressive effect of cancer-chemotheraputic agents. Smith-Kline is developing chemotherapy for cancer patients, and they want to know what the suppression of the immune system is as a side effect, and they use the "T" cell. They developed this test to develop cancer theraputic drugs and it turns out that the A.I.D.S epidemic hit at the same time they developed this technology.

As far as I know this really is the first hard data on a single patient with amalgam-where we could actually measure an increase and then a decrease doing it in reverse. (Dr. Eggleston is referring to the 'T' Cells-Editor)*

Q. Is Smith-Kline only in L.A.?

A. No, they have labs across the country. The one I am using is in Woodland Hills.

THE SMITH-KLINE "T" CELL TEST-WHAT TO ASK FOR

If you want the "T" cell test run, ask for what they call the Immune Deficiency Evaluation (IDE). It requires a vena puncture and drawing 4 test tubes of blood and a peripheral smear from the ear lobe or from the end of a digit. Cost $125.00

To get the"T-4"/"T-8"ratio that is another $145.00 in addition to the $125.00. It is a totally separate test. You don't want to run the "T-4"/"T-8" ratio until you determine that there is a suppression of the "T" cells. Use the $125.00 as a screen and then run the "T-4"/"T-8".

I haven't run the T-4/T-8 ratios yet. All the data we are collecting is strictly T cell level. Before we publish we will have to run some T-4/T-8 ratios, just to avoid the criticism that we are not using the ultimate state of the art test.

*This study was published in the Journal of Prosthetic Dentistry, Titled: Effect of Dental Amalgam and Nickel Alloys on T-lymphocytes: Prelimary Report- May 1984, page 617

I would like to know on dental materials, whether we are suppressing the "T-4" or the "T-8" or both. Again, it doesn't occur on every patient with amalgam. Before we change the amalgam we run the "T" cell test. If the "T" cells are normal then we only change the amalgam for any other reason; mechanically they need replacing, or the patient is worried about a future problem with it.

Q. How did she respond to the Dermatron?

A. We measured her with the alloys in place and we had a rather significant indicator drop, which was neutralized with the homeopathic preparation for amalgams. Then when we took out the amalgams we measured her at that time. Before we took out the amalgams she had the drop and as soon as we took it out, she had no drop.

<u>I feel within a couple of years the ADA will be forced to put a warning on amalgam that it cannot be used with patients with auto-immune disease or allergy type problems. That's forthcoming</u>.

<u>NICKEL</u>

WE are doing the same testing with nickel. I have a patient now who had no restorations in his mouth whatsoever. He broke off a central incisor, and we made 2 crowns for him. One with the all-porcelain cerestor crown, and another one with a nickel based crown. We just sent it out to a commerical lab and got a nickel crown made. We are going to run him through the same way. Put in the nickel. We will check him again with the nickel in place.

When this nickel alloy goes in the mouth we see this drastic change in these meridians. The nickel effects everyone. It caused an increase in the reading on everyone we have tested with the nickel. But it causes an indicator drop on only a percentage of those. So, not everyone has an indicator drop created by it <u>but everyone has an elevated or inflammatory type of response from it. It is universal</u>.

Q. Can you diagnose nickel under a crown with electro-acupuncture?

A. We can't completely. We put on a homeopathic dilution of nickel and we see if it improves the measurement. Again, that is a research level technology. But the problem is that we could get that to occur on someone that might be sensitized by nickel in jewelry and so forth. It's not specific to dental nickel. The patient could be sensitized from jewelry and we can neutralize that with a nickel dilution, whether it is coming from their dental nickel or some other source.

Because nickel is ubiquitous, it just occurs everywhere. It's in our water. in our cosmetics, in our dyes, in our teeth, it is just everywhere. Everyone is exposed to it to some degree. So, it is not uncommon to find an improvement when we use a serial dilution of nickel. We can't do a differential diagnosis to show that it is coming from the teeth. We can get a pretty good idea.

There are two tests coming up to check for nickel in the mouth. One is a dye that you place on the nickel. You paint it on the nickel. You paint it on the nickel and it changes color because nickel is continually being given off, or corroded off, the alloy. If you paint it on something where no nickel is coming to the surface, or leaching out, then it won't change color. That is one way of testing for nickel. The other way (Insurance Companies are concerned because they know that 80% of all the crowns made are being made with nickel based alloys), yet the majority of crowns being submitted for payment are porcelain fused to gold. So, either the dentists are unaware of what they are putting in the mouth or there is out-right fraud. That is a whole other problem that the ADA is going to start to deal with. So, the insurance companies are developing an instrument whereby shining a light on the metal, by the reflection of the light, they can tell a specific gravity. So, they can tell if a precious or non-precious alloy was used, just by shining the light on it. We can tell if nickel is in the mouth, but not with a Dermatron.

I don't feel dentistry as a health profession, has a right to put mercury in the mouth or nickel. I am getting hard line on that. We should do the research first to prove that it is safe, before we use the material rather then do the research to prove that it is harmful

NOTE: FOR DENTISTS & PHYSICIANS:LIFE SCIENCES CENTER PROJECT is doing research in electroacupuncture point measurement devices-For further information call (714) 664 4711.
See March 1985 issue of East West Journal regarding the COMPUTRONIX - a computer interface to simplify diagnosis & treatment of Electro-Acupuncture according to Voll, call or write COMPUTRONIX, 25825-104th Ave., S.E., Suite 302, Kent. Wa. 98031- (206) 630-4331. P.S. This adjunct to E.A.V. puts the use within grasp of your technician who has less training than yourself!

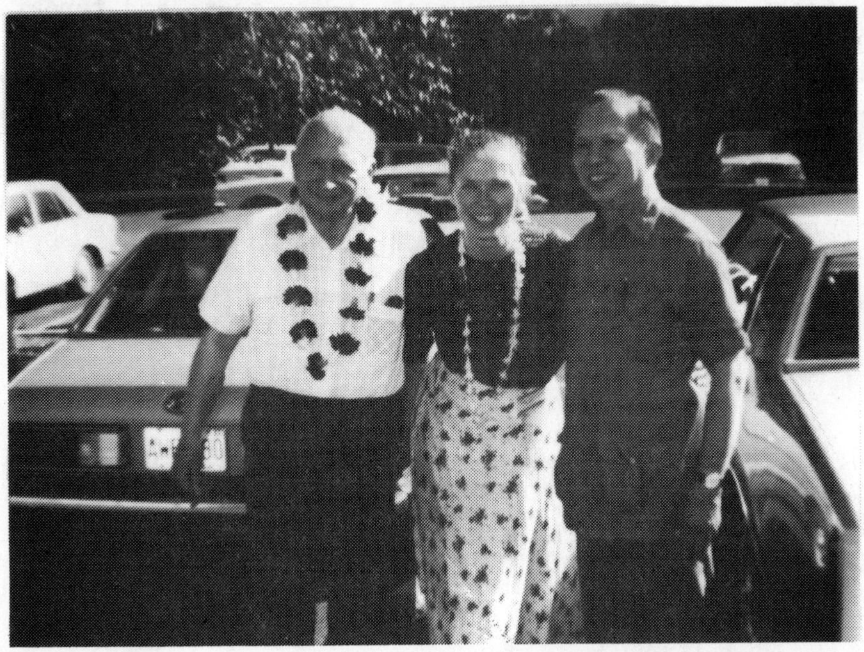

Betsy poses with Dr. R. Voll, M.D. & Dr. W. Khoe, M.D. at Voll Seminar in Hawaii. Both Dr. Voll & Dr. Khoe were Candidates for Nobel Prize in Medicine 1984.
August 1984

XIV

DENTAL GALVANISM—LEUKOPLAKIAS—CANDIDA

THE CONNECTION BETWEEN GALVANIC CURRENT, LEUKOPLAKIA-CANDIDIASIS, AIDS AND CANCER

GALVANISM

Galvanism is a condition in which burns and other soft tissue changes such as gingivitis, bleeding, are caused by a potential difference created by dissimilar metals in the oral cavity, with saliva serving as the electrolyte. ...."Galvinism results from the production of an electric current." (Cheraskin, E. DDS.:THE DYNAMICS OF ORAL DIAGNOSIS 1956)

LEUKOPLAKIA

Leukoplakia is the formation of white, smooth spots or patches, irregular in size and shape, on the mucous membrane of the cheek. The lesions are usually benign, but may become malignant. (New Webster's Med. Dictionary 1981)

HYPERPLASIA & LEUKOPLAKIA

Symptoms of galvanism: Pathogenic changes in the blood and kidneys causing hyperplasia (excessive increase in the number of normal cells in the tissue of an organ, resulting in an increase of its size), and leukoplakia of the soft tissue which may finally become malignant in extreme cases in which the metallic restorations are of radically different electropotentialities. J.A.M.A. 100:717 (March 11) 1933 (See two pages over for entire article)

Once this irritation (Leukoplakia) of the mucous membrane is established and continuous (because of silver/nickel fillings) the fungi, Candida, will then make its home in this area and flourish in the mouth and throat area. Once Candida is given full reign through improper diet (sweets), irritation in the mouth area, improper 'ph' balance and improper bowel functioning (sometimes caused by Candida), this can in turn overpower the thymus, paralyzing it from maturing and releasing the 'T' Cells which protect the body from foreign invaders. You then have the shutting down of the immune system and the opening up of the body to any opportunistic organism, such as cancer, etc. Editor-

---

Inovay, J. and Banocyz, J.: The role of electrical potential differences in the etiology of chronic diseases of the oral mucosa. J.D. Res. 40-894-889, 1961

"Measurements were made on 69 subjects, in which the following clinical diagnoses could be established: leukoplakia, 22 cases....."

Because of the simultaneous use of dissimilar metals is common in modern dentistry, their practical importance in the etiology of oral diseases is great.

Potential measurements in the oral cavity were performed in 109 instances on 69 patients who suffered chronic disease of the mucous membrane and did not respond to the usual treatment. In some cases, remarkable improvement was noted when harmfully high potentials were eliminated.

Solomon, Harold A.: The possibility of precancerous oral lesions from electrical causes. The Dental Digest. 39:142-144, April 1333

Among the many sources of irritation which can be considered as possible factors in the production of precancerous lesions in the oral cavity may be included the electrical irritation effect produced by some combinations of metals used for filling teeth and constructing other dental restorations. Bloodgood states, "Now and then a patch of leukoplakia can be produced by the irritation of a tooth, especially one with a metallic filling.

Our observations as well as those of other investigators indicate the possibility of production of benign, precancerous, and malignant oral lesions from the effect of electrical irritation of some combinations of metals used for restoring lost tooth structure.

Schriever, Wm.: Electromotive forces and electric current. Journal of Dental Research. April 1952

Since 1933 several papers have appeared in which are described cases of stomatitis, leukoplakia and oral cancer which were believed to have been caused by electrogalvanic action of dental restorations.

Cheraskin, E.: Dynamics of Oral Diagnosis. The Year Book Publ. Company 1956

Erythema with congestion of the soft tissue, blanching of the mucosa, divided patches with ulceration, and even areas of leukoplakia may be noted. The patient may complain of burning sensation especially related to the eating of spiced foods.

Treatment- Once the diagnosis has been established, and this is not always a simple matter, therapy consists of removal of the metallic restorations.

Silverman, Sol: Oral Candidiasis in the Healthy and Compromised Patient Lecture: For University of California-San Francisco, Sept. 21, 1984; "John Gurley Memorial Lecture"

Dr. Silverman, Professor and Chairman, Division of Oral Medicine, University of California-San Francisco, stated, "Candida can increase Leukoplakia which can go into cancer."

CANDIDIASIS: AN INFECTIOUS DISEASE OF INCREASING IMPORTANCE
Maxwell G. Shepherd: New Zealand Dental Journal 78:89, July 1982

With the increases use of antibiotics, corticosteroids, and immuno suppressive agents there has also been an increase in the prevalence of Candidiasis. There are several forms of oral Candidiasis including oral thrush, denture stomatitis, speckled oral leukoplakias, and angular cheilitis.

Published In

Journal of American Medical Association, Mar. 11, 1933

Reprinted in Dental Digest 1933

Electrogalvanic Lesions—*Lain*

I. NEWLY DISCOVERED ORAL CAVITY PHENOMENON:

"The human saliva is a good electrolyte and dissimilar metallic dentures* constitute the necessary electrodes; therefore, within every oral cavity containing dissimilar metallic dentures there is a complete galvanic battery."

II. SYMPTOMS

A. Objective—Changes in Metallic Dentures
1. Discoloration
2. Areas of erosion
3. Disintegration
4. Loosening of restorations
5. Possible maladjustment of dentures

B. Objective—Changes in Oral Tissues
1. Acute or chronic inflammatory, blanched or grayish patches, erosions, or ulcers
2. Leukoplakia on the gingival or buccal membranes beneath, adjacent to, or surrounding the metallic dentures
3. Metallic pigmentation of the mucous membranes

C. Subjective
1. Metallic or salty taste
2. Increased salivary secretion
3. Burning tongue
4. Dryness or tickling sensation in the throat
5. Nerve soreness, nerve shocks, nervous irritability
6. Indigestion and loss of weight
7. Pathogenic changes in the blood and kidneys causing hyperplasia and leukoplakia of the soft tissue which may finally become malignant in extreme cases in which the metallic restorations are of radically different electropotentialities

III. FACTORS INFLUENCING ELECTRIC CURRENT

A. Total surface or volume of the dissimilar metals
B. Chemical variation of the saliva
C. Resistance of tissues and distance between dentures
D. Duration—time since the restoration of the first and the subsequent dissimilar dentures
E. Relative position of the dissimilar metals in the electromotor series (most important)

IV. CONCLUSIONS

A. Infections, tobacco, and other causes of oral lesions must first be eliminated before a positive diagnosis of electrogalvanic phenomenon is made, although these other causes may augment electrogalvanic injuries.

B. Positive cases of electrogalvanic injuries are promptly relieved by removal of the offending dentures and substituting others that are of uniform electropotentiality.

C. In order to avoid the serious pathologic changes resulting from the electrogalvanic phenomenon, manufacturing dental laboratories are urged to offer to the profession satisfactory denture materials that are of the same electropotentiality.

—Lain, E. S.: Electrogalvanic Lesions of the Oral Cavity Produced by Metallic Dentures, J.A.M.A. 100:717 (March 11) 1933.

*Editor's Note: In this communication the author uses the term "dentures" in a sense not usually accepted as good dental usage; that is, he includes all metal restorations, plates, bridges, crowns, or fillings under the term "dentures."

Please Note: Editor's note on bottom left of article states, " In this communication the author uses the term "dentures" in a sense not usually accepted as good dental usage; that is, he includes all metal restorations plates, bridges, crowns, or fillings under the term "dentures".

CHRONIC ORAL CANDIDIASIS AND LEUKOPLAKIA

R.A. Cawson, M.B., B.S., B.D.S., F.D.S., M.C. Path., London England
Department of Dental Medicine, Guy's Hospital Medical School
Oral Surgery 22, 582 (1966)

Findings

Among 138 specimens of leukoplakia, 15 showed evidence of candidiasis,

Addendum

It may be of interest to note that since the period covered by this article (that is, in little longer than one year) no fewer than fifteen additional cases of chronic candidiasis have been seen or the diagnosis has been made on biopsy specimens.

OCCURANCE OF CANDIDA IN ORAL LEUKOPLAKIAS

Grete Renstrup: Dental Department, University Hospital, Copenhagen, and Departments of Oral Pathology and Oral Surgery, Royal Dental College, Copenhagen, Denmark

Biopsies from 235 patients with oral leukoplakias were investigated, (83 speckled leukoplakias, and 152 homogeneous leukoplakias). A candidal invasion was found in 23 per cent of the leukoplakias (in 61 per cent of the speckled leukoplakias, and in 3 per cent of the homogeneous leukoplakias.

THE PREVALENCE OF ORAL CARRIERS OF CANDIDA IN PATIENTS WITH TONGUE ABNORMALITIES

Journal of Dentistry, 11, No. 4, 1983 pp 313-317 Printed in Great Britain
A. Kullaa-Mikkonen, DDS
R. Kotilainen, DDS
Institute of Oral Surgery, Department of Dentistry, University of Kuopio, Finland

ABSTRACT

The prevalence of oral carriers of Candida in patients with tongue abnormalities was investigated among 51 patients and 23 controls. The salivary sample technique was used; salivary pH was measured. In the control group and in the fissured tongue group negative fungus growth was prominent. A positive culture was found in 16.6 per cent of the patients with filiform atrophy. Patients with geographic tongue had the highest carrier rate (90 per cent) compared with all the other tongue groups. A positive culture was found in 66.7 per cent of the patients with hairy tongue. A relationship between oral yeasts and salivary acidity was found, candidal carriers had a lower salivary pH than non-carriers.

ORAL "HAIRY" LEUCOPLAKIA IN MALE HOMOSEXUALS: EVIDENCE OF ASSOCIATION WITH BOTH PAPILLOMAVIRUS AND A HERPES-GROUP VIRUS

The Lancet, October 13, 1984: D. Greenspan, M. Conant, S. Silverman, J. Greenspan, V. Petersen, Y. De Souza: Department of Stomatology, (Divisions of Oral Medicine and Oral Biology), Dermatology, and Pathology, Schools of Dentistry and Medicine, University of California, San Francisco, California, USA

Summary: An outbreak of a new form of oral leucoplakia, found principally on the lateral borders of the tongue, is reported in male homesexuals in the San Francisco area. Many of the patients showed evidence of immunosuppression, and candida (26 of 37 cases) was often found in the lesions. ....This leucoplakia may presage AIDS, may be associated with both papillomavirus and a herpes-type virus.

Discussion: Harry leucoplakia appears to be a new entity found, as yet exclusively, in the mouths of male homosexuals. It fits the definition of leucoplakia currently used and we have added the adjective "hairy" because of the clinical and histological features. There is evidence that the patients are immunosuppressed and that a substantial proportion progress to AIDS.

The lesion is of interest for at least three further reasons. Firstly, recent reports suggest a previously unsuspected and possibly widespread role for papillomavirus in oral epithelial hyperplasia, dysplasia, and even oral carcinoma. Several cases of oral cancer in male homosexuals have been described.....

STATISTICS ON DENTAL GALVANISM REPORTS

1879 US	1961 HUNGARY
1880 US	1969 SWEDEN
1902 CANADA	1974 HOLLAND
1933 US	1977 US*
1933 CANADA	1977 US**
1933 US	1978 SWEDEN
1941 US	1980 US***
1952 US	1980 SWEDEN
1952 US	1980 GERMANY
1954 US	1982 SWEDEN
1956 US	1982 SWEDEN
1957 US	1981 SWEDEN

Upon scrutinizing the published Journals concerning research on oral galvanism, it was found that all publications concerning this subject seemed to have ended in the US in 1957 except for the *1977 US report (stating views do not reflect US Government views) and the ***1980 US report on chromium-type alloys only (No report on silver or copper); and a **1977 US report which indicates using silver nitrite on galvanic current.

SOME RESULTS OF DENTAL GALVANISM REPORTED FROM THE ABOVE JOURNALS

#1	1961 Hungary	Cancer
#2	1980 US	Adverse Tissue Response
#4	1978 Sweden	Harmful effects on tissue
#5	1980 Sweden	Corrosion
#6	1933 US	Cancer
#7	1957 US	Corrosion
#8	1952 US	Cancer
#12	1880 US	Mercury Vaporizes into body
#13	1969 Sweden	Skin disease
#15	1956 US	Leukoplakia
#19	1933 US	Cancer (AMA Report)
#25	1965 Sweden	Soft Issue Irritations
#22	1980 Germany	Irritation of Nervous System & psyche

	Date	Material Written In	Title and Journal or Book Material Published In
1.	1961	Hungary	The Role of Electrical Potential Differences in the Etiology of Chronic Diseases of the Oral Mucosa Journal of Dent. Research
2.	1980	US	Electrochemical Behavior of Surgical Alloys (Refers to Vitallium & Ticonium metals only) Military Medicine
3.	1977	US	Dental Pain of Galvanic Origin: Report of One Case Journal of Endod.* *Note at end of article: "The views expressed herein are those of the authors and do not necessarily reflect the views of the United States Air Force or the Department of Defense.
4.	1978	Sweden	Potential and Polarization Measurements in Vivo of the Oral Galvanism Scand. J. Dental Research
5.	1980	Sweden	Galvanic Curents Between Gold and Amalgam Scand. J. Dent. Research
6.	1933	US	The Possibility of Precancerous Oral Lesions From Electrical Causes The Dental Digest
7.	1957	US	Electrolytic Action in the Mouth and its Relationship to Pain Journal Dental Research
8.	1952	US	Electromotive Forces and Electric Current Journal of Dental Research
9.	1902	Canada	Electric Currents of the Oral Cavity Dominion Dental Journal
10.	1954	US	Electric Currents in the Mouth Science of Dental Materials
11.	1941	US	Corrosion of Amalgam JADA
12.	1880	US	Oral Electricity and the New Departure Dental Cosmos
13.	1969	Sweden	Allergy to Copper Derived from Dental Alloys as a Possible Cause of Oral Lichen Planus Sweden

14. 1933 Canada Dissimilar Metals in the Mouth as a Possible Cause of Otherwise Unexplainable Symptoms
The Canadian Medical Association Journal

15. 1956 US Dynamics of Oral Diagnosis
The Year Book Publishing Company

16. 1879 US Filled Teeth as Galvanic Batteries
The Dental Cosmos

17. 1974 Holland Dental Amalgam - A Poison in Our Mouth
Toxicology

18. 1952 US Electromotive Forces and Electric Currents Caused by Metallic Dental Fillings
Journal of Dental Research

19. 1933 US Electrogalvanic Lesions
Journal of American Medical Assoc.

20. 1982 Sweden Intraoral currents and taste thresholds.
Swed. Dent. Journal

21. 1981 Sweden Oral galvanic action after treatment with extensive metallic restorations.
Swedish Dental Journal Supplement

22. 1980 Germany Resistance to therapy
Medical Practice

23. 1982 Sweden On intraoral potential-and polarization. measurements of metallic restorations
Acta Odontologica Scand.

24. 1977 US Report of the Committee on Scientific investigation of the american academy of restorative dentistry.
J. Prosthet. Dent.

25. 1965 Sweden Studies of the transport of metal ions from gold inlays into environmental tissues.
Acta Odont. Scand.

GALVANIC CURRENT

Excerpts from 1983 Lecture-Holistic Dental Convention
Dr. D. Eggleston, D.D.S.

"Galvanic current can occur between dissimilar metals in the mouth, that's the way a battery works. You've got two different metals and a battery and we get a flow of electrons from one metal to the other; from one metal that has a high potential to another that has the low electrical potential. So, when you have dissimilar metals you have the possibility of this galvanic flow of electrical current. When we have metals in the mouth we have this dissimilar metal phenomena and this galvanic current. It's created quite a bit of research and discussion among dentists and it can create tooth sensitivity. If you place a gold restoration in the mouth that has a lot of amalgams, some of that tooth sensitivity may be due to this galvanic current. A person doing most of the research on this is a Dr. Wolf at the National Institute of Dental Research in Bethesda, Maryland. If you write to him he will send you a series of articles he has published and that he has on file. There are articles in the literature that demonstrate this. He says he is measuring people around 17 microamps of current.

I bought a potentiometer which is nothing more then an AMP meter and a Volt meter and we will measure some people here today.

I had a patient in within the last week who did go off the end of the meter. This meter goes up to 30 microamps. I have no idea what her total microamps or current is. It is a patient that has been in chronic pain for years with her dental work. We do have indication that this galvanic current can be harmful and Voll and Dr. Thomsen (dentist in Hamburg)has reported that anywhere over 2 or 3 microamps can create a problem.

The mouth should be isoletric. There should be no current going through the mouth. All major acupuncture circuits go through the teeth. We mentioned that the central lateral incisors, upper and lower relate to the kidney and urinary bladder. The cuspids relate to the liver and gall-bladder. The lower molars and upper pre-molars relate to the large intestine and lung. The lower bi-cuspids and upper molars are-spleen, pancreas and stomach. The third molars are heart and small intestine. So, all these teeth relate to acupuncture circuitry.

The Chinese thousands of years ago traced the lung and large intestine meridian and the large intestine meridian went over the face, over the lower molars and the upper bi-cuspids. Those charts go back thousands of years. So, disruptions with those teeth can effect those particular meridians.

Another interesting factor is that a lot of these patients have gold in one arch and silver opposing it in the other arch. I think that some of these patients whom we put in an occlusal splint and see this improvement, are really doing well. Then we take out the the splint and we equilibrate them and they just go right back to square one. We put the splint in and they do better. We may be insulating with the splint a galvanic problem between the upper and lower teeth. You have to consider the possibility that they won't get better after your equilibrate them."

To lease this instrument call:

Toxic Testing
(800) 327-8885

POTENTIAL (POTENTIOMETER)

Current and Voltage Measuring Instrument
with electronic storage for current measurement

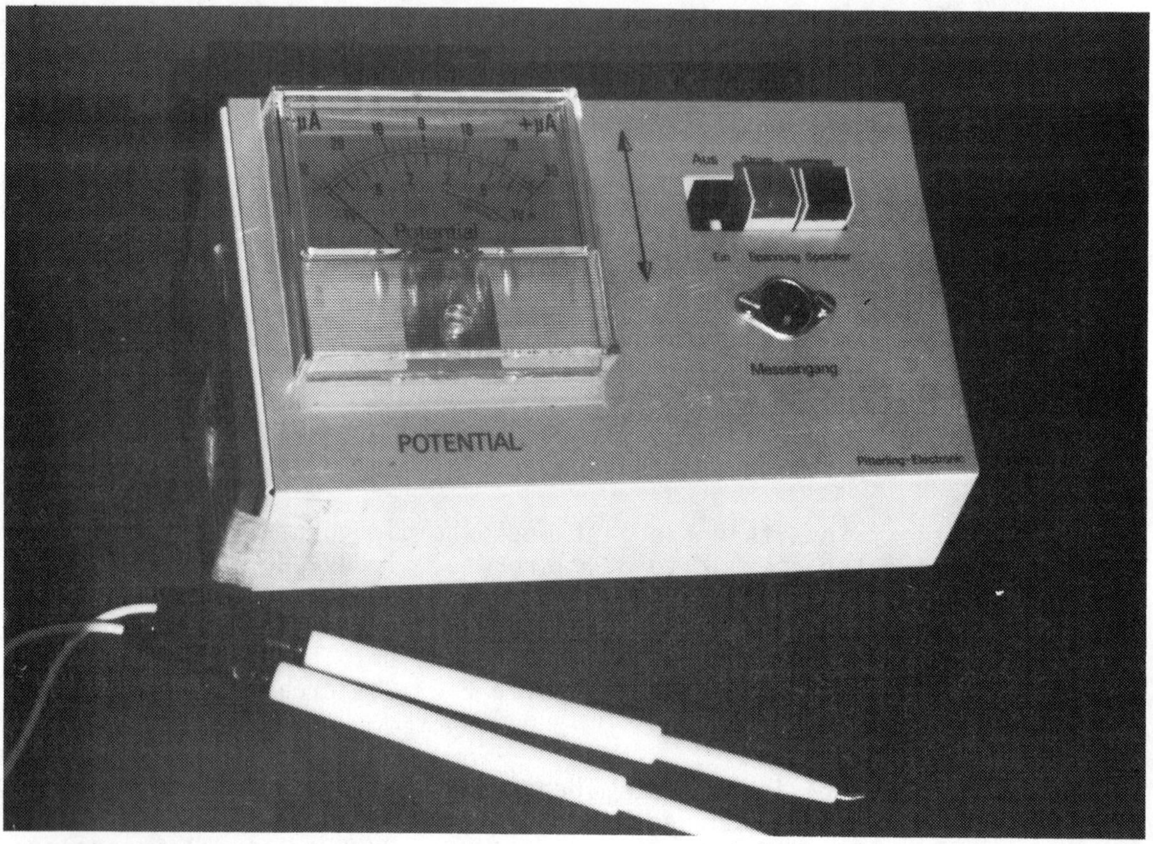

Principle:
Metals in the mouth can cause the formation of electric current. Especially in case of silver amalgam and in connection with gold work considerable voltages can be generated.

* Note: Dr. Robert G. Hansen, D.D.S., Dean of Oral Roberts University states, "It is important to realize that two types of instruments are used in assessing the effect of mixed metals and possibly toxic materials in the mouth. One type tests for vapors and the other tests for electrical energies caused by metals in the mouth." The above instrument, "The Potential Meter", measures electric current, and the other, "The "Jerome Mercury Vapor Analyzer" tests for mercury vapor in the mouth. (For a description of this instrument, see Chapter XVII)

XV

CANDIDA CAN SYNTHESIZE METHYLMERCURY IN THE INTESTINES THROUGH THE USE OF SILVER (mercury) FILLINGS

Wood, J.M.: Kennedy, F.S.: Rosen, C.G.: Synthesis of Methyl-mercury compounds by extracts of a Methanogenic Bacterium. Nature. Vol 220. October 12, 1968 173-174

It therefore seems that dimethyl-mercury could be the product of biological significance in mercury poisoning, and methyl-mercury could be an artefact of isolation procedures.

Apparently transfer of methyl groups from Co to Hg in biological systems may also occur as a non-enzymatic process. If this methyl-transfer reaction is significant in biological systems, then it will be enhanced by anaerobic conditions and by increasing numbers of bacteria capable of synthesizing alkylcobalamines. This means, for example, that pollution of a body of water with nutrients (that is, sewage) will increase the rate of formation of methyl-mercury at a certain concentration of Hg. Methyl-mercury could be formed by both enzymatic and non-enzymatic reactions, thus making this cumulative poison available for incorporation into various organisms in the aquatic environment, and secondarily into terrestrial predators. The cumulative nature of mercury poisoning can be titrated in fish. The extensive survey performed in Sweden has prompted legislation on the use of organomercurials in addition to close control of mercury pollution. Similarly in Japan legislation was brought into effect after the Minamata disaster. We feelthat the example set by these two countries should be followed elsewhere before concentrations of mercury reach a point where methyl-mercury is being titrated in humans as well as fish.

Jernelov, A. "Conversion of Mercury Compounds", Chap. 4 in Chemical Fallout (C.C. Thomas Publ., 1969). Publ. by. M.W. Miller.

Abstract-It has been shown in Sweden that fish contain methylmercury in instances where the original discharge contains other types of mercury compounds. Mercury discharge in the form of metallic mercury, inorganic divalent mercury, phenylmercury and alkoxi-alkylmercury can all be converted in nature to methylmercury.

It was shown by Jensen and Jernelov that large amounts of dimethylmercury was formed from either divalent inorganic mercury or from methylmercury during the anerobic putrefication of fish.

Discussion- Norseth: Have you tested the intestinal tracts of animals for conversion from inorganic to organic mercury?

Jernelov: Dr. Westoo has done such experiments.

Westoo: The rat does not convert injected inorganic mercury to organic mercury. But we have fed hens with inorganic mercury salts, phenylmercury salts, and methoxymethylmercury salts and in all cases observed some conversion to methylmercury.

International Conference on Environmental Mercury Contamination, University of Michigan, 1972. "Factors in the Transformation of Mercury to Methylmercury-Arne Jernelov

In many experiments where elementary mercury has been added to aquaria or other systems, we obtained the same methylation rate whether elementary mercury or inorganic bivalent mercury was added. This indicates that for elementary mercury the last step in the reaction, the biological methylation, is the rate-determining one. When mercuric sulfide is added, a much smaller amount of methylmercury is formed within the same period than if we add inorganic bivalent mercury.

When there were only microorganisms present, methylmercury was found and released only when the mercury-rich layer was on the surface. When we added macroorganisms to the system, we found that mercury-rich layers down to a depth of 2cm contributed to the formation and release of methylmercury.

The importance of anaerobic and aerobic conditions on the methylation of mercury is another much discussed factor.

The first system that was described for the methylation of mercury was the methylation from methyl cobalamine (methyl Vitamin B12) as described by Wood and his collaborators. This is a strictly anaerobic process that will occur only in the absence of oxygen. Another possible method for the methylation of mercury within the cell is from a complex between inorganic bivalent mercury and homocysteine.

Mercury in the environment: A toxicological and epidemiological appraisal by L. Friberg and Jaroslav, V.: Editors; Stockholm, November 1971

Conversion of deposits of inorganic mercury into volatile organomercury compounds could be a more effective way of transporting mercury into the geocycle. Jansen and Jernelov, 1969, reported that an unidentified microorganism in sludge from aquaria can methylate inorganic mercury.

CONVERTING INORGANIC MERCURY INTO HIGHLY TOXIC METHYL MERCURY IN THE BODY

1. Greener, Evan H.: Amalgam-Yesterday, Today, and Tomorrow Operative Dentistry; 4,24-35: 1979

...."problems of mercury possibly associated with poor standards of amalgam hygiene. One of the most dramatic findings was presented by Dale and coworkers, of the University of Glasgow, who found six times higher concentration of methylated mercury in the dental population and who have hypothesized that methylated mercury may be synthesized from the mercury vapor by micro-organisms in the gut.

2. Goolvard, Dale & Ferguson: Serum in organic methyl mercury levels in dental surgeons: Journal of Dental Research-Special Issue- 56 Annual Meeting: British Division: Abstract #144

Previous work has shown that dental surgeons and their assistants have greater concentrations of mercury in hair and nails. However, these findings can be complicated by direct adsorption.

Serum was obtained from a group of dental surgeons and their clinical assistants as well as from a control group of individuals not exposed to mercury. The inorganic mercury levels were measured using neutron activation analysis and the methyl mercury concentrations by gas liquid chromatography.

The results indicated that workers exposed to inorganic mercury not only had significantly higher amounts of inorganic mercury but also had greater quantities of methyl mercury.

This suggests that methylation of mercury occurs in vivo in humans and that certain of the clinical manifestations of poisoning may be attributed to methyl mercury, a known neurotoxin.

3. Carrel, A.B.: Mackowiak, Elaine: Chialastri, A.J.: The Accumulation of the Base Metals (Copper, Zinc and Mercury) in the Human Body Journal of Dentistry for Children: 30-33 September-October 1979

...."inorganic mercury must be converted to the organic compound by an intermediary such as fish, algae or industrial processes, to become detrimental to one's health."*

*According to some scientists human beings have certain anaerobic bacteria (those that live without air) and can convert inorganic mercury into highly toxic methyl mercury compounds. (Comment by "How Safe ore Silver Fillings"

4. Treptow, Richard S.: Amalgam Dental Fillings, Parts 1 and II Chemistry, April 17:30, May 15: 19, 1978

A Summary-

According to Dr. R. Treptow, Associate Professor of Chemistry at Chicago State University, "Early opposition to dental amalgam was bases in part upon the question of toxicity. Throughout the 150 years of domination of amalgam as a restorative material, the question has recurred continually. Scientists have discovered that certain anerobic bacterial (those that thrive without air) on the bottom of the sea can convert inorganic mercury into highly toxic methyl-mercury compounds. Human beings also have this kind of bacteria in our digestive tracts and we are at present exposed to an ever increasing variety of toxic substances. We know that many of these are synergistic-that is, their toxic effects are greater when one or more is combined.

Treptow goes on to say the mixture of tin and mercury is not as stable as it might be in contact with the saliva which of course, bathes the filling constantly. Oxidation of the filling tends to occur, especially in the presence of sulfides (which might be eggs) or citrate (which might be oranges). A by-product of the corrosion of tin and mercury is mercury. Dr. Treptow further states, "Upon release, free mercury combines with (silver and tin) according to setting reaction, and goes directly into the digestive tract." The professor tells us that the amount emitted from one square centimeter of filling, if it could be inhaled and assimilated through the lungs it would just about equal the amount of mercury in two grams of tuna fish containing the maximum allowable concentration of mercury which is 0.5 parts per million. The finished amalgam restoration contains on the average 45% to 50% mercury.

5. Merfield, D.P: Taylor, A: Gemmell, D.M.: Mercury Intoxication in a Dental Surgery Following Unreported Spillage British Dental Journal 179- : 1976

Mercury is the heaviest of the transitional elements and in its metallic state is comparatively innocuous unless finely divided, when it may become toxic owing to the inhalation of dust or vapor. It is probable that in the lung and the intestine the mercury dissolves in the fluid surfaces and is then absorbed. It's biological action results from readily formed covalent linkages with sulphur which inactivate sulphhydryl enzymes, thus interfering with cellular function.

6. Stofen, D.: Dental amalgam - apoison in our mouth. Toxicology 2:355-358 December, 1974

..."extracted teeth have proved that silver-tin fillings undergo mercury losses in the marginal layer under conditions existing in the mouth. There is evidence for the hypothesis that the lost mercury is partly vapourized and inhaled. Swallowing of ionized mercury derived from dental fillings also seems possible."

7. Koller, L.D.,,Methylmercury: Effect on Oncogenic and Nononcogenic viruses in mice. American Journal Vet. Res., 36 (10): 150-1-1504 1975.

Methylmercury is an environmental contaminant of both industrial and natural origins that accumulates in the food chain. Inorganic and organic mercury from industrial waste disposed in lakes, rivers, or the sea may be transformed into methylmercury and is often found in fish. Contaminated flour used for making bread, meat from animals and game birds fed wheat seed treated with methylmercury fungicide, and vegetation grown from soil contaminated with methylmercury are sources of human mercury poisoning. Methylmercury compounds are almost completely absorbed from the gastrointestinal tract, readily pass the blood-brain barrier to damage nerve cells, and pass the placental barrier. ....Results emphasize that methylmercury not only poses a threat to public health as a toxic agent, but at subclinical concentrations it may augment infectious agents to produce disease.

8. Heintze, V., et al. Methylation of mercury from dental amalgam and mercuric chloride by oral streptococci in vitro. Scand. J. Dent. Res. 91 (2): 150-152, 1983.

Abstract - The capacity of the oral bacteria Streptococcus mitior, S. mutans and S. mutans and S. sanguis to methylate to mercury was investigated in vitro.. Mercuric chloride and pulverized dental amalgam in distilled water, respectively, were used as sources of mercury. Methylmercury was found in the bacterial cells of all three tested strains. The results indicate that organic mercury compounds may be formed in the oral cavity.

Dental amalgam is the most used restorative material in dentistry. This material has been considered relatively stable in the oral environment. However, mercury is released from amalgam in various aqueous solutions. Furthermore, mercury may gradually migrate from a restoration into the enamel, dentin, pulp tissue and the adjacent gingival tissue and accumulate. Microorganisms from various sources, including the human intestine, have been found capable of methylating mercuric ions both under aerobic and anaerobic conditions.

....When considering our results from a clinical point of view, the following should be borne in mind. The experiments were carried out with pure cultures under favorable growth conditions. Moreover, several strains of bacterial and yeasts are capable of degrading methylmercury to inorganic mercury

9. Rowland, I.R., et al. The methlylation of mercuric chloride by human intestional bacteria. Experientia, 31: 1064-1065. 1975

Summary: Most strains of staphylococci, streptococci, yeasts and E. coli isolated from human faeces, could synthesize methylmercury compounds. In contrast, few strains of obligate anaerobes could do so. Up to 6 ng methylmercury/ml were fromed in 44 h from 2 ug mercuric chloride

Methylmercury synthesis by intestinal bacteria

Microorganism	No. tested	No. positive	Range (ng CH_3HgCl formed/ml/44 h)
Streptococci	6	4	2.1-5.8
Staphylococci	10	6	0.5-5.0
E. coli	5	3	0.9-3.0
Yeasts	9	4	0.7-1.7
Lactobacilli	9	1	0.5
Bacteroides / Bifidobacteria	10	3	0.4-0.6

XVI

CALIFORNIA DENTAL ASSN. JOURNAL
REPORTS ON SILVER (mercury) FILLINGS

UNIVERSITY OF CALIFORNIA DENTAL PROFESSORS WRITE CONFLICTING REPORTS-COMMENTS ON THREE REPORTS FROM THE CALIFORNIA DENTAL ASSOCIATION JOURNAL AND ONE REPORT FROM ORAL SURGERY CONCERNING MERCURY AND AMALGAM RESTORATIONS

I find it interesting that Dr. J. Bauer, DDS who reported on 136 articles she researched for the CDA Journal and who is on the dental staff at UCLA found after researching these articles that silver fillings were not harmful to the mouth. I researched 100 of these same articles and found that for the most part, the articles state silver fillings are harmful to the mouth.

The conclusion of the article states, "A review of the literature indicates that the use of mercury in dental amalgam is relatively safe"...

Also of interest in the same CDA Journal June 1982, Dr. Malcolm Jendersen, DDS wrote an article on 'Mercury in Dental Amalgam: Is it Safe?' and he comes to the same conclusion as Dr. Bauer. Dr. Jendersen is also on the staff of Restorative Dentistry at the University of California San Francisco.

Dr. Louis Hansen DDS, Professor and Chairman, Division of Oral Pathology, University of California San Francisco, wrote an article on "Amalgam Pigmentation (amalgam tattoo) of the Oral Mucosa; Oral Surg. Journal 49:139-147, 1980. His conclusion was that 17% showed a macrophagic reaction and in 38% there was a chronic inflammatory response to amalgam. The conclusion drawn was that there was over 50% of the implanted amalgam showing adverse tissue response. A direct quote from his article, "Although some textbooks of oral pathology have stated that amalgam does not evoke an inflammatory or giant cell response, our study has shown that, in fact, there is a wide histomorphologic spectrum of tissue response to dental amalgam."

Dr. Hansen then wrote another article in June of 1982 in the CJA Journal "Localized Tissue Reaction to Implanted Amalgam." In this article Dr. Hansen states in the body of the article, "After implantation, the pigmented areas may increase both in size and intensity of color, simulating its most serious differential diagnosis, the malignant melanoma. One explanation for this change may be that amalgam fragments disintegrate as a result of corrosion and/or by the action of macrophages, giant cells, etc." In the conclusion of the article Dr. Hansen states, "Our present knowledge of the response of tissues to implanted amalgam, based on the available clinical and experimental findings, suggests that there is no reason to believe that any actual or potential localized hazard results from the use of silver amalgam.

The articles on "Amalgam Pigmentation & "Localized Tissue Reaction to Implanted Amalgam" by Dr. Hansen in 1980 and 1982 show the body of the material presented in both articles to be similar in thought concerning implanted amalgams and amalgam tattoos and their possible harm to the human tissues.

When the conclusion or summary of both of these reports are drawn both indicate silver amalgam and/or amalgam tattoos are not dangerous to human tissue. The conclusions drawn by Dr. Hansen in 1980 & 1982 are not consistant with the body of these two reports.

Dr. Bauer's report throughout the body of her article quotes many journals stating silver fillings are harmful to the human body, yet in the conclusion Dr. Bauer states silver fillings are <u>not</u> harmful to the mouth. *

One interesting idea is that most dentists don't have the time to read these lengthly articles let alone research the same material. They turn to the conclusion or summary of an article and note what is stated there, fully trusting the researcher. If the dentists see an article stating silver fillings, etc., are not harmful, they will continue to practice using mercury in their dental practice, poisoning themselves, employees and patients alike.

I leave it up to the reader to wonder why the dentists must report the opposite in the conclusion of an article, rather then report a conclusion that is in keeping with the body of the report.

I would like to leave you with a final thought. A university as large as the University of California operates to a large extent on government grants (Military-Industrial Complex). <u>We are all aware of the fact that what government funds, government controls!</u>

*See following page on chart on 100 of the 136 articles Dr. Bauer researched. This chart clearly shows the articles for the most part were negative to Silver Fillings. Yet the conclusion drawn by Dr. Bauer was that silver amalgams are safe.

A CHART SHOWING NEGATIVE AND POSITIVE RESPONSE TO MERCURY FILLINGS

			NEGATIVE TO SILVER (MERCURY) FILLINGS	POSITIVE TO SILVER (MERCURY) FILLINGS	OTHER
1.	JADA 1953	1953	x		
2.	J. Periodontol	1974	x		
3.	Acta derm.ven.	1968	x		
4.	J. Oral Med.	1973	x		
5.	Amer. J. Card.	1964	x		
6.	Arch Envir Health	1968	x		
7.	Arch. Dermat.	1966		*x	
8.	Int'l J. Derm.	1975	x		
9.	Oper. Dent.	1979	x		
10.	Odonto. Revy	1974	x		
11.	Swed. Dent. J.	1978	x		
12.	JADA	1959	x		
13.	J. Prosthet. D.	1968	x		
14.	Acta Odont.Scand.	1962	x		
15.	Br. J. Derm.	1970	x		
16.	Oral Surg.	1980	x		
17.	Scand. J.Dent Res.	1974	x		
18.	Scand. J.Dent Res.	1979	x		
19.	Histochem. J.	1976	x		
20.	J. Pathol.	1977	x		
21.	Acta Odont Scand.	1965	x		
22.	J. Dent. Res.	1979	x		
23.	JADA	1974			x
24.	Arch. Derm.	1974			x
25.	JADA	1974	x		
26.	JADA	1976	x		
27.	Lancet	1982	x		
28.	JADA	1976	x		
29.	JADA	1976	x		
30.	JADA	1976		x	
31.	JADA	1976		*x	
32.	JADA	1971			x
33.	JADA	1970	x		
34.	JADA	1974			x
35.	NY State Dent. J.	1979	x		
36.	Arch Derm. & Syph	1938	x		
37.	J. Dent. Res.	1964	x		
38.	J. Prosth. Dent.	1977	x		
39.	J. of Oral Therap.	1965	x		
40.	Brit. Dent. J.	1971	x		
41.	Brit. Dent. J.	1973	x		
42.	Dent. Asst.	1974	x		
43.	J. Prosth. Dent.	1968	x		
44.	Dent. Survey	1973	x		
45.	Dental Survey	1973	x		
46.	Arch Envir. Hlth.	1968	x		
47.	Toxicology	1974	x		
48.	Oper. Dent.	1978			x
49.	Annals NY A. Sci.	1957	-x		
50.	Acta Odont Scand.	1965	x		

*Study was funded by Grant by Federal or State
-Body of article is different than conclusion

(continued on next page)

			NEGATIVE TO SILVER (MERCURY) FILLINGS	POSITIVE TO SILVER (MERCURY) FILLINGS	OTHER
51.	New Eng. J. Med.	1959	x		
52.	JADA	1976		x	
53.	JADA	1971		x	
54.	Dent. Mat. 4th Ed.	1954			x
55.	Int.Dent. Jour.	1969	x		
56.	J. Pediat.	1943	x		
57.	JADA	1935	x		
58.	South. Med. J.	1978	x		
59.	J. Dent. Res.	1929	x		
60.	Arch. Oral Biol.	1973	x		
61.	Dental Asst.	1976			*x
62.	Oral. Surg.	1972	x		
63.	Brit. Dent. J.	1976			
64.	Acta Odont. Scand.	1965	x		
65.	JAMA	1928	x		
66.	New Zealand D.J.	1971	x		
67.	Arch. Env. Hlth.	1968		*x	
68.	J. Dent. Res.	1977		*x	
69.	JAMA	1926	x		
70.	J. Dent. Res.	1980	x		
71.	J Dent. Children	1979		*x	
72.	J. Dent. Res.	1967		*x	
73.	Oral Surg.	1968	x		
74.	J. Dent. Res.	1975	x		
75.	JAMA	1938	x		
76.	JADA	1951	x		
77.	Acta Derm. Ven.	1969	x		
78.	JADA	1976		x	
79.	JADA	1976		x	
80.	Derm. Soc.	1966	x		
81.	Annals NY A. Sci.	1957	x		
82.	JADA	1941	x		
83.	Brit. Dent. J.	1969	x		
84.	JADA	1962	x		
85.	Brit. D. Jour.	1962	x		
86.	JADA	1974			x
87.	Annals NY A.Sci.	1957	x		
88.	Oper. Dent.	1979	x		
89.	JADA	1966			*x
90.	SSO	1973	x		
91.	SSO	1977		x	
92.	Dtsche Zeit	1980	x		
93.	Dtsche Zeit	1975			x
94.	Dtsche Zeit	1967	x		
95.	Dtsch. Stomat.	1963	x		
96.	Dtsche Zeit	1971	x		
97.	SSO	1972	x		
98.	Dtsche Zeit	1964			x
99.	SSO	1967	x		
100.	Arch.Env.Hlth.	1969	x		

*Study funded by 'Grant' from Federal or State level.

*CONNECTIONS BETWEEN ACADEMIC SCIENTISTS SERVING ON GOVERNMENT COMMITTEES AND AMERICA'S MAJOR CORPORATIONS

Charles Schwartz, professor of physics at the University of California Berkeley, has published a detailed study of the linkages between academic scientists serving on government committees and America's major corporations. While 55 members were classified as "pure academics," a closer investigation by Schwartz found that over two thirds of them were actually directors of or consultants of giant corporations, receiving remunerations of five thousand to ten thousand dollars or more for their affiliation.

There is also the prestigious National Science Board, which sets policy for the National Science Foundation, the government's science agency, whose purpose is to represent and fund 'pure' academic research, independent of the influence of industry. Again, Schwartz has found that of the 78 scientists who served on this committee from 1957 to 1973 62 were officially listed as "academics" when in fact more than half were also directors or consultants of giant corporations.

Perhaps the best example of how industry has come to dominate science in this country can be found in a close-up examination of the prestigious National Academy of Science. The NAS was set up by an act of Congress in 1868. According to its charter, "the Academy shall, whenever called upon by any department of the government, investigate, examine, and report upon any subject of science and art." While the expenses incurred by the Academy in doing reports were to be paid by the federal government, the institution itself was to remain independent and autonomous. A former NAS president characterized the Academy as "a Supreme Court of final advice" whose work is "wholly in the public interest, uninfluenced by any elements of personal, economic or political force."

Despite its claims to independence and objectivity in the name of pure science, the NAS has been attacked in recent years by a growing number of critics who believe that it has become a mere rubber stamp for establishment institutions. Former Secretary of the Interior Steward Udall charges that the Academy has become a "virtual puppet of the US government in a fashion that leaves little room to serve as an independent critical voice.

Still, according to critics, the Academy's interest in 'serving' the federal government is secondary to its interest in serving the American business community. Phillip Boffey, in his authoritative book on the NAS, entitled, "The Brain Bank of America", catalogues story after story of NAS complicity with the direct relationships to the giant corporations of the country.

Many of the NAS units receive much of their financial support directly from industry, which gives the business community the leverage it needs to influence the findings of reports and to determine what kind of studies are undertaken in the first place. This symbiotic relationship is particularly evident in the Drug Research Board, the Agricultural Board, Computer Science, Food and Nutrition, and the Building Research Advisory Board.

*From the book, WHO SHOULD PLAY GOD? by J. Rifkin, 1977-Dell

Then there is the Food Protection Committee, which has become a target of jokes even within the Academy membership. The committee is financed largely by the food, chemical, and packaging industry and is "biased as heck for industry," according to Dr. Marvin Legator, the FDA's former chief for genetic toxicology.

Given the incestuous ties between the corporate world and the scientists who compose the various committees of the national academy of sciences it should come as no surprise that of the nine financial sponsors of the NAS's first forum on recombinant DNA and genetic engineering, six were the very drug companies that are tooling up for entry into the genetics market.

Much of the success of the drug industry can be attributed to the hold it exercises over the American Medical Association and other large health organizations.

Biochemist, John Yiamouyiannis, Ph.D. was Editor of Chemical Abstracts Service. When he revealed the facts that fluoride causes cancer he was fired. See excerpts from Dr. Yiamouyiannis' new book, Fluoride, the Aging Factor in the chapter on Fluoridation.

Dentist, David Eggleston, within the past year was arrested in his own office and taken to jail handcuffed. Dr. Eggleston was arrested because he practices 'holistic' dentistry. Dr. Eggleston was released within a short period of time. Dr. Eggleston is on the teaching staff at the University of Southern California, and in private practice in Newport Beach.

Dentist Isadore Imber was on the teaching staff at the University of California Los Angeles. He was teaching 'holistic' dentistry. He was told to leave his position 'quietly'. Dr. Imber's is in private practice in Reseda, California.

There are many more out there who are being harrassed by the government every day and are doing nothing but practicing alternative methods of healing which do no harm to the body.

XVII
THE MERCURY AND NICKEL PATCH TEST KITS

Directors at the[1] Toxic Element Research Foundation urge that research methodologies be expanded to include biocompatibility studies already shown to be effected by toxic metal placement in the human. Studies they recommend for mercury are as follows:
(Other metals can be tested the same way.)

1. Urine mercury (or)
2 Whole blood mercury
3. Complete blood count
4. Immune differential
5. Oral electropotential
6. Patch hypersensitivity test
7. Patient oral temperature
8. Blood pressure
9. Blood profile
10. Electrocardiogram
11. Electroencephalogram
12. Hair analysis for toxic elements
13. Psychological testing
14. Physical history
15. Mercury vapor analysis as emitted from fillings
16. Retinal fundus photography

Many of these tests are beyond the scope of a general dental practice, but some tests are simple, easy, quick, inexpensive, and highly informative. It has become imperative that we be able to differentiate between the sensitive (everyone) and the hypersensitive patient. The hypersensitive patient is the one who develops untoward reactions classified as numerous diseases, that reverse upon amalgam and base metal removal.

Four tests that meet these criteria are oral temperature, blood pressure, the patch test, and electrical testing of the teeth.

The following information on the Mercury and Nickel Patch Tests shows how inexpensive, simple, easy, quick and highly informative these tests can be. (See Following pages)

If your dentist or physician doesn't have them they can be ordered from Tox Supply ---- - P.O. Box 620492 Littleton, Colorado 80162
(303) 985-4529

INSTRUMENT FOR MEASURING URINE, BLOOD AND HAIR FOR MERCURY

Chemical Analysis Test (Model 511)
Jerome Instrument Corp. (800) 952-2566
P.O. Box 336
Jerome, Arizona 86331

TO LEASE: Toxic Texting (800) 327 8885
303 E. Altamonte Dr.
Suite 232
Altamonte Springs, Fla. 32701

INSTRUMENT FOR TESTING MERCURY VAPOR GIVEN OFF BY SILVER AMALGAM FILLINGS

Gold Film Mercury Vapor Analyzer (Model 411)
P.O. Box 336
Jerome, Arizona 86331

TO LEASE: Toxic Testing (See Address above)

This machine is a precise and sensitive instrument and is 10 times more sensitive than other mercury detectors. In 1981 NASA used this instrument for mercury detection in a space shuttle. This same model was used in the submarine Trident to determin mercury levels. Dr. R.H. Roydhouse, Professor, Dept. of Restorative Dentistry-University of British Columbia endorses this Model No. 411.

1 Dr. H. Huggin's Research Foundation

THE MERCURY AND NICKEL PATCH TEST KITS

The Mercury and Nickel Patch Test Kits are other screening devices used to predict mercury and nickel hypersensitivity. They do this by placing a chemical solution of the metal being tested directly on the patients's skin. Depending on the patient's reaction within a 24-hour period or less, an indication of hypersensitivity can be suggested. Increases in pulse, blood pressure, blood white cell count, redness, lymph nodes swelling and many other reactions suggest affirmative patch reactions.

Each patch test kit contains 14 samples of the solution plus all necessary documentation forms and a complete set of instructions. Patch testing for metal hypersensitivity should be a routine examination for all patients to protect both the profession from litigation and the patient from harm. The test can be easily performed by auxiliary personnel.

1. Before the patch is placed, take the patient's: (1) pulse, (2) blood pressure, (3) temperature, and (4) any other tests you normally perform.

2. Peel off the protective layer from the patch. Squeeze the test solution from the packet onto the patch and place it on the underside of the forearm.

3. Give the patient the "Health Questionnaire" to fill out.

4. After the patient has completed the form, have an auxiliary check with them for untoward symptoms and to be sure they have an appointment scheduled in 24 hours.

5. At the second visit retake the original records (pressure, pulse and temperature) and, AT THIS TIME, ask them questions from the Doctor's Questionnaire and Record. Utmost significance is attached to changes in blood pressure, pulse, and temperature, for these may indicate endocrine malfunctions. The use of silver-mercury amalgams is discouraged in people who demonstrate positive reactions to the Mercury Patch Test. For people who have hypersensitive reactions to the Nickel Patch Test, nickel castings, like the metal under ceramic (porcelain) crowns should be avoided

NOTE: ALWAYS CAUTION THE PATIENT should an OVERT reaction occur, such as racing of the heart, constant buring or itching of the site, tremors or anything the patient feels is abnormal, instruct them to remove the patch, scrub the area with soap and water, and discontinue the test. These patients can be considered positive reactors without further testing.

See following page for Health Questionnaire and Doctor's Questionnaire and Record.

The Merc-Kit (14 tests) $35.00
The Nick-Kit (14 tests) $35.00

(These two tests are the same as the Mercury Nickel Patch tests & Dentists & Physicians can purchase them through Tox Supply P.O. Box 620492- Littleton, Colorado 80162)

PROTECTING THE MERCURY HYPERSENSITIVE PATIENT DURING AMALGAM REMOVAL*

Removal of amalgam from the hypersensitive patient may produce ntoward reactions. Whatever symptom a patient has had as a result of mercury sensitivity may appear in an exaggerated form. Headaches may turn into migraines. Rashes may become redder. Tempers may become hyperirritable.

Several things can be done to help moderate these reactions. The severe patient can be helped by receiving Vitamin C intravenously. Details of this procedure are available upon request. Vitamin C intravenously seems to have 2 effects. First, it can increase the cell membrane permeability allowing the mercury to be removed from the cells. Second, it presents a ligand with which the mercury can attach for excretion.

Most people do not show positive responses to mercury removal until more than half the amalgam is removed. After the last one is out reactions may occur. We have found that in the HYPERSENSITIVE--not just preventive patient--there is less of a reaction if amalgam is removed a quadrant or 2 quadrants at a time with 2 or 3 days in between. If all amalgams must be removed at once for time reasons, it is not dangerous, just potentially uncomfortable for patients as they respond with their "withdrawal reaction". Supplementation can be a great aid in these cases.

Another point of interest is that the immune system has several 'cycles . One of these is a 21 day cycle. How it effects the dental patient is that 21 days after amalgam removal the patient is apt to have a bad day. They just generally don't feel good. Nothing severe. Some people describe it as thinking they are catching the flu, but they get over it soon.

If the patient has 2 sessions of amalgam removal a week apart, he will probably have a down day 21 days after the initial removal, then another one a week later. Strange, but we maintain supplementation for at least 30 days to minimize these reactions.

*Doctor Huggins, has list of vitamins for removal of silver amalgam fillings. You may write to him for details at:

Dr. Hal Huggins, DDS
1715 Monterey Road
Colorado Springs, Colorado (303) 473/4703

Selenium as Food & Medicine by Richard A. Passwater, Ph.D. - Keats Publishing

"Several nutrients, including selenium, help protects us against heavy metal poisoning. ...In one study, they found that rats given water containing 10 parts per million mercury died within six weeks, while similar rats that were also given 0.5 part per million of selenium survived."

XVIII

SEXUAL MATURITY, ARTIFICIAL LIGHT & THE ENDOCRINE SYSTEM

POLLUTED LIGHT?

HOSPITAL PRACTICE
January 1969

Through the invention of artificial light man has lengthened his workday, increased industrial productivity, and extended his recreation time. But can the light he created - like environmental air and water - become a source of pollution? What does this mean and what are its consequences? The concept of "light pollution", mentioned by Dr. Wurtman in his article on the pineal gland, merits attention by the medical and lighting profession.

....Natural light from the sun and sky may be considered as unpolluted and serve as our criterion of environmental light. ....Light pollution, if defined as gross deviation from the spectral balance found in natural light, is visually apparent under today's most common artificial illuminants.

Too much sunlight is reportedly a causative factor in human skin cancer, but a small amount will provide the daily requirement of vitamin D and cure rickets. Most urban workers are deprived of the weekly equivalent of even 20 minutes of noon, summer sunlight. Is this a matter of concern to the physician? Should it be to the illuminating engineer?

One thing is certain: Light has physiologic effects upon people. Yet this fact has hardly been considered in the design of our artificial lighting environments. Man has declared himself independent of the ocean of light surrounding him without understanding the nature of his own dependency.

....Concern on the part of the medical profession over the possible effects of light pollution might help.

The framework of a light pollution control program may exist in Public Law No. 90-602, passed October 18, 1968, which is designed to study and control "electronic product radiation." While apparently stimulated by such problems areas as x-radiation from television sets, the law encompasses all electromagnetic radiation, ionizing or nonionizing. Physicians and engineers should lend their full support to the proposed study, and Dr. Wurtman's article should spur the inclusion of environmental lighting in the program.

Luke Thorington, Director
of Engineering for the
DuroTest Corporation
North Bergen, N.J.

HOW ARTIFICIAL LIGHT AFFECTS YOUR HEALTH

A Reader's Digest Reprint
Reprinted from the February 1981 issue

By Lowell Ponte

"Recent scientific investigations indicate that there is a dark side to light, particularly the types of light used so widely in our schools, factories and offices.

Little has been done to protect citizens against potentially harmful or biologically inadequate light, say Wurtman. "Both government and industry have been satisfied to allow people to serve as the unwitting subjects in a long-term experiment on the effects of artificial-lighting environments on human health.

In fact, light can enhance health, prevent disease and even heal. Blue light can help cure one kind of jaundice in premature babies. Herpes can be treated with low-intensity white fluorescent light. And psoriasis can be remedied by giving a patient a drug that increases his sensitivity to light and then exposing the skin to special ultraviolet radiation.

We are only beginning to understand how light, natural and unnatural, affects our health. What steps should we take now, as individuals and as a society?

1. The public should be informed of the potential hazards of artificial light. The FDA's tests have confirmed that radiation from fluorescent lamps can increase the risk of skin cancer in sensitive individuals.

2. Offices, factories & schools could minimize the hazards of lighting by using broad-spectrum fluorescent lamps instead of narrow-spectrum "cool white" fluorescent bulbs in common use."

FLUORESCENT LIGHTING CAN MAKE YOU ILL, EXPERT WARNS

"When man created artificial light he upset the natural-scheme of things. There may be low-level health risks involved in constant exposure, says Dr. F. Alan Anderson, a biophysicist with the U.S. Food and Drug Administration in Rockville, Md.

Nobody knows yet what the long-term effects of artificial light will be".

Studies by Anderson and other photobiologists - scientists analyzing the link between light and living organisms - warn that unshielded fluorescent lights may add up to 5 percent to the total weekly dose of radiation the average person receives, mostly from the sun.

In the case of susceptible individuals, this may be enough to cause skin cancer. Also, research shows artificial light may have an effect on human sexual developemnt, according to Anderson.

LIGHT & THE ENDOCRINE SYSTEM

"A happy accident stemming from my TV appearances now occurred and it came in the form of a letter from a viewer. He was a biology teacher in Chicago doing research with fish eggs and he wanted to experiment with time-lapse pictures. Delighted to help, I moved one of my time-lapse units right into his laboratory. Acting on a hunch, I suggested that we hang some of the various fluorescents used on the pumpkins over two or three of the fish tanks. Each fixture held two 40-watt fluorescent tubes placed about ten inches above the water equipped with morning and evening timers.

Three different types of tubes were used-cool white, daylight white and pink. The aquariums were not located near any window, so the fish were being subjected entirely to fluorescent light. The first thing that happened was that the fish completely stopped laying eggs. Unhappily, because the teacher needed eggs for his work. On the other hand, it did indicate that light possibly did have some effect on the fish. After two weeks the light intensity was cut in half by removing one of the fluorescent tubes from each fixture. Still no egg production. Gradually we shortened the length of time the lights were left on. When the duration was down to eight hours a day, the fish began producing eggs.

Ordinarily, the sex of certain fish can be determined by the development of the secondary sex characteristics in much the same way brilliantly colored plumage is more noticeable on most male birds. We waited and watched the pinhead-sized fish grow larger day by day as the weeks went by. One day the biology teacher moved all the aquariums and lights from their location alongside his desk to another room. Several days later he told me that the young fish were all beginning to look suspiciously like females, but it was still too soon to be certain. We waited approximately a month past the time the sex can normally be determined, and one evening he called me and said he had carefully checked each fish. He couldn't believe it, but all the ones under the pink light were definitely females. This was just the opposite from what might have been expected after the results with the pumpkin flowers. We waited another ten days, and then I told a few people about this first experiment with the fish. Although this was only one incident, and could not be given any scientific significance until repeated many more times, it was interesting that all fifty fish hatched from eggs of different parents appeared to be female.

The very next day....the phone rang....and the biology teacher was quite excited-or possibly I should say upset-for now some of the fish he was certain were females were beginning to show faint signs of masculine coloration. We waited several weeks more, and the final results were that 80 per cent of the fish definitely turned out to be females and 20 per cent were questionable. <u>They appeared to be males, but the development of the secondary male sex characteristics had been materially retarded.</u>

Word of the preliminary results reached the newspapers, and articles appeared in several magazines. As a result, a letter came from a lady in New Jersey who wrote as follows:

My sixteen year old son, who has a very keen interest in science, drew my attention to an article in a magazine regarding your experiments with light rays and their possible effect on sex determination.

I happen to be a chinchilla breeder and at the present time I am trying to establish a sizeable herd with sufficient breeding animals to enable me to start pelting within the next few years.

The loss of two excellent producing females in the last eight months, plus the fact that for the past three years my few breeding animals have yielded one female and nine males prompts me to write this letter to you.

I realize that perhaps you are not too familiar with chinchillas, but females are at a premium since one good male can serve several females thereby increasing the herd more rapidly plus cutting down on the costs of feeding, cages and space required. My interest in your experiments is more than passing. Since I am in a position whereby I could benefit greatly if it were possible to produce more females than males.

Chinchillas have very dense fur and are very sensitive to extreme heat, thriving best in cool, dry temperatures of between 65-70 degrees. Even in this temperature, chinchilla books state that they can be overcome withhh heat if they happen to be in a cage where bright, warm sunlight strikes them through a window for several hours during the day....

It is very, very discouraging to wait anxiously for three and a half months for a litter to be born only to discover that the offspring are all males....

I wrote and asked for all the details and particulars regarding the lighting conditions of the location where she was keeping her animals. She advised me that she was keeping the chinchillas in cages in a basement playroom. The room had one ceiling fixture with a regular 75-watt incandescent light and a small window at one end of the room. She also advised me that one baby female chinchilla was born of the animals in the cage at the end of the row nearest the window.

....I purchased two 100-watt daylight incandescent bulbs and sent them to her, one with the clear bluish glass that you can see through compared to the painted, frosted type that makes it impossible to see the filaments.

At last I received another letter from the lady in New Jersey: The blue light bulbs arrived on November seventh, and I want to thank you for them.... The first litter just arrived on January third. I am not in the habit of handling new babies until they are a week old unless it is absolutely necessary, but yesterday I couldn't control myself any longer, and I still find it hard to believe that I found three female baby chinchillas....

Again this was only one isolated instance, but a very interesting one. Another matter of particular interest was that the blue lights did not arrive until somewhere between one-third and one-half way through the period of gestation. If the lights did have anything to do with the controlling of the sex of the baby chinchillas, it would indicate the controlling factor had to do primarily with the female parent. It would also indicate that the sex of the offspring could be influenced well along during the pregnancy. Several months later another letter came advising that the next litter from other parents was all females. This was doubly interesting.

Once, while reflecting on some of the unusual results that seemed to be associated with light, it suddenly occurred to me that the various growth responses that I had produced or controlled were from using different types of artificial light containing a peak of energy in specific narrow bands of wavelengths. The normal growth developments that I had prevented, such as the apple not ripening, were the result of filtering certain wavelengths from natural sunlight. This positive and negative way of acting certainly emphasized the importance of specific wavelenghts of light.

Possibly a picture in one of my films might hold an answer or at least a partial explanation of all this. I found a microscopic time-lapse picture showing the streaming of the protoplasm within the cells of a living leaf of a plant. This activity goes on in connection with the process of photosynthesis in which the leaves respond to the energy of sunlight. They combine air and water with the minerals taken by the roots from the soil to create the food energy that supports all life on this earth. When the sun sets and it gets dark, this process of photosynthesis stops. It is a process of photochemistry through which chemical changes take place within the cells of the leaves of plants as they produce chlorophyll, carbohydrates and other chemical substances. Inasmuch as light is the source of energy that brings about these different chemical changes, it then seems reasonable to assume that by changing the characteristics of the light, the resulting chemical changes would likewise be altered.

This could explain the control of plant growth in response to the wavelength energy of light, but how could light affect the fish and the chinchillas? Here, the fact that the poultry industry knows that light received through the chicken's eye stimulates the pituitary gland and increases egg production might be a very important clue. The pituitary gland is the master balance wheel of the entire glandular system, not only in chickens but in other animals and humans as well. If this is so, and the entire glandular system can be affected-or glandular actions modified-by light received through the eye, the resulting consequences and possibilities of what this might mean are utterly fantastic. Possibly the basic principles of photochemistry in connection with the process of photosynthesis do carry over from plant life into animal life, but in a greatly improved way. If the basic chemistry of the human body responds to glandular actions controlled by the pituitary gland responding to light energy, then-as with plants-the characteristics of the light energy would be a very important factor. Different types of light and lighting conditions ranging from natural unfiltered sunlight to various kinds of artificial light, or natural sunlight filtered through different kinds of glass, or light reflected from different colored interior decorations in a room could affect the physical well-being of an individual.....

by John N. Ott
Health & Light
Pocket Books 1973
Reprinted with Permission

THE PINEAL AND ENDOCRINE FUNCTION

Wurtman, Richard J.: Hospital Practice, January 1969

Dr. Wurtman is associate professor of endocrinology and metabolism in the department of nutrition and food science at Massachusetts Institute of Technology, Cambridge.

Recognition that levels of hormonal secretion vary markedly from day to night has triggered intensive investigation into the influence of environmental light upon endocrine function. These studies have pointed to the pineal gland as a major mediator of a wide variety of hormonal responses involving the gonads, thyroid, and pituitary, and the hypothalamus and other regions in the brain.

It is becoming increasingly evident that a number of such biologic rhythms, notably those involving the neuroendocrine apparatus, are activated or synchronized by a source that is rarely considered by physicians - environmental light. In fact, with the exception of food, it appears that the day-night cycle represents the only physiologic input that can exogenously activate endocrine rhythms. And it now has been experimentally substantiated that this exogenous signal (light-dark) is mediated in part by the pineal gland, a structure that until very recently was thought to be vestigial.

The physiologic role of the pineal was entirely unknown until about 75 years ago, when several cases of precocious puberty were reported in boys with tumors that had destroyed the pineal. Soon afterward, the notion arose that the pineal was a gland and that it played some part in regulating or inhibiting gonadal function.

....The role of pineal cells appears to be to convert a neural input controlled by an exogenous factor (light) to an endogenous glandular output (its hormone).

....Dr. Virginia Fiske of Wellesley College had observed that constant light increased, and constant darkness inhibited, the growth of the ovaries in the rat. And in 1961 she reported that the reverse was true of rat pineals- continuous light was associated with decreased pineal weights, while darkness produced enlarged pineals.

After learning about Dr. Fiske's experiments, I began to speculate that perhaps photic activation of the gonads was secondary to inhibition of the pineal, i.e., perhaps light stimulated the gonads by inhibiting the formation of a gonad-inhibiting substance in the pineal. Some tentative experiments indicated this hypothesis might be correct.....

We placed a number of rats in either constant light or constant darkness for two weeks, then removed and weighed the pineals and analyzed their HIOMT activities. The animals kept in constant light had small pineals with very little HIOMT: those in constant darkness had large pineals and high HIOMT activity. We could now speculate that the effect of light-dark on the gonads was mediated by the pineal - that light inhibited melatonin synthesis and thereby reduced the amount of the hormone available to inhibit the gonads.

....Although the pineal originates embryologically as part of the brain and remains firmly connected to the brain in lower vertebrates, in mammals this connection disappears almost entirely by birth or soon thereafter. Instead the pineal receives its neural messages from rather unlikely source - the sympathetic nervous system.

LIGHT
photosynthesis, the occulo-endocrine system
AND DENTAL CARIES (Excerpts)

John Ott, Sc D Hon

"In the past, the primary interest in different artificial light sources in the dental office has been associated with matching white enamel surfaces or being able to see into the back of the patient's mouth. Recent studies, however, point to another much greater cause for concern about the type of artificial lights used not only in the dental office but wherever patients spend any considerable time in-doors.

Light entering the eyes, in addition to vision, is now known to stimulate activity in both the pituitary and pineal glands[1 2] and possibly other areas of the mid-brain region that control the endocrine system and the production of hormones. Thus light energy exerts an influence on our body chemistry as we know it does through the process of photosynthesis in plants. Recent experimental[3 4] studies have indicated that abnormal growth responses develop when any part of the natural sunlight spectral energy is blocked from entering the eyes, and these include dental caries and tooth decay[5] in both laboratory animals and school children.

Sharon et al[18] have shown that immature golden hamsters that were fed a cariogenic diet developed a significantly greater incidence (5-fold increase) of dental caries when raised for a period of 15 weeks under conventional Cool-White fluorescent lighting than hamsters raised for the same period under fluorescent lighting that simulated natural out-door light (Full-Spectrum lighting). Carious lesions were very extensive in the former groups and the crowns of the teeth were virtually destroyed in many cases. Other associated changes included retarded testicular development, resulting in immature seminiferous tubules and no spermatogenesis by the end of the time period, and immature ductal epithelium and lobular architecture in the submandibular gland tissue.

A Study of the effects of these two types of lighting, as well as radiation shielding, was performed on first-grade school children in four windowless classrooms in a Florida school.[19] The results of this five month study indicated that hyperactivity was decreased in the two rooms with Full-Spectrum lighting and radiation shielding increased in the two rooms with conventional Cool-White lighting. In addition, there were strong indications that the experimental conditions played a role in the attainment of academic achievement to a degree much greater than that seen in the control Cool-White classrooms. This pilot study, performed between January and June of 1973, was continued throughout the school year of September, 1973 to June, 1974.

The results confirm the work of Sharon et al in that there was higher incidence of cavities in those children who were in classrooms containing Cool-White fluorescent lighting.

CAVITIES MAY BE RELATED TO AVAILABLE SUNSHINE HOURS

Feller, R.P. Burney, S.W., Sharon, I.M., Some Effects of Light on the Golden Hamster. 1970 Paper presented to meeting of the International Association for Dental Research, New York 1970

VA Outpatient Clinic, Boston, and School of Dentistry, University of the Pacific San Francisco

Studies correlating human caries incidence to sunshine, latitude and winter temperature have shown that caries may be inversely related to the available sunshine hours. Increased vitamin D synthesis mediated by the UV portion of sunlight has been considered responsible. This study investigated some biological implications of two floursecent lights, distinct in UV wave length characteristics. The caries incidence in the golden hamster served as the primary indicator. The lights used were cool white, meager tin UV light, and experimental, abundant in UV light, orange and red. Caged, male hamsters were raised under one of the lights and fed a cariogenic diet, containing 61% sucrose. The animals were sacrificed at 15 weeks, carious teeth were scored and the testes, adrenals, kidneys, submaxillary glands, liver and spleen were removed. The animals raised under the cool white light had an average of 10.9 carious teeth, the experimental animals averaged 2.2 carious teeth. ....This study suggests that caries is related to gonadal development (sexual maturity) which may be affected by different wave lengths of light.

TOOTH DECAY=DIFFERENT COLORS OR WAVELENGTHS OF LIGHT

Ott, John, Sc.D. The Influence of Light on the Retinal Hypothalamic Endocrine System. 1969 Annals of Dentistry, Vol 27, May, No. 1: 10-16

Preliminary results of a pilot experiment conducted jointly with the Zoller Dental Clinic of the University of Chicago indicated a significant difference in the amount of tooth decay in rats kept on the same caries inducing diet but under different colors or wavelengths of light.

In the January 30, 1967, issue of the Journal of the American Medical Association a group of investigators at Baylor University Medical School in Houston, Texas, report alteration of the normal light-dark cycle of the twenty-four hour day causes disturbances in the human biological clock that can effect fine motor and sensory responses.

CHANGE YOUR Ph & BODY CHEMISTRY
THROUGH THE "KIVA" LIGHT!

ARTIFICIAL LIGHT & THE IMMUNE SYSTEM VERSES A PROPERLY BALANCED LIGHT

MANY CHANGES TAKE PLACE WHEN LIGHT TOUCHES (Excerpts)

by Orie Bachechi

THE EFFECT OF LIGHT ON FOOD AND WATER

"It is known that as food and water go through the digestive system of the body, the acid foods create an alkaline product in the body, while alkaline foods create an acid product. It is also known that in an alkaline field, bacteria grow abundantly. For instance, if you eat food in which the alkalinity has been lowered by light, and you consistently eat that food all the time, the body will slowly go into an alkaline zone.

Since bacteria can grow in an alkaline field, the body then becomes an incubator and can grow anything from a common cold to any disease you wish to name.

It is known that the body should be slightly on the acid side to fight off any invaders. The body's immune system has not been allowed to function properly, however, because of exposure to the wrong type of light that has negated the p^H values of the water and food that have been ingested.

Medical practitioners using drugs, and nutritionists using vitamins and foods are trying to bring about a balance in the human body. It has not occurred to anyone that light could be the cause of the imbalance. We do not have a device that can tell us just how much energy each mineral possesses. Since we don't know how much is contained in the food we eat, we could be eating food that is of a lower energy value than the energy value of the body itself. This, then, would cause the body to eventually function at a lower energy rate, bringing on tiredness and other ailments. Natural light imparts energy to all minerals and substances, which in turn provides life-giving ingredients for all life. When food is energized by natural light that is balanced, it will receive optimum energies from the sun. The food, in turn, is at a higher energy value, thus imparting a higher energy value to the body. When vegetables do not receive any light of any kind, the plants die. All plant life and all animal life need light for survival. If the light were to have a balance spectrum, all life would be greatly benefited.

The theory of balanced light shows that each wave of light consists of a balanced spectrum, and each color has a balanced spectral density. Man-made light may be full spectrum, but not a balance full spectrum. Nature has everything in balance, and when consituent parts are combined they are combined in proper portions to keep things in complete balance. Man-made light is out of balance with the sun, thus creating an unbalanced environment. A substance that is irradiated by any kind of light reacts to the components of the waves. The imparted energies received by the substance will excite the molecular vibrations and change the properties of the substance. These changes will be in direct proportion to the vibrations of the spectral color densities. Hense, a substance irradiated by natural light will differ from that of man-made light. When water that has many minerals dissolved in it is irradiated with natural light, these minerals will be highly energized. If one then drinks the water, the energized minerals will impart this added energy to the body. On the other hand, if the same water is irradiated by man-made light, since it will have been energized by an unbalanced light source, it will impart an unbalanced supply of water and minerals. This will be the case whether the water is found in a kitchen, restaurant, hospital, research lab, or whatever.

If we now extend to all situations the theory that light is a source of irradiation, the same results would be evident. If the wrong light source is used, the results will be wrong, or at the least, very misleading. In any place that uses man-made lights, which are not a balanced full spectrum, all things whether they are people, plants or minerals, that are exposed to these lights will be greatly affected by their exposure to this unbalanced environment. This unbalanced environment will produce different anomalies in people, plants, animals and minerals.

These facts should be thoroughly investigated in the food industry in order to safeguard the foods that people eat. In another instance, in the field of medicine, for example, if light were to change the strength of a product which has been prescribed according to the laboratory test specifications, and the product is sold by a drug store to an individual who takes it according to directions, how well will the medicine perform if it is then exposed to another unbalanced light source? Is the individual taking what has been described or is he now taking something else? If the strength has changed, it could appear to be the wrong product since the laboratory specifications were set up under one source of light and the ingestion of the product took place under a different source of light. This type of situation could be very dangerous and a potential health hazard to those whom the product was intended to help.

....Take any one ray of light, follow it through a cell point, and note the change it will show. Take a man-made light source and note the Kelvin rating (°K) of the lamp -- this will indicate its highest point and why certain lamps perform special duties. Example: When babies are born and are taken to the nursery they are under "10 cool white" lamps with a Kelvin rating of 4500 °K, it has been found that some infants develop yellow jaundice or bilirubin after seventy-two hours in the nursery. The medical profession, in order to correct the anomalies that have shown up in the babies, has employed a blue lamp with a 15,000 °K rating to offset the "10 cool white" lamp.

This has changed the Kelvin rating of the room to an alkaline field, 7125 °K, thereby offsetting the Kelvin rating of 4500 °K, an acid producing field. This not only changes the field, but also changes the food that the babies must eat. The babies have to remain under these blue lights for forty hours. The average baby will eat twenty times during this period of time. In theory, the milk or formula has been stored and formulated under 4500 °K, which has destroyed any alkalinity within the milk or formula. As this adulterated food, (which is lacking in alkalinity) goes through the digestive processes of the body, the body begins to change from hi-alkaline to lower acid, thereby killing the virus that can host yellow jaundice. In addition, as the light shines on the baby, it can also through its effect on the pineal gland, cause the baby to become very hyper and very tender to the touch.

To show what I feel is happening inside the cell from the point of light, I use color. It can be translated into any form, any action, or any formula that can be used. For the purpose of discussion, let's say that a cell is composed of three parts. RED - BLUE - YELLOW, enveloped in white.

When one color of light, blue for instance, is shown upon a cell, the BLUE inside receives blue light -- it is seen as blue in a true manner. But at the same time, the RED part of the cell turns violet, and YELLOW GOES TO green. With a yellow light, we have a different change: BLUE turns green, RED turns orange, and YELLOW becomes a stronger yellow. With a red light, another change takes place. BLUE goes to brown, YELLOW goes to orange, and RED becomes a stronger red. When looking at the cells, you should take into consideration the fact that each of these lamps have other parts of the spectrum built into them at all times. In order to balance this, all three colors must shine at the same time so as to strengthen each part of the cell. Now, if these three colors are coming through the pineal gland, they would be giving the correct electrical force to the cell. When food is in balance and is eaten and passes through the digestive system and sent forth to all of these cells, the cell can then utilize the correct amount it needs. When everything that enters the body is balanced, the immune system can operate correctly. If everything were kept at this high level of energy, the body could ward off anything having energy of lesser value. The associate pH values must be in accordance with the energy values. By eating proteins that are in proper balance one could clear up anything from a cold to cancer."

"We in Albuquerque, New Mexico, have discovered that all artificial (man-made) light changes the flavor of water (coffee, tea, etc.). This change in flavor corresponded to a change in pH. This change in water when utilized in the manufacture of bread, changed the amino acids present, thereby giving us a higher protein value bread. Simultaneously, friends of ours found that many changes took place in their bodies when they began using what is now called the Kiva Process.

This process involves the use of a properly balanced LAMP*, and the knowledge of how to use this lamp, in conjunction with food and water. Depending on the degree to which a person stays with the process, minor or major physical balances have been established. With so many diverse problems aided, we believe that the immune system has been stimulated to respond more efficiently to allow the body to cleanse and heal itself more naturally."

*48" T-12 Bipin Fluorescent Tube

LIGHT DEVELOPED BY KIVA FOR USE WITH WATER AND FOOD

KIVA PROCESS

This lamp is built to a specification of 5500 degrees Kelvin plus or minus 1 1/2% under patent No. 3,670,193. The owner of this patent does not in any way lay claim to this process nor do they in any way endorse this process.

KIVA, INC. recommends the use of a 48" fixture and lamp because:

1. It is portable and can be used in any room
2. This size lamp has been found to be most effective when utilized over an area where food is prepared and stored, as prescribed under the KIVA PROCESS.

This lamp is a lamp designed to put, as close as possible sunlight in your kitchen. The light is as close as man can make it to give you the rays that are as close as the sun produces in the shade of a tree.

FOR FURTHER INFORMATION WRITE TO: Oreste Bachechi
c/o KIMO'S INTERNATIONAL
VITALIZED ASSOCIATION, INC.
1311 Tijeras NW
Albuquerque, New Mexico 87102

NOTE: Private testimony given to Editor regarding the use of the KIVA lamp by an R.N. who had Candida. After using the lamp for sometime along with other modalities she has regained her health.

WHERE TO WRITE FOR INFORMATION ON RADIATION EMISSION STANDARDS

You may write to Mr. Villforth concerning the radiation emission rulings on T.V.'s, microwave ovens, flourescent lights, dental & chest x-rays, screening devices at airports, video display terminals, computers, etc., and you may want to ask how the rulings in this country compares with the rulings in other countries of similar populations.

Address: John C. Villforth, Director-Center for Devices & Radiological Health-5600 Fisher's Lane, Rockville, Maryland 20857 - Tel: (301) 443-1228

TV VIEWING HITS NEW RECORD

TV Viewing Per Home Tops 7 Hours Daily

By Fred Rothenberg
Associated Press

New York

America's television fixation reached an all-time high in 1983, with average daily TV viewing per household breaking the seven-hour mark.

A.C. Nielsen's numbers revealed that TV watching per home averaged seven hours, two minutes, an increase of 14 minutes over 1982's record.

It was the sixth consecutive year of record-setting TV viewing, and the 14-minute increase tied 1964 for the biggest rise ever. Network ratings stabilized after a period of decline, while overall viewing for independent and cable stations increased.

Viewing for 1983 was up every month, except for January, although the seven-hour, 38-minute consumption level for January 1983 turned out to be the year's highest monthly average. In comparison, January 1982 had an average of seven hours, 47 minutes.

February, another cold-weather month when viewers gather around the TV set, ranked second in 1983 with an average of seven hours, 33 minutes. The low consumption level, six hours, 23 minutes, came in both June and July.

Viewing was up for all age groups, except children 2-11, said Nielsen.

By breaking the seven-hour barrier by two minutes, 1983 joined 1956 and 1971 as history-making years. In 1956, the five-hour level was reached and, 16 years later, viewing surpassed six hours.

"No one factor accounts for the tremendous jump," said Jeremy Handelman, a CBS researcher. "In general, this additional viewing is likely to come from a variety of groups, watching a variety of programs. All the bits and pieces add up."

Among the reasons cited by industry observers are:

■ The increase in cable penetration. It was in 31 percent of the nation's more than 80 million TV homes in January 1982, 35 percent one year ago and nearly 40 percent today. Cable not only increases TV options, it improves the reception of previously fuzzy independent and PBS stations.

Over a 24-hour broadcast day for the first 11 months of 1983, Handelman said the average number of households watching TV at any given minute was 33.9 percent in homes with pay-cable, 28.1 percent in homes with basic cable and 27.2 percent in non-cable homes.

■ An increase in homes with multiple sets. Figures released this week by the Electronic Industries Association show a 23 percent rise in sales of color TV sets, pushing the total of all TV sales for 1983 to a record 19.7 million sets.

Extra sets in the home accounted for Nielsen's TV breakdown totalling more than 100 percent. The year's prime-time viewing through November had 78 percent watching network stations, 12 percent watching independents, 6 percent watching pay-cable (HBO, Showtime), 4 percent watching cable-originated stations (MTV, ESPN, CNN), 4 percent watching PBS and 3 percent watching superstations (Atlanta's WTBS, Chicago's WGN).

■ More effective major programming. "Programs like the 'M*A*S*H' finale (CBS), 'The Day After' (ABC), 'Thorn Birds' (ABC), 'Winds of War' (ABC) and 'Kennedy' (NBC) attracted the non-habitual TV viewer," said John Sisk, senior vice president for network broadcasting at the J. Walter Thompson ad agency.

■ Change in Nielsen sampling size. Nielsen went from 1200 test homes to 1700 in 1983, and Joel Segal of the Ted Bates ad agency thinks the new surveys have picked up more TV addicts. He called it his "main reason. The increase in viewing could be an aberration," Segal said.

AMERICA'S TV HABIT KEEPS GROWING

AVERAGE VIEWING HOURS PER DAY

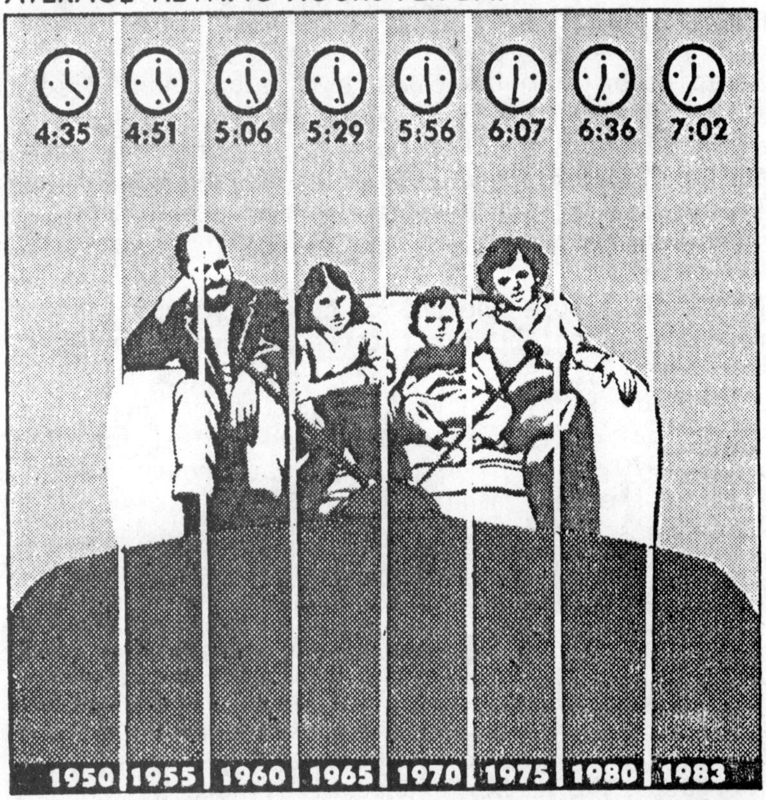

Chart by John Boring

TERROR IN THE TUBE-ALONG THE FRONTIER OF MADNESS

October 20, 1975, FDA informed Zenith Radio Corporation that over one million of their color TV receivers, manufactured from Spring 1974 through Spring 1975, needed "corrective action" because of capacitor failure, in which case the viewers might be exposed to radiation ranging from five to ten milliroentgens. The Federal Standard limit is 0.5 millirads per hour (mr/hr).

X-radiation from the picture tube of your TV set is like a time-bomb with radiation that is cumulative in the body and can alter the physical and mental growth of infants and effect the general health of children and adults, exerting a genetic influence on unborn generations. "Of all living things, the developing embryo and fetus are by far the most sensitive to radiation," write the authors of Silent Slaughter...

TV x-rays expose the unborn child through the entire nine months of development including the first three months of greatest sensitivity...The odds are probably one in ten that a color set manufactured before 1970 will be giving off x-rays above the limit from one side or another. It was always known that T.V. had the potential for giving off harmful x-rays, but it wasn't until 1970 that this situation was brought under any kind of legal control. Most of the sets manufactured during the 40s and early 50s were black and white sets in the low voltage ranges between 16 and 20 kilovolts (kv) and the x-rays they produced were generally too weak to penetrate the glass of the screen, but the high-voltage color sets produced in the 50s had no such built-in safe-guard.

Any electronic tube will emit x-rays when the voltage applied to it exceeds about 5 kv. A TV set is a low voltage x-ray machine. TV tubes operate anywhere from 8 to 25 kv or higher. A small increase in voltage greatly increases the number and penetrating power of the x-rays, and under certain circumstances, in the new sets, the radiation is able to shoot right out the front and reach the viewer. What made the situation worse was that color sets employed two additional x-ray-emitting tubes in addition to the picture tube - the shunt regulator and the voltage rectifier.

The December 15, 1975 EHLRI NEWS (Environmental Health and Light Research Institute) reported that over 1,300,000 new color TVs have been recalled this year-more than any other year. Random checks showed that 20 percent of sets gave off excessive radiation, some dangerous amounts. EHLR's experiments showed that exposure to a color TV screen would kill laboratory mice within 12 days, while those mice protected from TV by a lead shield showed no physical changes. To date, despite documented demonstrations proving that TVs and fluorescent fixtures can be made completely safe, manufacturers haven't made any attempt to rid their products of radiation emissions. (Update: Vita-Lite & the KIVA light are acceptable lights)-Ed.

Dr. John Ott patented a TV radiation shield which uses a mirror device to achieve zero-level radiation. The mirror reflects the picture, while it absorbs the radiation, and the viewer no longer looks directly into the cathode ray gun of the picture tube. But no manufacturers of TV sets have adopted the shield, they simple aren't concerned because they are already complying with government standards based on the 1960 "recommendations" which weren't adequate in the first place.

Rep. Paul Rogers would like to know why N.C.I. turns a deaf ear to the reports of doctors at six major medical centers indicating that light has a direct influence in the tumor development of their lab animal studies.

Excerpt from:
"A Report to the Consumer"
by Ida Honorof
January 1976

MUST YOU GET ZAPPED BY COLOR TV?

You have probably never thought of associating the way you feel with the number of late late shows you yawn through...All of these seemingly unrelated events have something in common. Along with the vivid colors, the laughter, excitement, or boredom, comes a dose of x-radiation from the picture tube of your TV set.

Because it spews forth radiation emissions that are cumulative in the body, television can actually alter the physical and mental growth of infants, can affect the general health of children and adults and can exert a genetic influence on generations yet unborn.

These dire warning were contained in a report by John Nash Ott, Executive Director of Environmental Health and Sight Institute....

Dr. Ott...performed experiments which indicate that radiation in amounts far smaller than what is considered safe by present standards, can affect glandular development, is dangerous to children and adults and disastrous to infants. "Nobody," he says, "and especially an infant, should remain within 15 feet of any part of an operating television set even if it is in another room. That doesn't mean that 15 feet is necessarily a safe distance..... It depends on the set. Many of them spew much more radiation than the law allows.

The baby asleep in his crib in the bedroom on the other side of the wall against which the TV set is placed is in the most critical position. "The infant receives the full effect of radiation from the least protected part of the set at a stage of its life when radiation could do irreparable damage," Ott warns.

Ott's experiments indicate that radiation from TV screens may be entering the pituitary gland at the base of the brain, through the eyes, causing excessive secretions into the endocrine glandular system which controls hormones, the chemistry of the body, and genetically, the future of the race.

Dr. Ott, who, after observing the effects of the accepted standards of e emission on the behavior of his laboratory animals and on the growth pattern of bean sprouts, was even more firmly convinced that the only safe dose of radiation is no dose.

When Ott placed young rats close to a color TV set with the picture tube covered with black photograpic paper, they became highly stimulated, then progressively lethargic. All died in 10 to 12 days. Plants showed a distorted growth pattern.

Other living things, like children, are also adversely affected by levels of radiation considered safe by government standards. A study done in Sarasota, Florida, school system, reported by Dorothy Stockbirdge in the SARASOTA JOURNAL (December 6, 1972) revealed that some of the most highly disturbed school children showed improvement in their behavior after they were made to sit back from the sets and were restricted in the number of hours of TV watching.

In the conventional TV set, the picture tube is horizontally mounted so that the viewing face is vertical and is viewed from the front of the set. As you watch your favorite TV shows, you are directly in the path of x-rays passing through the tube face. Since the x-rays reduce their intensity as they pass through the air, your exposure varies according to your distance from the tube.

Dr. Ott and many scientists maintain that even minute radiation may be harmful since it is the cumulative dosage that affects the gonads and other vital body organs.

Dr. Ott set himself what was considered an impossible goal: breakfast with the "Today" show without radiation emissions belting you in the eyeballs and chest....Dr. Ott put his inventive genius to work and came up with a design for a TV set that has zero radiation emissions for the viewer. A U.S. patent for the invention has already been awarded to him.

If your set were built according to Dr. Ott's new design, the picture tube, which is the source of radiation emissions, would be aimed not at you but at a special mirror which would reflect the picture to you while it absorbed the radiation. Radiation passing through the mirror reflector would be absorbed by a lead shield placed on the back of it. Additional shielding around the radiation source would absorb the remainder of the radiation leakage.

IS TV HARMING OUR CHILDREN?

Rexford Daniels, expert in electromagnetic side-effects, consultant to the Defense and Navy departments and chairman of the President's committee to study the effects of electromagnetism in everyday life including radiation from television, has been studying similar theories that lend support to Ott's suspicions. Daniels said Ott's is a serious scientific work.

"....every year as many as 29,000 people die in the United States as a result of radiation. We know that an overdose of x-ray may cause cancer. We know that the effect of radiation is cumulative, that it builds up in the body over the years. We know, too, that all radiation is essentially the same whether its source is a fallout from nuclear fission, whether it's from radar beams, ultrasonic devices, x-rays to which we are so often exposed for dianostic purposes or television.

The radiation from as little as one x-ray picture can start the chain of events in an embryo developing in its mother's womb that may eventually lead to blood cancer, says Dr. Eugene J. Sternglass of the Westinghouse Research Laboratories (J. Nutrition 47, 289, 1952)

We have been able to ascertain from a radiologist, Dr. David O. Williams of Allentown, Pennsylvania that the average dosage to the abdomen of a pregnant woman for a diagnostic x-ray is about one roentgen. The question arises. How much TV time has the same effect as one x-ray?

SUGGESTED READING ON TELEVISION

The Drug-In Plug
Four Arguments For the Elimination of Television
Zapping of America
Health & Light
Radiation, Light & You
Let There Be Light (Cancer Control Journal)
Co-Evolution Quarterly #16 1979
My Ivory Cellar

Radiation Protection Manuel-1986 $5.00 + $1.00 shipping
by Lita Lee, Ph.D.
2639 Garfield Ct.
San Mateo, Ca. 94403

Note: Permission has been granted to reprint portions of Cancer Control Journal, Let There Be Light, in this Chapter.

XIX

RADIATION OF THE ORAL CAVITY, DENTAL X RAYS & CANDIDA

Lecture: Current Trends in Oral Oncology by: Sol Silverman, D.D.S. Professor & Chairman Div. Oral Medicine University of California-San Francisco	Lecture given to: Amer. Assoc. of Med. Dosimetrists; 2nd Annual Meeting-Region 1 September 28, 1984-San Francisco, Calif. Golden Gateway Holiday Inn

Effects of radiation on Candida in the oral cavity

a) Candida is a constant problem with patients who receive radiation
b) Before radiation 22% had Candida. After radiation 49% had Candida.
c) Radiation causes pathological Candida infections in the mouth.
d) Radiation causes dry environment in the mouth which leads to oral candidiasis.

Other effects of radiation in the oral cavity

a) Radiation causes dental decay
b) Radiation causes pyorrhea
c) Radiation causes diminished saliva and interferes with quality of saliva, making it difficult to swallow
d) [1]Radiation diminishes enzymes
e) Radiation causes loss of taste(which can never be recovered after radiation)[2]
f) Radiation causes teeth to decalcify faster
g) Radiation causes plaque
h) Radiation is reflected off metals in the mouth (gold and silver) causing burns of the gingiva tissue.

[1]Hyrodgen Peroxide is discussed in earlier chapters (through the journals) as being a compound that heals. Here again it is appropriate to state:

a) malignant cancer cells are anaerobic (live without oxygen) and-as shown by Otto Warburg, twice a Nobel prize winner-die in the presence of a properly functioning oxygen (02) mechanism.
b) Hydrogen peroxide can kill the bacteria, viruses, and/or parasites associated with most serious diseases.
c) Hydrogen peroxide does not harm the body

-Editor.

In McGraws Hills's Encyclopedia of Science & Technology (5th Edition) 1982, page 747, under the heading HYDROGEN PEROXIDE it states, ..."ionizing radiation gives off hydrogen peroxide." My question to you the reader is why not use the actual hydrogen peroxide for healing in cancer patients rather then ionizing radiation? -Editor

2 Dr. Silverman states, "Many die after they lose their taste, because they refuse to eat."

(Notes at this seminar taken by Editor.)

RADIATION-DENTAL X-RAYS AND YOU!

*"Up to 30 percent of the 278 million medical and dental diagnostic x-rays made yearly really aren't needed, and since any x ray increases a person's risk of getting cancer, these excess radiations are an unnecessary peril to public health." So says FDA's John C. Villforth, director of Center for Devices and Radiological Health. (See Chapter-Sexual Maturity, Artificial Light & Endocrine System for address of Mr. Villforth for article, "X-Raying of America" FDA Consumer, Dec. 79- Jan.-80.)

A single errant radioactive atom or ray can damage the structure of a cell and its "message center". The genetic coding by which normal growth is regulated.

If its gene structure is mutated, a single cell can multiply out of control. Instead of reproducing normally, the damaged cell goes wild, creating millions of useless, malignant cells like it, crippling the body and eventually leading to a cancerous death.

Radiation can also injure the genetic coding in sperm and egg cells, leading to defects among unborn children.

Though the government continues to contend that there are "safe" levels of exposure, scientific studies by Doctors Victor Archer, Rosalie Bertell, Irwin Bross, Martha Drake, John Gofman, Thomas Mancusco, Thomas Najarian, Ernest Sternglass, Alice Stewart, Arthur Tamplin and others indicate otherwise.

The attack of radiation on our cells is cumulative.

Biological Effects of Radiation

Toxin Production
Enzyme Inactivation
Protein Destruction
Alteration in Cell Permeability (Membrane Damage)
Altered Cellular Metabolism
Morphological Changes
Mutations
Retardation of Cell Division
Total Inhibition of Cell Division
Abnormal Cell Division

Comparing Radiation Exposure of Jet Flights and Dental X-Rays

A commercial pilot may receive several hundred millirems exposure in the course of a year from coast-to-coast jet flights. Whereas a full set of dental X-rays could easily result in a dose of 1,000 millirems to the face. Medical radiation is by far the greatest man-made source of radiation.

*Dr. Bruce Halstead, M.D (Toxicologist)stated in a Lecture given before the Cancer Control Society , July 4th, 1986 that the U.S. Goverment was suppressing information on Radiation Protection.

Radiation and Human Health by Dr. John Gofman, M.D.

In the chapter "Dental X-Rays and Brain Cancer", Dr. Gofman states, "It appears to the author that the place to which one should direct serious attention, in the case of dental X-rays is the dose to the brain itself.

Many people are considerably concerned about thyroid doses and thyroid cancer from dental X-ray procedures. The brain is of far more concern per rad delivered, as these specific-organ cancer doses demonstrate. Eyes are of concern, for example, with respect to cataract or corneal injury, but are of far less concern than the brain with respect to cancer death risk."

Dr. Gofman goes on to say, "Dental examinations are often performed on children, repeatedly. We must emphasize that the specific-organ cancer doses will be some four times lower for very young children than the values listed above, or on the order of 2,000 to 2,500 organ-rads.

If a young male child received 1 rad to the brain, he receives 1 brain rad. If it takes 2,000 brain-rads to guarantee 1 fatal brain cancer, then the delivery of 1 brain rad gives him a risk of fatal cancer of 0.0005, or 5 chances in 10,000. Stated otherwise, 5 out of every 10,000 male children given 1 rad to the brain will eventually die of brain cancer.

One rad to the brain constitutes a high risk, in the author's opinion, in exchange for the benefits of dental X-rays in general. So does 0.2 rad to the brain, which means that 1 out of every 10,000 children so " "examined" will die of brain cancer. Given that techniques are very different from office to office, and locale to locale, we should not be surprised al all to find a 100-fold range in brain exposure from dental X-rays.

There are undoubtedly good reasons for dental examinations; the decision is up to the individual adult or the family of the individual child. But the dental profession has an obligation to provide some serious estimate of brain radiation dose for the procedures and equipment which are being used. The public should demand this information."

Dr. Gofman's remedy: "A better solution, consistent with liberty and dignity, lies in the widespread education of the medical community, the legal profession, patients, and jurors (the general public) about the hazards of ionizing radiation."

SUGGESTED READING:
Radiation Protection Manual
Lita Lee, Ph.D. ($5. + $1.)
2639 Garfield St.
San Mateo, Ca.94403

FOR RADIATION PROTECTION:
COENZYME Q_{10}
Biotics Research Corp.
5731 Savoy Lane
Houston, Texas 77036
(800) 231-5777

MONTMORILLIONITE
P.O. Box 945
Sequoia West
San Carlos, Calif.

CABBAGE JUICE* - See Chap. VIII
WHEAT GRASS JUICE " " "
SUPER OXIDE DISMUTASE (S.O.D.)
*See Gov. Report "Reduction of X-Radiation Mortality by Cabbage and Broccoli-U.S.Army QM Food & Con
Dec. 2, 1958

XX

THE JAW JOINT, HYPOGLYCEMIA & CANDIDA

THE TEMPOROMANDIBULAR JOINT

The temporomandibular joint is also known as the jaw joint or TMJ. The TMJ is the hinge at the side of the face that connects the jaw, or mandible, to the temporal bone of the skull. It is located just in front of the ear and is the joint from which all jaw movements take place.

Approximately 40% of the nerves leave the cranium through the TMJ. If these nerves are suppressed or restricted in any manner through the TMJ being out of alignment, this can cause serious and far reaching health problems.

Since the TMJ problem is a cumulative disorder, you might notice such early signs as feature imbalance, pain radiating up the side of the head from in front of the ear; muscle cramps and pain in the shoulders and neck; earaches & toothaches despite the absence of infection. You might notice symptoms of pain arising in the arms, lower back and legs.

SELF EVALUATION FOR THE TMJ PROBLEM

Gently insert the ends of your little fingers into your ears and press forward, toward the front of the ear, while opening and closing your mouth several times. If your TMJ is normal, you will feel nothing unusual. If your jaw is unbalanced, however, you will feel the head of the jawbone, pushing against your finger. This will be quite noticeable on the side which is most severely out of place. Any pain you may feel is further indication of trouble.

TMJ MOST IMPORTANT JOINT IN THE BODY

Dr. John Diamond, M.D., of Valley Cottage, New York stated in an address given to the International College of Applied Kinesiology in June 1976, "The Temporomandibular Joint is the most important joint in the body." Any uncorrected imbalance in the jaw joint can lead to symptoms and illnesses anywhere in the body.

Dr. Harold Arlen, M.D. states the TMJ syndrome is a physical problem but eventually affects one psychologically. Patients with ear pain, fullness, hearing loss, loss of equilibrium have a disorder of the TMJ associated with the spasm of the muscles of mastication.

George Goodheart, D.C. stated the TMJ is the most important joint in the body and it actually can cause circulation problems, lymphatic blockage and could have psychological influences.

Dr. Allen Shore, DDS states in the October 1970 issue of Dental Survey that approximately 20% of the population is afflicted with some form of TMJ dysfunction; the condition is mis-diagnosed in a majority of cases. Kinesiological and Dermatron methods show that the figure is closer to 40%.

FUNCTION OF THE TMJ

The TMJ is a primary intersection for the circulation of blood to and from the brain. Most headaches are a result of a disturbance in blood supply to the brain, and oral stress causes the neck to tighten, restricting circulation. This area is also a crucial pathway for the transmission of neural impulses. To have this center and the major muscle groups that operate the mouth and lower lower jaw in a constant state of stress leads not only to physical tension but to abnormal changes in hormonal and chemical balance as well.

It is also known that four bio-electromagnetic circuits pass through the TMJ area. These are: Small Intestine Circuit, Gall Bladder Circuit, Stomach circuit &(1)Endocrine circuits. An abnormal TMJ affects all structures on these circuits resulting in clinical symptoms.

THE BRAIN, THE JAW AND THE EAR

Dr. Harold Arlen, M.D. suggests neural patterns are established within the brain stem in which the jaw-bone and ear-bone movements are integrated.

This is the key to the relationship between the jaw and ear dysfunction that is plaguing modern man, along with the deterioration of other parts of the jaw and dental apparatus. Dr. Arlen goes on to state, "We must look into the disturbances in neuromuscular joint dysfunction. This takes us into the central nervous system.

MORE SYMPTOMS OF THE TMJ SYNDROME

TMJ pain in ear,
Backache, neck problems
Headache
Weak muscle
Shoulder problems
Ear ache
Tinnitis
Middle and inner ear problem

Sinusitis
Scoliosis
Equilibrium problems
Leg length abnormality
Muscular weakness & imbalance (MS)
Stomach problems
Small intestine abnormality
(2) Endocrine abnormality and irregulariti

(1) and (2) refer to Endocrine. Included in the Endocrine system is the 'Thymus'. If the TMJ is out of alignment this will in turn effect the Thymus cutting down on the nerve stimulation sent to it in order for it to function properly. Again, when the Thymus is working improperly the 'T' cells are not released in full strength and this in turn sets up the foreign invader to come in and take over as the 'T' cells are unable to fight these invaders.

HYPOGLYCEMIA QUESTIONNAIRE

Directions: Check each symptom according to its severity:

Column 0 indicates that the problem never occurs
Column 1 means that it is mild and occurs occasionally
Column 2 is moderate and/or occurs at least once a week
Column 3 means that is is severe and occurs frequently

PART A

0	1	2	3	
				Tired all of the time
				Hungry between meals or at night
				Depressed
				Insomnia, awakening with inability to return to sleep
				Wake up after a few hours sleep
				Fearful (Overwhelmed by people, places or things)
				Can't decide easily
				Can't concentrate
				Poor memory
				Worry frequently
				Feel insecure or have a low self image
				Highly emotional
				Moody
				Cry easily, or feel like crying inside
				Fits of anger
				Magnify insignificant details (mountains out of molehills)
				Eat candy, cake, or drink soda pop
				Eat bread, pasta, potatoes, rice, or beans
				Consume alcohol
				Drink more than three cups of coffee or cola drinks daily
				Crave candy, soda, or coffee between meals or mid-afternoon
				Can't work well under pressure
				Headaches
				Sleepy during the day
				Sleepy or drowsy after meals
				Lack of energy
				Reduced initiative
				Can't get started in the morning
				Eat when nervous

PART B

0	1	2	3	
				Stomach cramps or 'nervous stomach'
				Allergies: asthma, hay fever, skin rash, sinus trouble, etc.
				Fatigue relieved by eating
				Suicidal thoughts or tendencies; feeling of hopelessness
				Bored
				Bad dreams
				Irritable before meals
				Heart beats fast (palpitations)
				Get shakey inside when hungry
				Feel faint if meal is delayed
				Ulcers, gastritis, chronic indigestion, abdominal bloating
				Cold hands or feet
				Blurred vision
				Bleeding gums
				Dizziness, giddiness, or light headedness
				Aware of breathing heavily
				Bruise easily
				Reduced sex drive
				Uncoordination (drop or bump into things)
				Sweating excessively
				Unsocial or antisocial behavior
				Muscle twitching or cramps
				Skin aches or itches
				Phobias (excessive fear of some thing or situation)
				Hallucinations
				Convulsions
				Trembling (shaking) of the hands
0				TOTALS (number of checks in each column times column number)*

TOTAL OF COLUMNS 1, 2, & 3: ________

* Add up the number of checks in a single column in Part A and Part B and then multiply that number by the number at the head of that column. For example, if you have 15 checks in column headed by the #3, multiply 15 times 3 and the total for that column is 45. Repeat this procedure for column numbers 1 & 2 and then add the three totals together.

GRAND TOTAL OF:
15 OR LESS INDICATES 5% PROBABILITY OF HAVING HYPOGLYCEMIA
15 - 20 INDICATES 15% PROBABILITY OF HAVING HYPOGLYCEMIA
20 - 25 INDICATES UP TO 50% PROBABILITY OF HAVING HYPOGLYCEMIA
25 - 35 INDICATES 75% PROBABILITY OF HAVING HYPOGLYCEMIA
35 - 45 INDICATES 90% PROBABILITY OF HAVING HYPOGLYCEMIA
45 - INDICATES 98% PROBABILITY OF HAVING HYPOGLYCEMIA

NAME________________ **DATE**__________ **SEX**______ **AGE**______ **WEIGHT**______ **HEIGHT**______

REFERENCE: Dr. Harold W. Harper, M.D.

SYMPTOMS OF HYPOGLYCEMIA
(from 1100 cases)

by Carlton Fredericks, Ph.D.

PER CENT	SYMPTOM
94	Nervousness
89	Irritibility
87	Exhaustion
86	Faintness, dizziness, tremor, cold sweats
80	Lack of motivation, lack of desire to take on projects, procrastination
77	Depression
73	Vertigo, dizziness, lack of balance
72	Drowsiness, especially P.M. and evenings
71	Headaches
69	Digestive disturbances
67	Forgetfulness
62	Insomnia (awakening and inability to return to sleep)
62	Constant worrying, unprovoked anxiety
57	Mental confusion
57	Internal trembling
54	Palpitation of the heart, rapid pulse
53	Muscle spasms
51	Numbness
50	Unsocial, asocial, antisocial behavior, lack of patience
50	Indecisiveness
46	Crying spells
44	Lack of sex drive (females)
43	Allergies
43	Lack of coordination
43	Leg cramps
42	Lack of concentration
40	Blurred vision
40	Twitching, jerking muscles
39	Itching and crawling sensation on skin
37	Gasping for breath
34	Smothering spells
34	Staggering
30	Sighing and yawning
29	Impotence (male)
27	Unconsciousness
27	Night terrors, nightmares
24	Rheumatoid arthritis
23	Phobias, fears
21	Neuro-dermititis
20	Suicidal tendency
17	Nervous breakdown
2	Convulsion

"Hypoglycemia is directly related with temporomandibular joint (jaw joint) disturbances through the electromagnetic system. Experience has shown that practically all TMJ syndromes involve hypoglycemia (low blood sugar). Correcting TMJ problems often result in improvement of or correction of the symptoms just listed."

James Ouye, D.D.S.

Jaw joint problems lead to an imbalance of the p^H in the saliva. This in turn will upset the balance of the intestinal flora. Not only will this cause functional disorders but also structural disorders which will in turn affect the ileocecal valve, perhaps causing it to remain in an open position, letting food particles re-enter the intestional tract, thus causing parasites, etc.

It is also important to know that one of the four "bio-electromagnetic" circuits which pass through the TMJ is the Endocrine Circuit, which regulates the Thymus. If this circuit is interferred with through Jaw Joint misalignment you will then have a Thymus dis-regulation.

From the above paragraphs, you the reader can now discern why Dr. R. Voll, M.D. of West Germany, (Nobel Prize Candidate for Medicine, 1983, 1984) stated that the jaw joint was the most important joint in the body. You the reader can now also see when there is jaw joint misalignment, hypoglycemia and then Candida follow in a natural sequence.

Editor.

Dr. David Eggleston, D.D.S. and Professor of Dentistry at the University of Southern California stated, "Malocclusion has generally been assumed to be genetic in origin. But genetics do <u>NOT</u> explain the dramatic increase in malocclusion in ONE GENERATION when a primitive society adapts a "civilized" diet and/or life style. It is common in the United States for people to have heart disease, diabetes, hypertension, dental caries, malocclusion...."

"Abnormal function of the nervous and endocrine system (Immune System is part of this system) with no underlying structural deformity of these systems is considered a functional disorder. When the patient is under distress the nervous system and the endocrine system send out their distress signals. When the person is under distress, the signals from these two systems are not normal and functional disorders occur."

"Abnormal endocrine, nervous and muscular system function creates poor digestion, poor blood and lymph-circulation, electrolyte imbalance, hormonal imbalance and low resistance to microbes. These are the major factors in the pathogenesis of dental and systemic degenerative diseases."

"Nutritional and/or environmental stressors can cause functional disorders. The abnormal neurology, endocrinology, and kinesiology (muscle function) can interfere with proper growth and development resulting in malocclusion. The malocclusion can become an additional stressor (structural distress) which perpetuates and aggravates the state of stress within the patient."

(In the above paragraph Dr. Eggleston mentions nutritional and environmental stressors which cause functional disorders-"jaw joint syndrome". Some of these nutritional stressors are the preservatives and chemicals in the food, and the pesticides being used on the soil. Some of the environmental stressors are of course fluoride which is in the drinking water and is being emitted through Nuclear Plants and other industrial cites. - Ed.)

"Any abnormal muscle function resulting from functional disorders (tongue thrusting, ileocecal valve spasm, etc.) will cause changes in skeletal muscle or soft tissue (malocclusion, colitis, etc.) These abnormalities can be perceived by the brain as a distress."

(Again Dr. Eggleston explains how having a jaw joint syndrome leads to a malfunctioning ileocecal valve. This of course can lead one to become a prime candidate for Candida. Refer back to Introduction on Dr. John Lubecki's book on "Body Balancing" and the consequences of a malfunctioning ileocecal valve. Ed.)

"Occlusal adjustment by the dentist will eliminate the distress of malocclusion but if the nutritional and environmental stressors remain at a level above the patient's distress threshold, the abnormal function will continue."

Summary: The following hypothesis has been proposed: Stressors-environmental and/or nutritional-can cause functional disorders. Functional disorders are abnormal neurology, endocrinology, and kinesiology without underlying organic pathology, The malfunction of these three systems is a major factor in the pathogenesis of systemic and dental degenerative diseases.

(Dr. Egglestons stresses that functional problems (jaw joint problems) lead to abnormal neurology, endocrinology (immune system) and kinesiology (muscle system) and that these problems are not genetic in orgin but from a daily stress of nutritional and environmental factors. Ed.)

The above article is from:

THE INTERRELATIONSHIP OF STRESS AND DEGENERATIVE DISEASES
The Journal of Prosthetic Dentistry
November 1980 Volume 44 Number 5
by Dr. David Eggleston, D.D.S.
(Excerpts)

For Reprint Requests write to:
Dr. D. W. Eggleston, DDS
1441 Avocado Ave., Ste. 508
Newport Beach, Calif. 92660

(The above article ties in with Dr. Carlton Fredericks' Symptoms of Hypoglycemia and the paragraph following, written by Dr. James Ouye, who relates that Jaw Joint syndrome or problems lead to Hypoglycemia. Over 50% of the population in the United States have jaw joint problems. This would mean that over 50% have symptoms of hypoglycemia. Ed.)

According to Dr. Luc De Schepper, M.D. and Acupuncturist the spleen is the master of the immune system & both Hypoglycemia and Candida are a spleen deficiency.

There are four bio-electromagnetic circuits which pass through the TMJ area. If the TMJ is out of alignment it will effect all of these circuits adversely. (One of these circuits is the Stomach circuit which corresponds with the "paired organ" - spleen-pancreas).

Summarizing the above, reason would follow that spleen deficiency can be caused by an imbalance of the jaw joint. The jaw joint is adversely effected through nutritional (chemicals, preservatives, pesticides, etc.) and environmental factors (fluorides and heavy metals, i.e., mercury & nickel). Editor.

The following excerpt from the book, THE REAL AMERICAN TRAGEDY, (with a forward by Dr. Royal Lee, D.D.S.) has a very interesting section on the jaw joint and fluoridation which will "tie" in with how jaw joint problems are formed in this country through environmental pollutants (read paragraph below).

"The official data reveals the aggravations of oral conditions in Newburgh: There is a radical increase in mal-occlusion, i.e., improper meshing of teeth of the two jaws when the mouth is closed. Furthermore, according to the University of the State of New York, in 1954, in Newburgh 3 out of every 5 children suffered from some oral trouble as compared with 2 out of 5 in Kingston, a neighboring non-fluoridated city chosen by PHS for a comparison. Another unexpected discovery was made. The dental arch of fluoridated children became deformed."

THE CONNECTION BETWEEN THE THYMUS, THE JAW JOINT, VERTEBRAE C1, C2 AND A.I.D.S.

C1 and C2 are the first two vertebrae in the neck area. The atlas and axis. The atlas is called the 'King Pin' (most important vertebrae). If these vertebrae are out of alignment, the entire structure will be out of alignment. Both of these vertebrae supply the THYMUS. Through mis-alignment, nerve flow from C1 and C2 to the THYMUS will effect its production of 'T' cells, which in turn will effect the function of the immune system.

REFERENCES OF DOCTORS WHO PRACTICE TMJ/CRANIAL THERAPY:

Harold Gelb, DDS
635 Madison Ave.
New York, New York

Dr. Brendan C. Stack, DDS
803 West Broad Street-
Falls Church, Virginia 22046
(or-Springfiled, Va.)

Dr. Lawrence Funt, DDS
Bethesda, Maryland

Dr. Charles Hulsey, DDS
Solana Beach, California

Dr. John Char, DDS
850 Kamehameha Highway
Pearl City, Hawaii 96782

Dr. Mark Abramson, DDS
853 Middlefield Road
Palo Alto, California

Dr. James Ouye, DDS
1660 Westwood Drive
San Jose, California

Dr. A. Landerman, DDS
7064 Corline Court Suite #1
Sebastopol, California 95472

Dr. Richard Robertshaw, D.C.
473 Pine Street
San Francisco, California

Dr. Dennis Steigerwald, D.C.
Solana Beach, California

Dr. Clyde Schultz, DDS
450 Sutter
San Francisco, California

Bruce H. Kinnie, DDS, P.A.
7007 Brookfield Road
Columbia, S. Carolina 29206

David G. Denton, D.C.
12381 Wilshire Blvd.
W. Los Angeles, Calif. 90025

Viola Fryman, D.O.
8030 Girard Ave.
La Jolla, California
(Children only)

Elliott Blackman, D.O.
1956 Union Street
San Francisco, California

Dr. Robert Ricketts, DDS
881 Alma Real Drive
Pacific Palisades, California

I. Imber, DDS
Reseda
San Fernando Valley
California

Dr. Robert J. Peshek, DDS
7759 California Ave.
Riverside, California

D.F. Hazelnus, D.M.D.
4414 N.E. Fremont Street
Portland, Oregon, 97213

Craig Foster, D.D.S.
450 Sutter Street
San Francisco, California

FOR HYPOGLYCEMIA- BIOGLYCOZYME FORTE. Bioglycozyme Forte contains all the B Vitamin fractions that are integral parts of carbohydrate metabolism, along with the necessary minerals to improve glucose tolerance. This product also provides complete glandular and enzyme support for a properly functioning endocrine system to enhance carbohydrate metabolism.

1134 $12.00/90 tablets
1135 $32.00/270 tablets (Purchased only through chiropractor, physician or pharmacist). Biotics Research Corp. 12117 Moorpark St., Studio City, Ca. 91604 1-800-722-0046

XXI

THE VAGUS NERVE

THE VAGUS NERVE, THE TEETH AND THE JAW JOINT (TMJ) IN RELATION TO THE THYMUS AND AIDS

According to Dr. Roger Williams, "Every organ and tissue in the body has a 'telephone system'; how these organs and tissues function depends upon the messages they receive. Since the distribution of nerves (telephone lines) is distinctive in each of us, just as is the distribution of blood vessels, this contributes greatly to the diversity which exists within our bodies."

NEUROLOGIC TOOTH INVOLVEMENT

The teeth and the entire mouth, like the jaw joint receive an abundant nerve supply out of proportion to the rest of the body. Because of this large supply there is a greater chance for noxious impulses to enter the 'computer-like' body. If an imbalance of function develops at this area, it can cause problems in any area of the body.

The teeth are related through meridians and nerves to the 12 cranial nerves (see following page for cranial nerve chart) and each tooth is directly or indirectly related to a specific organ of the body.

Teeth can actually be filled with a filling causing a neurological allergy to one of the twelve cranial nerves, which in turn can cause one of the organs of the body to mal-function. (e.g., silver fillings and/or gold crowns with silver underneath). An example would be: teeth 20 and 28 are related to cranial nerve No. 10 (the vagus nerve). These fillings could cause particular organs associated with this nerve to mal-function.

The organs associated with the vagus nerve are: heart, lungs, stomach, blood vessels of abdomen, liver & ducts, gall bladder, small intestine, large intestine and the thymus gland. (See Vagus Nerve Chart this Chapter)

Dental appliances or fillings can cause an allergy thus sending noxious impulses to the brain causing mal-functioning organs. The jaw joint may also then become involved and mis-aligned thus impinging in some way on the vagus nerve and in turn slow down its process of sending nerve stimulation to the thymus.

Since the vagus nerve supplies the thymus gland, and this is the gland that manufacturers the 'T' Cells for the immune system, this cranial nerve #10 can become in-active through dentistry and/or cranial fixation, accident, etc, then the body can come down with any type of disease, as the immune system ceases to protect us from the fungi, e.g., 'Candidia', which can then multiply and completely paralyze the thymus from maturing the 'T' cells and releasing them to fight foreign invaders. Thus the body succumbs to any infection and this is known as AIDS.

Mercury/ Silver fillings affects the lymphatic system with all its membranes and glands, and the thymus.

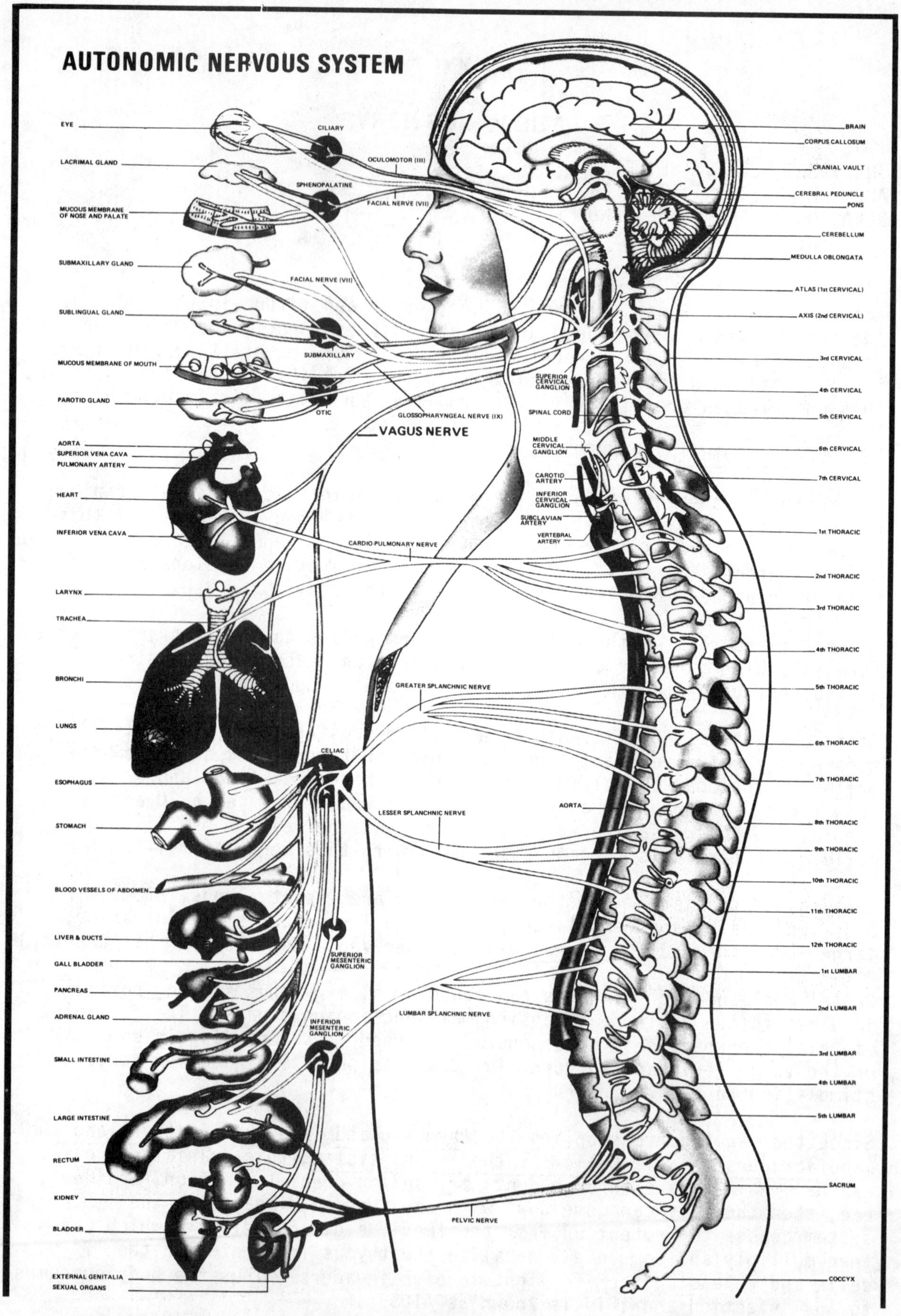

The above chart shows the vagus nerve connecting with the major organs of the body. The vagus nerve also supplies the thymus gland which is not shown here in the chart.

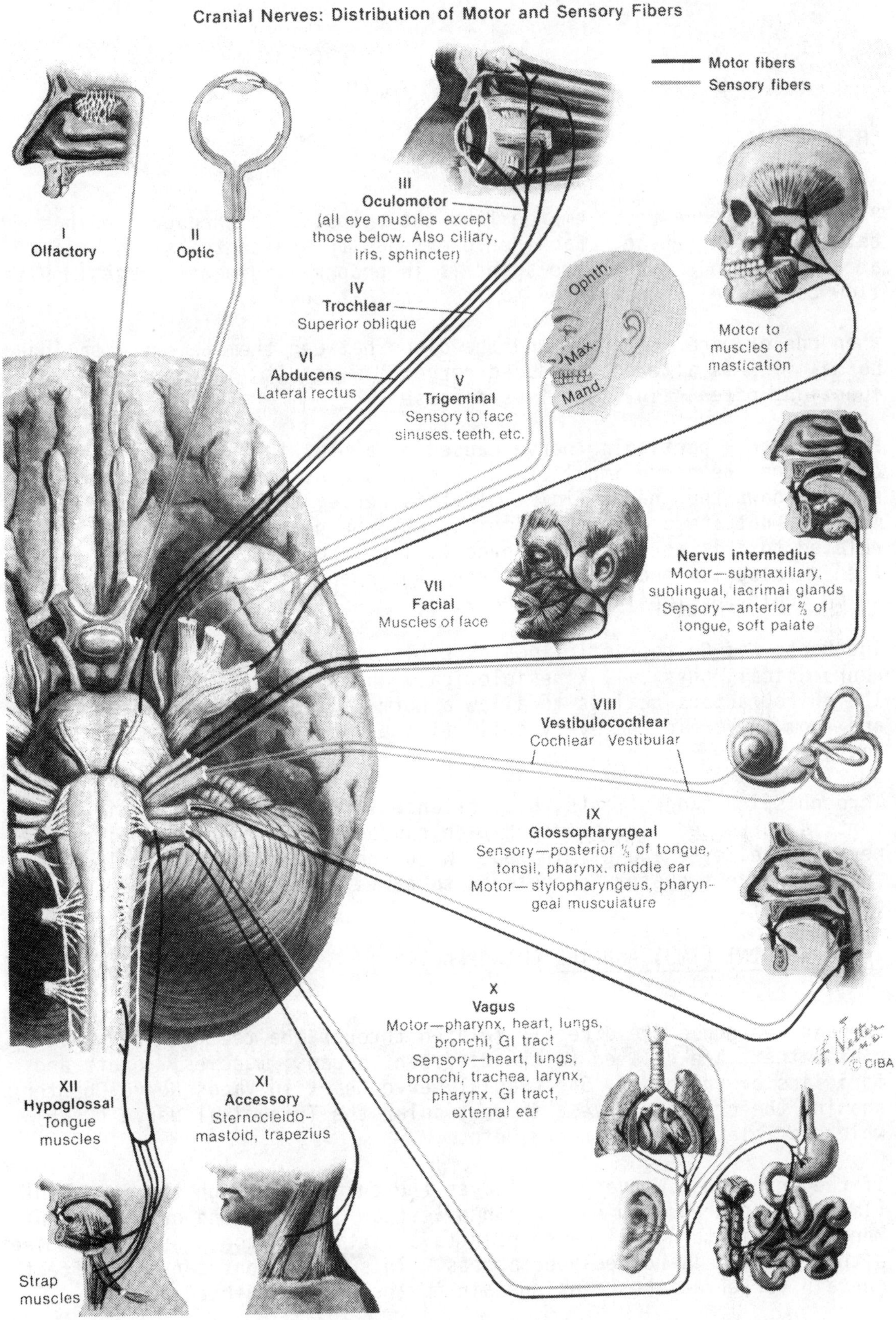

Ten of the 12 cranial nerves are associated with the temporal bone. If this bone is out of alignment through accident, birth, dentistry (malocclusion or holding jaw open for long periods of time) this can affect the related organs of the body.

XXII

CHIROPRACTIC

CHIROPRACTIC

31 pairs of nerve roots emerge from the spinal cord through openings between the vertebrae. Each nerve extends to and controls a specific area of the body. When the spine is in proper alignment, nerve-impulse flow can travel unrestricted to its destination.

When one or more vertebrae and the discs between them become misaligned normal flow is altered. Reduced nerve flow results in impaired function, often pain, sometimes disease.

Pressure on a particular nerve caused by a blow to the head or spine can change the nerve impulses to various organs, thus stopping or slowing down the 'nerve flow'. If this nerve, through vertebrae alignment, is not freed from this impingment, the particular organ related to this nerve will be greatly impaired. The person will then develop low energy and further impairment of the body which could develop into a disease.

The Doctor of Chiropractic locates subluxations through orthopedic, neurological, physical, kinesiological, and spinal examinations. The chiropractors goal is to allow a normal flow of communication to and from the brain and every cell, tissue, organ, and system in the body; a pre-requisite to health.

Through spinal adjustments, body balance is restored, spinal mis-alignment is corrected, and the condition caused by the pinched or irritated nerve is relieved and eliminated. When the correction is completed and the nervous system is restored to normal function, the body will cure itself.

THE JAW JOINT (TMJ) AND THE CHIROPRACTOR

Certain vertebrae are directly related through the teeth. The nerves of the teeth are related to the different organs, muscles, joints and meridians of the body. See Cranial Nerve Chart in Vagus Nerve Chapter showing the cranial nerves, in particular the Trigeminal Nerve (No.5) which is related to the teeth, etc.

If the Trigeminal Nerve which leaves the cranium through the jaw joint (TMJ) is impinged upon by the condoyle (jaw joint) being out of alignment, this in turn will cause pain to a particular tooth or several teeth, although there is no decay or abcess. This impingment can also effect certain vertebrae thus causing pain in the related vertebrae.

Until the jaw joint is corrected, the adjustments by the chiropractor will not be permanent.

Our bodies are structural, nutritional, spiritual and electrical. The jaw joint is not only held in place by muscles and tendons, but functions electrically as well. If per chance there are noxious impulses being fed into the cranial nerves through allergic fillings, (silver/mercury), the jaw joint will not stay in place, nor the vertebrae associated with the teeth of the allergic fillings.

CRANIAL CERVICAL SYNDROME

Structural imbalance of the joints and muscles of our head and neck causes related functional imbalance of the nervous system.
Cranial cervical syndrome is treated by a program of gentle adjustments and re-alignment of the cranial, spinal, face and jaw structure by a cranially trained chiropractor, osteopath, or dentist.

THE ATLAS AND AXIS

The Atlas and Axis (cervical vertebrae 1 & 2) if out of alignment can adversely affect the jaw joint and the entire nervous system as these top vertebrae are the "king pins".

REFERENCE

Dr. Dennis Steigerwald, D.C. of Solana Beach, California is a member of the Holistic Dental Association and gives seminars to various groups of dentists and chiropractors

According to Dr. D.W. Kelley DDS, there is a group of dentists who use a new method called Mandibular Equilibration to re-shape the skull, take stresses from the brain, and in this way effect very profound neurological changes. Note: In order for treatment to work and put the jaw back in alignment and the vertebrae, one of the important things to remember is that all allergic fillings must be removed from the mouth in order to make the adjustment permanent. Also a diet high in grains and greens must be adhered to.

THE SPINE AND NERVOUS SYSTEM

"The nervous system controls and coordinates all organs and structures of the human body." (*Gray's Anatomy*, 29th Ed., page 4). Misalignments of spinal vertebrae and discs may cause irritation to the nervous system and affect the structures, organs, and functions shown below.

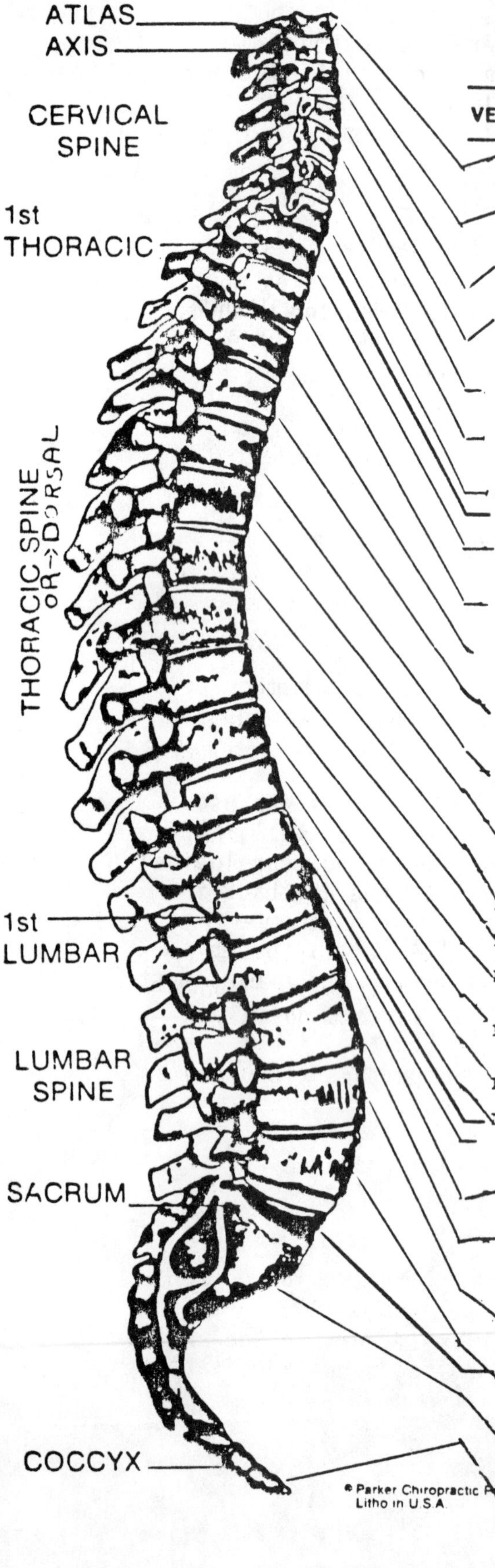

VERTEBRAE	STRUCTURES, ORGANS, AND FUNCTIONS AFFECTED
C-1	Cranial bones, scalp or head, parts of the brain, optic tracts, EAR & Atlas itself
C-2	Posterior part of skull, external ear, orbital region, brain & cranial bones,
C-3	Nasal passages, retina, teeth, orbital region, cheeks, & ears
C-4	Retina, eyelids, orbital region, eustachian tubes, naso pharynx, nasal passages, external nose, hyoid bone, hard & soft palates of the mouth, gums, teeth, bones of the face, salivary glands, cervical glands, & the tissues of upper cervical region
C-5	Retina, nose, face, teeth, posterior & lateral muscles of the neck, thyroid gland, parathyroid glands, & shoulder joint
C-6	Trachea, thyroid gland, lower tonsils, hyoid bone, larynx part of pharynx, anterior part of shoulder, arm, forearm and hand
C-7	Trachea, bronchi, muscles of lower part of neck, tonsils, thyroid glands, larynx, tissues of throat, the shoulders, arms, forearms & hands
D-1	Bronchi, Sternum, clavicle, Including muscles attached to clavicle & scapula, shoulder, arm & hand
D-2	Heart, pericardium, aorta, arm, forearm, hands, bronchi, sternum, shoulders, 2nd pair of ribs, muscles & skin of this region
D-3	Lungs, pleura, lower part of heart, sternum, mammary glands, 34d pr. of ribs, muscles & skin of that region, posterior part of shoulders, internal side of arm & forearm and hand
-4	Liver, gall bladder, bele duct, lower part of lungs, 4th pair of ribs, muscles & skin of that region
D-5	Esophagus, cardiac region, stomach, liver, gall bladder, lower part of pleura, & sometimes arms, sometimes temporal
D-6	Esophagus, stomach, tongue, glands of throat, sublingual, sub-maxillary & parotid glands, eyeballs, pharynx, 6th pr. of ribs, & skin and muscles of that region
D-7	Lower part of stomach
D-8	Duodenum, gall bladder
D-9	Common Bile duct, pancreas, spleen, diaphragm, lower part of liver, 7th & 8th & 9th pairs of ribs & muscles and skin of that region
D-10	Supra Renal Glands, upper part of kidneys, eyelids, 10th pr. of ribs, muscles & skin of that area, sometimes spleen
D-11	Kidneys, 11th & 12th pairs of ribs,
D-12	Skin & muscles of that region, eyelids & upper part of ureters.
L-1	Peritoneum, lower part of Kidneys, small intestine, ureters
L-2	Peritoneum, ileocecal valve, lower part of small intestine, cecum, appendix, ovaries, skin & muscles
L-3	Lower Part of small intestine, cecum, vermiform appendix, muscles of lower abdomen, lower part of peritoneum, bladder, testes, ovaries uterus, broad ligament, lg. intestine, prostrate, muscles of front thigh & knee joint
L-4	Bladder, testes, uterus, vagina, lg. intestine, innominate bones, & Bones of lower extremities, prostate, rectum, muscles of back of thigh, leg & foot
L-5	Buttocks, bladder, uterus, lower part of ureters, prostate, rectum, back of thigh
Sacrum & Coccyx	Buttocks, & generative organs, sacroiliac articulations, sacrum & sacral muscles, rectum, leg & foot
Coccyx	Anus & tissues of coxxyx, rectum

XXIII

FLUORIDE DAMAGES THE IMMUNE SYSTEM

25 September, 1983

Excerpts from-
A Letter To 'Spotlight' Newspaper
FLUORIDATION IMPLICATED IN "AIDS"

The fluoridated cities of New York, San Francisco and Miami have four times more AIDS (Acquired Immune Deficiency Syndrome) cases than non-fluoridated Newark, Houston and Los Angeles. In cases per 100,000 population New York leads with 31.6 followed by San Francisco with 24 and Miami with 19.1 as of September 24, 1982 from Center for Disease Control Morbidity and Mortality Weekly Report, Vol. 31, #37, pg. 513. The three cities not fluoridated are Newark with only 7.6 cases per 100,000, Houston with 5.2 and Los Angeles with only 4.9.

These extremely significant statistics are not, however, surprising to scientists and researchers familiar with the highly reactive element, fluorine- the most electronegative of all elements and most reactive. The exact mechanism, at the molecular level, of how fluoride damages enzymes has been known since the work of Emsley and co-workers of King's College, England was reported in the Journal of the American Chemical Society, January 14, 1981. They discovered that the second strongest hydrogen bond ever known is that of the fluoride ion with the hydrogen of the amide radical forming amino acid chains which form proteins. Enzymes are proteins and function by making and breaking of loose bonds. Thus the fluoride ion in forming this very strong bond stops the function of the enzyme. Without enzymes life cannot exist. The conclusion is easily drawn that there is no such thing as an optimum or safe dose of Fluoride. Only one ion can destroy an enzyme.

Since fluoridation has also been proven in court to cause at least 10,000 to 40,000 cancer deaths annually, causes kidney damage, diminished sight and hearing and a host of other problems, including tooth and bone damage and there is hardly a cell in the body which cannot be damaged by this highly toxic poison, it is not surprising that it also damages the white cells- THE IMMUNE SYSTEM! When the enzyme and immune systems are functioning properly infections and cancer are prevented or overcome quickly.

....When fluoride destroys this immune system, ANY opportunistic organism can multiply at will and destroy the now helpless host. This means that anyone can succumb to the so-called AIDS depending on: (1) total ingestion of fluoride from all sources (food, air, water), (2) nutritional state, (3) heredity (which is also affected by nutrition and pollutants) and/or (4) other enzyme or immune system pollutants.

Thus the underlying cause of AIDS is an immune system destroying poison, quite possibly mainly fluoride as the statistics so graphically show. The precipitating cause then may be any infectious organism, or, in the absence of sufficiently numerous or virulent organisms, the degenerative effect of the toxic poison may manifest itself as cancer.

Since gays are more intimately in contact with disease organisms, and their lifestyle may not include proper nutrition, and since drug users have damaged body chemistry and exposure to germs from needles, these two sub-cultures are most often affected by AIDS. The nutritional state of the Haitians is usually very poor due to the almost starvation conditions in Haiti, so that when they are then subjected to the immune system destroyer, fluoride in Miami and other fluoridated areas many of them succumb to the so-called AIDS even though this is very rare in unfluoridated Haiti.

Thus it is, that those who so self-righteously blame AIDS entirely on gays and claim it is God's punishment for their lifestyle, may themselves eventually be victims since fluoride is now escalating in the environment at an ever increasing rate, and thus more and more people will have less and less ability to fight off <u>any</u> organism.

It is now obvious that fluoride can, and is, destroying America, and must be stopped very soon. Yet, in spite of knowing the AIDS statistics are significantly related to fluoridation, the California Legistlature recently passed, with very few dissenting votes, a Resolution to form a "Task Force" to study the "<u>benefits</u>" of <u>mandating</u> fluoridation in the state of California. One must certainly question what powerful forces or what intimidating methods are being used on our legislators to make them turn their backs on the safety of their constituents and themselves. Or is it merely greed and lust for political power? The AMA, ADA and all those in the 'sickness business' have much money to further their own interests since this "sickness business" is now nearly, if not actually, our greatest GNP at 10% of the total, and continually increasing. The medical professions and the forces behind them are actively promoting the toxic poison fluoride as a "nutrient"- an unconscionable fraud!

....In practically all of Europe fluoridation is banned or has never been considered. What is the matter with America? Must we force a highly toxic poison in ever escalating amounts into the entire population? Obviously, this can lead to only one result - the demise of America as we know it. What powerful forces wish to destroy America for their own greedy purposes in such a slow, insidious, diabolical way? FLUORIDATION MUST BE STOPPED!

FOR THOSE INTERESTED IN FIGHTING FLUORIDE IN THE STATE OF CALIFORNIA AND THE UNITED STATES, WRITE TO THE ADDRESS GIVEN BY MS. MACMARTIN

Marie MacMartin, R.N.
National Health Researcher
859 Juniper
Nipomo, California 93444
(805) 929-5539

THE CONNECTION BETWEEN THE THYMUS AND FLUORIDATION

Fluoride confuses the immune system and causes it to attack the body's own tissues.

The Center for Disease Control in Atlanta, Georgia, 1982 lists 6 major cities of cases (AIDS) per million population. The first three cities listed with about 3 times the number of cases are all fluoridated! The last 3 are not fluoridated. (See following page for statistics)

YEARBOOK OF AGRICULTURE-REPORT FOR 1939-by Margaret & Howard Smith

Fluoride is poisonous to human beings in very small amounts. It affects the teeth, producing mottled enamel, and structural weaknesses. (p.21)

YEARBOOK OF AGRICULTURE-REPORT FOR 1942-by Department of Agriculture

Fluorine is a cumulative poison, and long-continued consumption of relatively small quantities produces chronic fluorosis in all farm animals and poultry.

The general symptoms of chronic fluorine poisoning are abnormal teeth and bones, stiffness of joints, loss of appetite, emaciation, reduction of milk flow, salt hunger, kidney damage, and injury to other organs, such as the liver, heart, adrenal glands, testes, and thyroid. (p. 338)

THE JAW JOINT AND FLUORIDATION

Book, The Real American Tragedy, published by Dr. Royal Lee, DDS 1960

"The official data reveals the aggravations of oral conditions in Newburgh: There is a radical increase in mal-occlusion, i.e., improper meshing of teeth of the two jaws when the mouth is closed. ...."in 1954, in Newburgh 3 out of every 5 children suffer from some oral trouble as compared with 2 out of 5 in Kingston, a neighboring non-fluoridated city chosen by PHS for a comparison. Another unexpected discovery was made. The dental arch of fluoridated children became deformed.

Dr. D.W. Eggleston, DDS: The Interrelationship of Stress and Degenerative Diseases. 1980

"Mal-occlusion has generally been assumed to be genetic in origin But genetics do not explain the dramatic increase in mal-occlusion in one generation when a primitive society adapts a 'civilized' diet and/or life style."

A LINK BETWEEN "A.I.D.S." AND FLUORIDATION?

CENTER FOR DISEASE CONTROL
ATLANTA, GEORGIA
REPORT OF SEPT. 24, 1982 (Vol. 31:No. 37; p. 513)
UPDATE ON ACQUIRED IMMUNE DEFICIENCY SYNDROME (AIDS) UNITED STATES
MORBIDITY AND MORTALITY WEEKLY REPORT

AIDS CASES PER MILLION POPULATION BY STANDARD METROPOLITAN STATISTICAL AREA OF RESIDENCE REPORTED FROM JUNE 1, 1981 TO SEPTEMBER 15, 1982, UNITED STATES

*FLUORIDATED AREAS

(1) MOST CASES PER MILLION POPULATION PER INCIDENCE OF AIDS

NEW YORK, N.Y.	31.6
SAN FRANCISCO, CA.	24.
MIAMI, FLA.	19.1

*NON-FLUORIDATED AREAS

(2) LEAST CASES PER MILLION POPULATION PER INCIDENCE OF AIDS

NEWARK, N.J.	7.6
HOUSTON, TEXAS	5.2
LOS ANGELES, CA.	4.9

*Editor's insertion
(1) THE HIGHEST INCIDENCE OF AIDS PER MILLION POPULATION WAS IN FLUORIDATED AREAS.
(2) THE LEAST INCIDENCE OF AIDS PER MILLION POPULATION WAS IN NON-FLUORIDATED AREAS. (In a ratio of approximately 3 to 1)

THE CONNECTION BETWEEN THE THYMUS AND FLUORIDATION

(a quote from the 1983 book "Fluoride the Aging Factor" by John Yiamouyiannis Ph.D.)

"Fluoride Tricks and Damages the Immune System

Fluoride confuses the immune system and causes it to attack the body's own tissues. In such cases, the clinical observations of skin rashes, gastrointestinal disorders, lupus, rheumatoid arthritis, etc. are to be expected. The cumulative effect of tissue damage by these fluoride-induced autoimmune responses is what is commonly recognized as aging.

Fluoride slows down and weakens those very cells which serve as the body's defense system and thus allows foreign agents such as bacteria, viruses, and chemicals as well as the body's own obsolete, damaged, or cancerous cells to wreak havoc throughout the body. Otherwise minor infections, now fighting an immune system weakened by fluoride, take longer to throw off and more serious illnesses result. Cancer cells which might otherwise be contained or destroyed end up taking the life of the victim.

This fluoride-induced weakening of the immune system explains the results of Dr. Alfred Taylor and Nell Taylor of the University of Texas who found that fluoride in the drinking water at levels of one-half to one part per million increased tumor growth rate in cancer-prone mice by 15-25%. This increased tumor growth rate can be attributed to the inability of the immune system of fluoride-treated mice to attack tumors

WARNING: Fluoride not only causes the immune system to act like the immune system of an "old" person, it causes autoimmune damage to the entire body and accelerates the aging process of that body. The low levels at which fluoride exerts its deleterious effects indicates that there is no safe level of fluoride."

CHAPTER 8 "Fluoride the Aging Factor"

"Disarming The Immune System

The immune system is the body's major defense mechanism against disease. It is composed of white blood cells *(which consist of 'T' Cells) and a number of tissues throughout the body that make or activate white blood cells. These cells serve as the body's surveillance system to recognize and destroy foreign agents such as bacteria, viruses, and chemicals as well as the body's own obsolete, damaged, or cancerous cells.

...Dr. Sheila Gibson from the University of Glasgow, showed that fluoride,

*The Editors Note

at levels comparable to those found in the blood of people living in fluoridated areas, decreased migration rate of human white blood cells. As can be seen from the following table, exposure of white blood cells to as little as 0.1 part per million fluoride for six hours decreased the migration rate to 79% of those receiving no fluoride. In other words, a 6-hour exposure of white cells to 0.1 part per million fluoride inhibits migration rate by 21%."

THE EFFECT OF FLUORIDE ON THE MIGRATION OF WHITE BLOOD CELLS

FLUORIDE CONCENTRATION	EXPOSURE TIME	RELATIVE MIGRATION RATE
0 ppm	6 hours	100%
0.1 ppm	6 hours	79%
0.5 ppm	6 hours	26%
1 ppm	6 hours	15%
2 ppm	6 hours	0%

University of California in cooperation with CBS Radio Network gives weekly updates of the latest scientific work around the nation.

The following quote may prove to be of interest to you. (Science Editor Transcript--Broadcast #10816, S.E. #1517) Tuesday, January 5, 1982.

...."a program at the Dental Institute he considers particularly exciting is the development of pea-sized carriers of fluoride that could be bonded to a tooth or attached to dental braces or other structures to give a continuous low-level infusion of fluoride."

There is much evidence now available pointing to the fact that fluoride and fluoridation are enzyme inhibitors and degenerate the cells causing systemic disease. -Editor

---

FLUORIDE TOOTHPASTE

Book: FLUORIDE THE AGING FACTOR
By: John Yiamouyiannis, Ph.D
Health Action Press 1983

Chapter 8 page 44

"Dr. Milton Saunders, a practitioner from Virginia Beach, Virginia, reported that acne-like eruptions also result from the mere contact of fluoridated toothpaste with areas around the mouth. In his report, published in the Archives of Dermatology, noted: "I requested that these patients switch, on a trial basis, from their fluoride toothpastes to a nonfluoride toothpaste. Within a period varying from two to four weeks, approximately one half of the patients thus observed cleared of their previously persistent acne-like eruption. Several of the patients, who were concerned about the dental health factors relative to fluoride and its exclusion, requested to resume use of a fluoride toothpaste. Without exception, each developed the same distribution of acne-like eruption that had previously occurred."

Chapter 8 page 45

"Drs. Howard Beerman and Bernard Kirschbaum from the University of Pennsylvania School of Medicine point out that substances such as fluoride constitute an important source of skin reactions because of their widespread use in many types of proprietary preparations (such as toothpaste). In addition, they state that some patients may experience aggravation of their acne by the ingestion of certain vitamins with minerals (e.g., fluoride-containing vitamins)."

Chapter 8 page 44

"In Chapter 3, it was pointed out that the recently found chemical properties of fluoride indicate that it has the ability to distort the conformation of the body's own protein so much that it sets off an autoimmune or allergic response.

It is well-documented that this allergic-type reaction occurs as a result of fluoride exposure. The 1983 Physicians Desk Reference, in discussing vitamin tablets containing only 1/2 milligram of fluoride, warns: "In hypersensitive individuals, fluorides occasionally cause skin eruptions such as atopic dermatitits, eczema, or urticaria. Gastric distress, headaches, and weakness have also been reported. These hypersensitive reactions usually disappear promptly after discontinuation of the fluoride." One-half milligram of fluoride is the amount of fluoride contained in only one pint of fluoridated water."

INFORMATION ON DR. YIAMOUYIANNIS FROM THE INSIDE COVER OF HIS NEW BOOK, FLUORIDE, THE AGING FACTOR.

Dr. Yiamouyiannis received his B.S. in Biochemistry from the University of Chicago in 1963, his Ph.D. in Biochemistry from the University of Rhode Island in 1967. He was Editor of Chemical Abstracts Service, the worlds largest chemical information center. It was here he became aware of the health damaging effects of fluoride. Dr. Yiamouyiannis is the world's leading authority on the biological effects of fluoride. He lives outside Columbus, Ohio with his wife and children on 35 acres. There lifestyle is devoted to living without fluoridation. In 20 years the doctor bills have been not over the sum of $500.00. The doctor is currently president of Safe Water Foundation. His address is 6439 Taggart Rd., Delaware, Ohio.

Commentary Thurs., Oct. 6, 1983 ☆ S.F. EXAMINER B3.

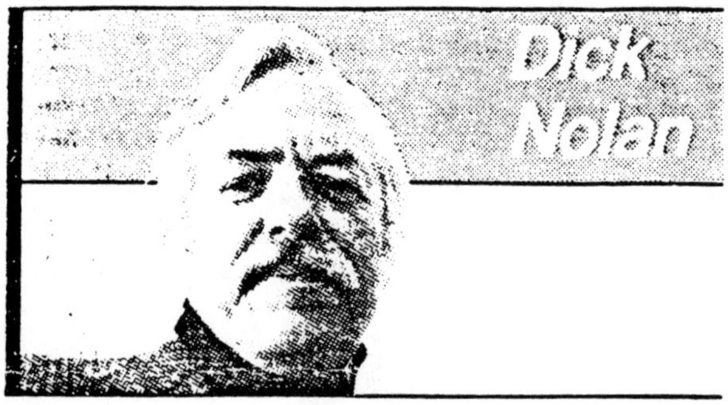

Fluoride treatment

All right, here's the question: Are we absolutely certain, after all, that adding fluoride to our public water supply is a procedure entirely without danger? I've been poking around for answers, and finding none that are at all satisfactory. We seem to be expected to take this on trust.

I got into this in an odd enough way a while back when Sam The Airedale got took with the itches and scratches for no obvious reason at all. Nope, he didn't have fleas or ticks. The best educated guesses zeroed in on poor Sam's diet. An allergy of some kind perhaps?

An interested reader proposed a clue. She submitted a heavy file of research data tending to suggest that heavy levels of fluoride in commercial dog food had caused all kinds of weird problems in kennels all across the country. Our vet didn't buy the fluoride theory, but he did prescribe a diet change. And Sam's coat did improve. So much for peripheral discussion.

But I was left with that sheaf of anti-fluoride documentation, and it was more than a little unsettling. The stuff is a poison. And it does accumulate in the body. And if it is entirely safe, why has fluoridation been banned or abandoned in such enlightened European countries as Norway, Sweden, Austria, Belgium, Holland, Denmark, France, Italy and West Germany?

A Dutch medical doctor, H. C. Moolenburgh, offered interesting testimony as to the effects of a brief use of fluoridation in the Netherlands, before that country outlawed it. It happened (he reported) that half his patients lived in a community receiving fluoridated water, while the other half did not. Within weeks he began seeing patients with all kinds of strange problems: mouth sores, headaches, dizziness, and recurrences of allergy problems that had not bothered these patients for years.

It was soon seen that the influx of patients with these curious ailments were those who were drinking the fluoridated water. When, on Moolenburgh's orders, they stopped doing so, their symptoms disappeared.

The doctor was moved by his experience to form a research group. After two years of study the Dutch doctors concluded that fluoridation caused a low grade poisoning which stays beneath the surface in most people, but in some, and especially in those whose health is deteriorating, produces clinical symptoms.

"It appeared that side effects in our patients flickered on and off," Moolenburgh reported. "When patients came back from holidays, relaxed and rested, there were few side effects, but when they were tired, nervous or were attacked by another illness, side effects abounded.

Our own medical and dental establishment (with many rebels dissenting) generally puts this sort of thing down. The official contention is that the low concentrations of fluoride used in treating public water supplies are harmless. It is also generally agreed (with many dissenting) that the treatment does improve the dental health of those who, from childhood, absorb fluoride with their drinking water.

The controversy here goes back to the early '50s, when, after furious debate, a fluoridation measure was adopted in 1952 by public vote. It was a time long before environmentalism had become a burning issue. As a top Water Department official put it to me the other day: "I don't think that measure would pass if it was up for a vote now."

At first, fluoridation was accomplished rather crudely here by feeding the dry chemical into the water supply. Now a potent liquid form of the stuff, hydrofluorosalycic acid, is delivered in big tank trucks and metered into the system. Our Water Department people, relying on the word of federal agencies, are sure what they're doing is entirely safe. But it has been a long time since anybody in an official capacity has even considered whether the process should be subjected to a fresh review.

COMMONWEALTH OF PENNSYLVANIA

SUPREME COURT
SIX GATEWAY CENTER
PITTSBURGH, PENNSYLVANIA 15222

JOHN P. FLAHERTY
JUSTICE

July 31, 1979

Sir Dove-Myer Robinson, Mayor
Auckland, New Zealand

Dear Sir Mayor:

I am in receipt of your letter of July 25, 1979, and thank you for it.

You are correct that I entered an injunction against the fluoridation of the public water supply for a large portion of Allegheny County, Pennsylvania. I did this after a very lengthy series of hearings on the issue. The trial brought into my court experts on the subject of fluoridation, and I meticulously considered the objective evidence. In my view, the evidence is quite convincing that the addition of sodium fluoride to the public water supply at one part per million is extremely deleterious to the human body, and, a review of the evidence will disclose that there was no convincing evidence to the contrary. Since my decision, I have received hundreds of letters, quite a few of which have been sent by physicians and dentists, all concurring with my decision. Contrary to your information, my decree has not been set aside by a higher court. Presently, the issue is on appeal to the Commonwealth Court of Pennsylvania, but the appeal involves merely the jurisdiction of the court--it does not involve the substantative merits of the case.

Prior to my hearing this case, I gave the matter of fluoridation little, if any, thought, but I received quite an education, and noted that the proponents of fluoridation do nothing more than try to impune the objectivity of those who oppose fluoridation. I seriously believe that few responsible people have objectively reviewed the evidence. If you are interested, I suggest that you review the twenty-eight hundred pages of testimony and all of the exhibits presented in this case.

Thank you very much for your inquiry.

Sincerely,

JOHN P. FLAHERTY
Justice
Supreme Court of Pennsylvania

JPF:pld

P.S. I enclose a copy of a letter I received from the Chancellor of Fairleigh Dickinson University, which is representative of the hundreds I have received.

J.P.F.

P.S. Since my decision on fluoride, I was elevated to the Supreme Court of Pa.

CHARO 2000: Clean Water System
Forever Living Product

The Charo 2000 Clean Water System will guarantee your family the safest, cleanest water possible.

Installation is simple and the entire operation is virtually maintenance free. No electricity is required to run the system. The special Charo 2000 filter and carbon block will last in most cases a full year before replacement is necessary.

Effective removal of the following: Fluoride, Pesticides, Asbestos, Viruses, Bacteria, Nitrate, Sodium Lead, Chlorine, Insecticides, etc.

Unit is self-cleaning, self-discharging of waste water.

Distributed by: B. Manning c/o Barber Associates, 6010 Main Street, Williamsville, New York 14221, (716) 632-7310 (day), or (716) 839-3007 (night). Cost $369.00 shipping included.

PURWATER Distributed by Charlotte Blacburn, P.O. Box 4130, San Rafael, Ca. 94903
Cost $250. and up.

The water you are drinking may be harmful to your health! More and more, throughout our nation, magazines and newspapers warn about the dangers of drinking polluted water.

Safe drinking water can no longer be taken for granted.

Is there a solution? The answer is YES! Through a purification method called reverse osmosis.

The process was developed at great expense by the U.S. Government, and is incredibly simple: Polluted tap water is forced against a proprietary semi-permeable membrane (Dept. of Interior License #3,417,870) using only water pressure as the power source. No electricity or other energy source is required. When water is applied under pressure, the properties of the membrane allow the pure water molecules, but not the pollutants, to pass through.

Can water be purified and still taste good? The answer is YES.

This unit will take out sodium, arsenic, lead, cadimium, potassium, sulfates, calcium (hardness), magnesium (hardness) phosphates, chlorides, fluorides, alkalinity, fecal bacteria, viruses, organics, trihalomethanes (THM) Trichloroethylene (TCE), dioxin, radioactive contaminants, chlorine, pesticides, sediment, unpleasant taste/odor.

Acqua Products- Reverse Osmosis- "Toaster Size", Non Electric. (You need 40PSI to operate). Guaranteed one year. Filter must be changed at this time, cost for this-$38.00. This product is known as the "Bottled Water Machine" It is an excellent product for someone who lives in small apartment or lives alone, (although can be used for more then one person). Makes 3 gallons a day. This is an excellent piece equipment for survival means since it requires no electricity. Cost $129.00 + $2.50 shipping charge. Write Kevin Manning, 2504 Cross Hill Road, Louisville, Ky.40205 (502) 895-7601

XXIV

ENVIRONMENTAL FACTORS THAT DISTURB THE BODY

BY Dr. James Ouye, DDS

In order to get well a patient thinks he must do two things; 1) see an orthodox physician, and 2) use the treatment of drugs and/or surgery. The real purpose of a physician or the sum total of what a physician should do (whether orthodox physician or a preventative, 'holistic' therapist) is to raise the resistance level of the body and to arm the immune system so that the body can fight the problem. No therapist heals a patient. The body heals itself.

Abnormality and Disease is caused by the lowering of the body's stress resistance and the lowering of the immune system which allows the disease to take hold and get an upper hand on the body.

The patient as well as the physician must become aware of the many things in the environment that serve to lower the body's resistance and the immune system. Not only does bacteria, chemicals and the traditional things cause disease, but there are other factors the orthodox medical establishment must become aware of.

These factors are what I call environmental factors resulting in lowering of stress resistance. It has been shown that many treatments done by orthodox medical doctors as well as the "holistic" doctors are not completely successful, and it can be concluded that this is so because the stress resistance and the immune processes of the body have not been raised high enough in order for the body to cope with the problem.

It is highly possible that a major reason for these failures even though the physician or therapist does raise the resistance level some, or even to a great amount is- the person is exposing himself to negative factors from the environment (including what he eats). These factors are counteracting or neutralizing what the physician has been trying to do, subsequently the lowering of stress resistance of the body. For this reason it is important that the patient, the therapist and the medical doctor become aware of disturbing things in the environment, so that the patient can free himself of the disease processes and abnormality.

It is known that the taking in of food additives such as, artificial flavorings, colorings and preservatives, can cause a person to become hyperactive, to become hostile and to become fatigued. By being aware of this fact, and by keeping away from these things, the stress resistance is raised high enough so that the body and mind function more normally.

There are many indications that people who are exposed to computers and computer terminals, video and video games are prone to disease processes. It is not known by the orthodox medical profession why this is so. If they were to examine environmental factors, such as microwave, nuclear radiation, electricity, plastics and their effect on the body, they would find that these environmental factors are oftentimes the main cause of disease process and if not they contribute to the failure to recover or the slowdown in recovery.

There is a national organization in the computer industry called "Nine to Five" and their purpose is to find out why people in the industry and those who work on terminals are having all kinds of medical problems. They need to know about negative environmental factors. The treatment or method to correct these problems is known. The physician must acquire the knowledge of the effect of these negative factors on the electromagnetic system of the body.

MAGNETIC FIELDS INFLUENCE HEALTH-by Andreas Marx (An Article)
Worldwide, many medical doctors and physicists have recently discovered and recognized a complete new problem of our civilized world and named it "geopathic disturbance." It is also sometimes referred to as "electric smog." For example, the case history of the following patient could represent thousands of people with a similar problem. It goes like this: The patient says, "Since we moved into our new house, I suffer from sleeplessness. A geopathic disturbance expert examined the patient's bedroom and discovered that the head of the bed was exactly at the side of the wall where the power supply and all the electrical wiring of the house was located. With a magnetometer, the expert measured an extremely high electro-magnetic field that radiated over the head of the bed.

It was recommended to the patient to move his bed into another position. Two days later, the patient and his wife had no more complaints about their sleeplessness. Other examples are by avoiding the use of electric blankets, waterbeds, telephones and electric quartz clocks that are too near the head of the bed, even removing televisions from the bedroom has caused patients to lose their pathological symptoms. Geopathic disturbances can often be found at one's working place. Some people suffer from electro-magnetic radiation when working near neon light tubes, electronic equipment, TV screens, and microwaves (microwave radiation leakage has been widely discussed as a possible health hazard). Scientists from the U. of Colorado reported that the death rate through Cancer, such as leukemia, is more than average high in people who live within 50 yard radius of outdoor power lines. In 1973, W. Ross Adey, at the brain research institute of the Univ. of California in L.A. exposed monkeys to electrical radiation with frequencies comparable to what we are exposed to in our daily lives and he documented abnormal behavior by the monkeys. The earth's natural magnetic field has a strength measured at only about 3/4 gauss. This magnetic field is one of the most important basics for all life on earth. In some areas in big cities especially in high concrete buildings, one is isolated from this natural life force. On top of this, these natural fields are blanketed by much stronger electro-magnetic radiation such as high voltage power lines which can create an imbalance in the biorhythm. The German physicist and researcher, Dr. Mersmann, discovered that people suffering under electromagnetic pollution have left spinning blood. The blood of cancer patients also shows a left spin. Healthy blood always spins to the right. Mersmann developed an electro-magnetic spin tester expecially for this test with this instrument and method, one is able to test almost every substance on this spin. It was learned that most healthy organically grown foods spins to the right.

THE BODY ELECTRIC by Robert O. Becker, M.D. 1985, William Morrow & Company.
...The admittedly sketchy evidence to date suggests that our electropollution is presenting us, and perhaps all animals, with a double challenge: weaker immune systems & stronger diseases. Reyes syndrome...Lyme disease...Legionnaire's disease...A.I.D.S....

SUGGESTED READING- ELECTROMAGNETIC DISTURBANCES AND THE "GEOPATHIC ZONES"
"Dr. Nieper's Revolution in Technology Medicine and Society."1985 $40.00 + $2.00 shipping
Cancer Control Society, 2043 N. Berendo St., Los Angeles, California 90027

XXV

BIBLIOGRAPHY

Yiamouyiannis, John, Ph.D. Fluoride the Aging Factor, July 1983 Health Action Press

San Francisco Chronicle, "Doctors Link Aids to Thymus Gland," June 3, 1983

Smudde, Roy, DDS: Cancer Control Convention-Doctors' Seminar. Lecturer on "Acupath & Dermatron Machines and How to Identify and Measure Energies," July 1983 (Excerpts)

Flannagan, Patrict, Ph.D.; National Health Federation. Lecturer on Electrical Energy Fields of the Body, etc. June 1983. (Excerpts)

Eggleston, D. DDS: Holistic Dental Convention. Lecturer on Electro-Acupuncture According to Voll (Dermatron), Electromagnetic Energy of the Body, Nickel/Silver Fillings, Thymus and 'T' Cells, Smith-Kline T Cell Tests, How.to measure Galvanic Current in the mouth. March 1983 (Excerpts)

Published by Royal Lee, DDS (lee Foundation for Nutritional Research 1960. The Jaw Joint and Fluoridation

US Dept. of Health and Human Services, Center for Disease Control. 'Update on Acquired Immune Deficiency Syndrome (AIDS) United States Morbidity and Mortality Weekly Report. Sept. 24, 1982 (Vol 31:No. 37; p. 513)

Yearbook of Agriculture-Report for 1938 by Margaret & Howard Smith (Fluoridation)

Yearbook of Agriculture-Report for 1942 by Department of Agriculture Research Team. (Fluoridation)

Eggleston, D.W. DDS, "The Interrelationship of Stress and Degenerative Diseases", 1980. 1441 Avocado Ave. Ste. 508. Newport Beach, Ca. 92660

University of California, Berkeley-In cooperation with CBS Radio Network (Science Editor Transcript-Broadcast #10816, S.E. #1517) Tuesday, January 5, 1982 'Down with Dental Decay!'

"Symptoms of Side Effects Through the use of Materials for Protheses (Stomatitis) Gasser, Von F.: Concerning foreign bodies in the mouth in research and practice
Translated from the German: Schweizerische Monatsschrift Fuer Zahnheilkunde (SSO) 77(4):307-323.April 1967

Battista, Al, N.P.: 'You can Stop Fungus Infections,' Health Express August 1983

USDA, Beltsville Research Center. Report on Pao D'Arco Tea by James A. Duke, Ph.D.: Tabebuia Spp.- Bignoniaceae -Pao D'Arco

Huemer, R. M.D.: Lets Live Magazine, Preventive Medicine-on Pac D'Arco Tea. Sept. 1983 p. 64

Lorenzani, S. Ph.D., 1982 Price Pottinger Foundation Seminar. Lecturer on "Candidiasis" (Excerpts)
Handouts on:
Candida Albicans Questionnaire
Dietary Suppression of Candida Albicans
Foods Containing Yeast

The Mercury/Nickel Patch Test by: Toxic Testing- 303 E. Altamonte Dr. Suite 232, Altamonte Springs, Florida 32701

Potential Meter- Frank Marrero, P.O. Box 546, San Rafael, Calif. 94915 (415) 492-9192 & Toxic Testing (See address above)

Instrument for Measuring Urine, Blood and Hair for Mercury
Chemical Analysis Test (Model 511) To Lease: Toxic Testing
Jerome Instrument Corp. (See Address above)
P.O. Box 336
Jerome, Arizona 86331

Chart: Dental Materials Containing Beryllium and Nickel, from the book: Metals '82, by Gordon J. Christensen, DDS, Ph.D.

A Healing Crisis-The Whole Body Approach to Cancer Therapy, By Jack Tropp.

Gasser, Von F.: Concerning Foreign Bodies in the mouth in research and practice. Schweizerische Monatsschrift Fuer Zahnnheilkunde (SSO) 77(4):307-323. April 1967 Side Effects of Metal-Inhomogenous alloys : precious metal with chrome, nickel and steel (Chart) 1
Side Effects of Amalgam (edited by 24 authors) (Healing through elimination) (Chart) 2

Bauer, Janet G., DDS, MS & First, Howard A., DDS.: The Toxicity of Mercury in Dental Amalgam 47-61. June 1982 California Dental Association Journal

Buchner, A. and Hansen, L.S.: Amalgam Pigmentation (amalgam tattoo) of the Oral Mucosa. Oral Surg. 49:139-147, 1980.

Hansen, L.S. and Silverman, S.: Localized Tissue Reaction to Implanted Amalgam: A Review. CDA Journal June 1982

Jendresen, Malcolm, D.: Mercury in Dental Amalgam: Is it Safe? CDA Journal: 31-32 June 1982

Wood, J.M.: Kennedy, F.S.: Rosen, C.G.: Synthesis of Methyl-mercury compounds by extracts of a Methanogenic Bacterium. Nature. Vol 220. October 12, 1968 173-174

Jernelov, A. "Conversion of Mercury Compounds:, Chap. 4 in Chemical Fallout (CC Thomas Publ., 1969) Publ. by M.W. Miller

International Converence on Environmental Mercury Contamination, University of Michigan, 19721 "Factors in the Transformation of Mercury to Methylmercury-Arne Jernelov

Mercury in the Environment: A toxicological and epidemiological appraisal by L. Friberg and Jaroslav, V.: Editors: Stockholm, November 1971

Greener, Evan: . Amalgam-Yesterday, Today, and Tomorrow. Operative Dentistry; 4, 24-35: 1979

Goolvard, Dale & Ferguson: Serum in organic methyl mercury levels in dental surgeons: Journal of Dental Research-Special Issue- 56 Annual Meeting: British Division: Abstract #144

Carrell, A.B.: Mackowiak, Elaine: Chialastri, A.J.: The Accumulation of the Base Metals (Copper, Zinc and Mercury) in the Human Body Journal of Dentistry for Children: 30-33 September-October 1979

Treptow, Richard S.: Amalgam Dental Fillings, Parts 1 and II Chemistry, April 17:30, May 15: 19, 1978

Merfield, D.P: Taylor, A: Gemmell, D.M.: Mercury Intoxication in a Dental Surgery Following Unreported Spillage British Dental Journal 179- : 1976

Stofen, D.: Dental amalgam - a poison in our mouth. Toxicology 2:355-358 December, 1974

Williams, Roger J. Ph.D.: You Are Extraordinary, Random House 1967

Lubecki, John, D.C.: Better Health Through Body Balancing. 1982
P.O. Box 412, Fair Oaks, Ca. 95628

Truss, C.O., M.D.: The Missing Diagnosis, 1982
P.O. Box 26508
Birmingham, Al. 35226

ORDER FORM

PLEASE SEND ME THE FOLLOWING BOOKS EDITED BY BETSY RUSSELL-MANNING.

_____copies CANDIDA, SILVER (mercury) FILLINGS AND THE IMMUNE SYSTEM, at $15.95 eaach + $3.00 shipping (UPS)

_____copies HOW SAFE ARE SILVER (mercury) FILLINGS? - HIDDEN HEALTH FACTS, at $39.95 each + $3.00 shipping (UPS).

_____copies WHEAT GRASS JUICE-GIFT OF NATURE at $2.95 each + $1.00 shipping UPS

_____copies HOW SILVER MERCURY FILLINGS AFFECT YOUR ENERGY SYSTEM at $10.00 each + $1.50 shipping (UPS)

_____copies MERCURY A POISON IN YOUR MOUTH (A political overview) at $6.00 each + $1.50 shipping (UPS).

NAME____

STREET____

CITY____

NOTE: Californians please add 6 1/2% Sales Tax
Please add $1.00 extra for shipping 2nd book
I can't wait for U.P.S. deliver. Here is $12.50 for next day delivery.

Write to one of the following:

Betsy Russell-Manning
c/o Greensward Press
1600 Larkin #104
San Francisco, California
94109

Cancer Control Society
2043 N. Berendo Street
Los Angeles, California
90027
(213) 663-7801